BARTRAM'S
NATURE'S
PLAN
for Your
HEALTH

BARTRAM'S
NATURE'S PLAN
for Your
HEALTH

The complete guide to nutrition, exercise and complementary remedies for total health

Line and tone illustrations by
David Dowland and Joyce Smith

Thomas Bartram

ROBINSON
London

Constable & Robinson Ltd
3 The Lanchesters
162 Fulham Palace Road
London W6 9ER
www.constablerobinson.com

First published by Blandford Press in 1984,
then by Grace Publishers in 1989

This revised edition published by Robinson,
an imprint of Constable & Robinson Ltd 2005

A copy of the British Library Cataloguing in Publication Data is available from the British Library.

ISBN 1-84529-164-6

Printed and bound in the UK

1 3 5 7 9 10 8 6 4 2

Contents

Acknowledgements

NO apology is offered for this book. It is an earnest attempt to assist the reader towards a healthy and satisfying lifestyle. It is offered as a guide to everyone who takes minerals, supplements and medicinal herbs. An understanding of the elements of nutrition may go a long way towards the well-being of mind and body. I hope it will appeal to the thoughtful man and woman who does not rely entirely upon conventional medicine but who wishes to take a measure of personal responsibility for their own health.

I am sorry I cannot prescribe for personal health problems. This book is not intended to replace or conflict with advice given by your doctor or health professional who have records of your medical history and general health. They are in a situation of forming professional judgement of each patient's individual case. Therefore I cannot accept responsibility for any liability arising from the use of this book.

Further information on herbal medicines mentioned in this book is available in *Bartram's Encyclopedia of Herbal Medicine*, also published by Constable & Robinson.

Recommendations are not intended to take the place of diagnosis and treatment by a medical practitioner or qualified medical herbalist. All information has a record of efficacy, though treatment cannot be expected to be always successful. Any condition that persists for more than ten days should be referred to a doctor, especially if it is not in the nature of a cold or influenza. All reasonable care has been taken in the preparation of this book. The author does not imply any guarantee of cure and cannot accept responsibility for adverse effects arising from the use thereof.

In the case of a known serious condition a doctor should be consulted.

All medicines should be avoided during pregnancy and lactation unless prescribed by a doctor.

Treatments in this book are intended to be used at the discretion of the reader and do not in the usual way produce side effects, but on rare occasions an allergic reaction may be possible.

Thomas Bartram

Preface

FOR over forty years my waiting room accommodated business executives, scientists, artists, lawyers, ministers and members of other professions.

For as long as I can remember I have had a passion for natural methods of healing. Orthodox medicine and surgery are indispensable. But there comes a time when sound manipulative therapy and gentle-acting, natural healing plants offer their unique ministry. Nature rises to tend her sick children when other methods fail.

As I look back on a busy professional practice, I recall over 500 plant extracts, tinctures, essential oils and homoeopathic remedies represented in my dispensary. We made extracts of most of the medicinal plants used in the practice. Over the years, we have proved for ourselves the efficacy and safety of Nature's pharmacy.

I believe an gram of prevention is worth a ton of cure.

However effective certain treatments might be, prevention is better than cure. Does our present lifestyle put us at risk? With a little self-help we can avoid many individual health problems.

In this book I have tried to cultivate a love of living instead of a fear of dying. Happiness is the elusive prize that becomes possible when we devote a few minutes each day to bringing out the magic of our bodies. In our search for strength and increased vitality, we need knowledge and enthusiasm to open the door to radiant health.

Treat this book as you would a friend. Wherever you are, there is always something new to learn. What a fascinating world it becomes when we discover the secret of a revitalizing positive lifestyle.

Is there a life without strain? Can we safeguard our own well-being and not let ourselves deteriorate so that surgeons can perform costly modern miracles on us? I believe we can. The business of life is joy, unspeakable, in every sense of the word.

Nutrition, recreation of mind and body, fostering happy relationships and a purpose in life are all part of the complete pattern for health. And if things sometimes go wrong, Nature has her remedies.

I have attempted a broad canvas in covering so many aspects of this fascinating subject. Readers may be led to make further discoveries of their own in specific areas. Recapture the thrill of living. Be glad you're alive.

Cordial acknowledgements are tendered to owners of copyright. Care has been taken to record copyright matter. If, however, any short excerpts have been printed without formal consent, the author begs the goodwill and indulgence of those concerned. I acknowledge with thanks the expertise of Mr Tony Purvis, his team at GreenShires Group Ltd., and all others engaged in the production of this book. I am grateful for the sensitive drawings by David Dowland and Joyce Smith, and to my wife for her patient forbearance during time spent in the writing. I am especially grateful to my friend, Terence Goldsmith, whose helpful advice and guidance was warmly appreciated.

Thomas Bartram

Introduction – The Marvel of the Human Body

'I believe in the sacredness of the human body; this transient dwelling place of a living soul. I deem it a duty to every man and woman to keep his or her body beautiful through right thinking and right living.'

Emerson

Your body is the most wonderful thing in the world. It is the most reliable of all machines. Unless misused by neglect or injured by accident, it will keep you perfectly adjusted to your environment day after day. It will do this under the most adverse conditions until worn out.

Your body is a miniature factory in which each single department fits together to create a perfect whole. Understandably, there are times when a part gets out of order. When we supply the wrong fuel, or fail to provide an adequate supply of oxygen to burn that fuel, the whole machine comes to a standstill. We are sick.

If the computer (brain and spinal cord) fails, messages cannot get through to the various departments. All is well as long as the factory is properly ventilated by fresh air taken in by the nose and mouth. Complicated chemical operations are performed in the laboratory – the liver and kidneys.

Your skin keeps the body at an even temperature, giving signals through its nerves of damage, heat and cold. It expels wastes by sweating, and forms the nails and hair. By means of a colour pigment, it protects us from concentrated rays of the sun.

Our sense of wonder deepens when we reflect that tiny blood vessels nourish every cell in the body. Built-in mechanisms shield us from excessive cold and heat. When blood is spilt in injury, it hardens on the surface, forming a clot to hasten repair of the wound.

The eye focuses light on a lens and flashes through a dark chamber before registering on a sensitive background – better than even the most advanced camera!

Muscles are only one means by which the body adapts to its environment. However relaxed, they are always in a state of tension poised to react immediately to messages from the head. From the instant a muscle responds to stimuli, there follows a complicated chain of chemical events.

In the event of pain, the telephone lines will be busy. Pain is a necessary signal that a part of the body is hurt. Blood is then diverted to injured tissue. Blood pressure rises and the heart beats faster. To cope with the emergency, the liver, the largest gland in the body, pours fuel into the bloodstream to provide more energy.

The most important organ in the body is the heart – a hollow muscular pump that lies in the middle of the chest behind the breastbone. Its shape is like a triangle, the apex of which is found below the left nipple where the its beat (approximately seventy per minute) can be felt pulsating.

This powerful organ pumps blood continuously around the body; first to the arteries where its oxygen is absorbed by organs and tissues; and secondly, to the lungs to replace oxygen. With its oxygen renewed, blood is returned to the heart for the circulatory cycle to begin again.

The wonder of the human body would not be complete without the world's most astounding transport system. Longer than any railway, your circulatory system has over 80,470 km (50,000 miles) of track. From birth to death its efficient flow is the nearest approach to perpetual motion we know. To millions of cells it conveys oxygen and nutriment. In return, it carries away wastes. It is when these wastes accumulate and poison the life-giving stream that the scene is set for chronic disease. From the circulation the vital components of our food are made available to replenish and rebuild decaying cells to provide body warmth and energy, and to ensure our good health.

Conversion of food into cell structures is one of the most enduring miracles of biochemistry. 'Our body intelligence knows more than the combined wisdom of all the scientists in the world,' says Frank Remington. 'In the most up-to-date laboratory, typical protein must boil for a minimum of twenty-four hours in a chemical solution before it is broken down thoroughly. The chemical system in our body completes the identical job in only four hours – and without temperatures.'

Truly, we are fearfully and wonderfully made.

A sound mind in a sound body

Our bodies are our health. Today's lifestyle has everything to do with our tomorrow. In pursuit of the whole personality, self-awareness is vital. When our values and aspirations are in line we achieve harmony between body, mind and spirit. But if one of these is ailing, the others must be off balance. Stress and tension rise when these three elements are not integrated.

High-level fitness emphasizes preventive health care through attention to a number of factors that foster a sense of well-being – nutrition, exercise, vitamins, minerals, relaxation, and meditation. Students of well-being will be quick to recognize sickness in the mind, which reveals an underlying neglect or rebellion. They will see the wisdom of cleansing himself of moral pollution, and will try to resolve wrongs by forgiveness and tolerance before they manifest themselves in the body as pathological symptoms.

If we observe a few simple rules we can enjoy a healthier, happier life. When we eat and drink too much, or smoke and take too little exercise, live too fast, we open ourselves to life-threatening habits.

When we are ill there are effective alternative natural therapies that can come to our aid, part of a system of medicine that treats the whole person rather than just isolated symptoms. Healing is wholeness – restoration to the created norm.

The whole man looks to himself for health, is involved in his own care, feels responsible for himself, is sensitive to his environment, expresses his talents and creative abilities freely, and deals with stress without the aid of drugs.

As we grow towards harmony and balance, we learn to accept ourselves, and to understand that spiritual resources are as essential as food and clothing.

The world about us

We share a kinship that joins us to all living things. When we identify with that world, we sense a purpose in everything. Whether we live in the country or walk through public gardens in the busy cities, we remember they are the homes of wild creatures and plants.

When did you last contemplate the thrush that sings in early morning? When we savour the fragrance of a wild rose or marvel at the life cycle of the honeybee we are engaged in an act of meditation. Finding time to stand and stare ought to be one of our top priorities.

Do we treat animals with indifference? If some people are cruel to them, they must expect Nature to retaliate. We all need a deeper concept of animals. Do we view them with compassion? From a world more ancient than ours, they survive to share with us the treasures and travails of this good earth. A fully mature person will be ever conscious of their welfare.

We should honour the earth and love her for the inspiration she gives, born of the beauty and mystery of the world. When we touch a tree or stroke an animal we express emotions of reverence to the Creative Intelligence behind all life.

Creation is with us here and now. It is the basis of our understanding of how Nature works, and gives us a deeper insight into her everlasting laws. All of God's laws are good. As you may have sensed, there is a timeless wisdom in the world of growing things. We need to recapture moments of child–like faith, listen to the songs of summer, and choose a lifestyle that takes account of all that Nature has to offer.

'Come forth into the light of things, Let nature be your teacher.'
Wordsworth

1

Nutrition in a Nutshell

The world's healthiest diet

Proper nutrition is one of the most important factors in a new lifestyle. How can we be healthy without whole foods, unrefined foods to which nothing has been added or taken away? What we eat must be intimately related to our sense of well-being.

Dr Robert McCarrison, the world-renowned British physician and surgeon wrote: 'I know of nothing so potent in maintaining good health as perfectly constituted food. I know of nothing so potent in producing ill-health as improperly constituted food.'

McCarrison found that when non-Europeans change their natural diet to an affluent Western diet they develop the common Western diseases – obesity, internal disorders, constipation, varicose veins, piles and non-infective chronic diseases.

His researches led him to the Hunzas of Northern Pakistan, a people unsurpassed in perfection of physique and freedom from disease. Their diet consists of whole foods, grains, vegetables and fruits, with a certain amount of milk and butter. They eat meat only on feast days.

They do not use white sugar or any of the refined carbohydrates that cause so much chronic disease in the West. Because of their singular lifestyle, the Hunzas are said to be extremely disease-resistant, healthy, intelligent and long lived. Rheumatism and high blood pressure are almost unknown. What they have been doing for centuries we can emulate with profit. Indeed, thousands of Western people today are living testimonials to the positive changes that occur when a person kicks the junk food habit and develops a respect for proper nutrition.

Wherever we live, we all want to preserve our eyesight, hearing, smell and taste as long as we can. So why do medical statistics reveal widespread deterioration in these senses?

We can find the answer if we look at the lives of long-lived peoples of Georgia (Russia), South America, the Polynesians, the Maoris and other isolated communities. Their foods are those on which rugged mountain settlers and sturdy plainsmen have for centuries survived the rigours of life in the raw. To them, your style of living would be like that of a king. Sociologists might describe them as 'under-privileged', yet they are noted for a physical hardihood and mental independence that would put many of us to shame.

Like the Hunzas, they have never been able to afford the elegant non-foods of the supermarket, but exist largely on a meatless diet. Never have they been deceived by white sugar dyed brown, cakes coloured yellow, frozen vegetables and canned peas stained all hues of green, or jellies stiff with texturizers.

They are so 'backward' they have no food packaging. So there are no labels on which to read, in the mysterious jargon of the West, of the glycerol monostearate (GMS), acetic acid (vinegar), butylated hydroxyanisole (BHA) and other allergy-forming chemical jiggery-pokery.

Hunza peoples do not have an over-abundance of food and yet John Tobe, natural-health researcher and world traveller who at thirty-nine was a phys-ical wreck but who was saved by a new lifestyle to live to a vigorous old age, said: 'It is crystal clear that they are among the healthiest people I have ever seen in my life, and I have travelled extensively.'

If you live in a modern industrialized society, it takes trouble and thought to select the right foods and eat properly. Food might even take a little longer to prepare. Besides, those foods that do you most good may not be easily available in the big stores. You might have to seek out a little shop – something special – at the other end of the town for organically-grown vegetables. But it would be worth it.

Nutrition is the most pressing health problem. We no longer face the threat of smallpox or tuberculosis, but a whole set of new diseases looms on the horizon because we have forgotten the way to eat.

To recover that essential knowledge we must return to what primitive peoples seem to have sorted out long ago – the relationship between acid-forming and alkaline-forming foods.

What are acid foods?

Acid-forming foods are meat, eggs, cheese, fish and game. They include starches such as bread, all kinds of flour and foods made from flour.

Cereals and foodstuffs manufactured from grain also come under this heading as well, of course, as sugar.

Ash from these foods contains sulphur, phosphorus and chlorine. These salts are necessary to form sulphuric acid, phosphoric acid and hydrochloric acid, all essential to efficient metabolism.

What are alkaline foods?

Alkaline-forming foods include all fruits and all green leafy vegetables such as Brussels sprouts, carrots, broccoli, potatoes (cooked in their skins, and their skins eaten) and parsnips. They include all fruits such as oranges, apples and pears.

Alkaline foods contain more water than concentrated foods such as meat and starch. They are more bulky. They leave an alkaline ash after digestion has taken place. Ash is the mineral matter left after foods have been broken down by oxygen. Alkaline foods are high in sodium and potassium.

We tend to label citrus fruits (oranges, lemons, grapefruit) 'acid' but this does not mean that they are acid-forming. In fact, their content of alkaline salts is high, the chief ones being calcium, magnesium and potassium. They are acid to the mouth, but alkaline to the blood.

A healthy bloodstream depends upon maintenance of an acid/alkaline balance. Blood is always slightly alkaline. Only slight variations on either side are compatible with life. When this vital balance is disturbed through faulty excretion of acids in the urine, carbon dioxide from the lungs, and faulty elimination of acid wastes, a condition appears known as acidosis, a known precursor of chronic disease.

Nothing deranges this delicate acid/alkaline balance more than the modern 'civilized' diet of large quantities of meat, eggs, cheeses, cereals and starches, which create excessive wastes and toxins. In excess, these increase the acid reaction of the blood, destroying its natural acid/alkaline balance. When elimination is imperfect, three things occur: firstly, the accumulation of noxious toxins; secondly, abnormal composition of the blood and lymph; and thirdly, a lowering of vitality.

Proteins and starches produce acid waste materials which need to be neutralized. It is the purpose of the alkaline foods (vegetables and fruits rich in organic salts) to neutralize and ensure healthy elimination.

We cannot stay well when acid-forming exceed alkaline-forming foods. In the healthy diet, the proportion of acid to alkaline foods is on the basis of one to four. For every one part of meat, eggs, cheese, fish, cereals, grains and all kinds of bread and flour, we should consume four parts green and root vegetables and fruits. It is important to know which foods are acid, and which are alkaline-forming in order to maintain the proper acid/alkali balance.

A high proportion of water and low proportion of solids seems to be a rule by which Nature maintains the acid/alkaline balance. When we look at milk and vegetables we see how she observes this law.

What are proteins?

Proteins are the bricks that build up our flesh and tissue. They are made up of small chemical units – consisting mainly of carbon, oxygen, nitrogen and hydrogen – called amino acids.

We get our protein mainly from animal and vegetable foods. That from lean meat is known as myosin, from eggs albumin, from flour gluten, and from peas and beans legumen.

At present there are twenty known amino acids required for good health. Twelve are synthesized in the body, but there are eight essential ones the body cannot make.

Any food containing all eight essential amino acids is called a first-class, or complete, protein. One containing perhaps only three or four is an incomplete protein. Lean meat and milk are first-class proteins. But before the body can build them into solid bone or soft tissue it has first to split them up into their various amino acids, using the digestive juices to do so.

When protein is digested, nitrogen is released, but it cannot be stored in the body. This is why we must take a little protein every day of our lives. Waste products of protein are conveyed by the blood to the liver.

Protein is the magic word today. It's in your hairspray, your shampoo and deodorant. These are probably the most expensive forms of protein you can buy, but the protein you eat does not have to be expensive. You can be healthy on a small budget. An omelette for eight costs about the same as a beef meal for four. Fish for two will cost a lot less than a fancy chocolate cake.

If you mix your protein from animal and vegetable sources, vary those sources for maximum nutrition. If you prefer a cheaper intake of protein, you need not eat regularly the complete, or first-class proteins. You can mix, say, peas and the legumes such as soya products with wholegrains, together with other foods in combinations to achieve a wider protein 'spread'.

With regards to the amount of protein you need a day, this depends on many factors including the stress level at which you live, the efficiency of your liver, the general state of health, and whether you do sedentary or manual work.

Sometimes there is a case for the 'mono-diet' (one food at a time) where combinations cause you to feel, think or be unwell.

What are the best sources of protein?
Most people think that animal flesh and organs are indispensable for a healthy body. The absolute necessity of a diet of meat, eggs, butter and dairy products has been instilled into us as far back as we can remember. Plant proteins, on the other hand, have always been considered incomplete. But now, researchers have found that some are a natural source of protein containing all the amino acids. The amounts are small but still sufficient to satisfy our normal requirements.

Plant proteins are being shown as a high calorie, low protein diet ideal for building and maintenance. Happily, where there are deficiencies of essential amino acids in one plant food, these may be offset by other plants containing the missing ingredients. The average American and European consumes more than twice as much animal protein as he or she needs. This over-indulgence increases the acid secretion in the urine that can impose extra strain upon the kidneys. Soon the blood becomes less alkaline and more acid, thus creating conditions for the onset of disease.

There is so much more to the process of nourishing the body than just eating.

Examples of food combinations

Legumes (peas, beans, lentils and peanuts) combine well with grains (brown rice, barley, rye, oats, wheat, buckwheat).

Nuts and seeds combine with legumes.

Eggs and dairy products go well with vegetable protein (soya flour, etc.).

Suggestions include: soy-beans and hazelnuts, brown rice and beans, wholegrain macaroni and cheese, pea soup with barley kernels.

It is not good to eat starchy foods, like bread, with acid fruits. Fermentation is caused by the fruit acid on contact with the starch and gastric discomfort is possible. Food should be varied during the day, but not at the same meal. The fewer foods mixed together at one meal the better.

What are fats?

All foods, including fruit, vegetables, whole grains, nuts and some pressed seeds, contain fat. Most fats consist of glycerol and fatty acids, and are made up mostly of energy-producing carbon and hydrogen. Glycerol (or glycerine) and fatty acids have an affinity for each other. In combination, they form calorie-producing materials known as triglycerides.

The glycerol (of fats) is stored as glycogen, a substance similar to starch, which may be used immediately for energy production or stored in the liver until needed. The simplest way of putting on unwanted weight is to build up such a stock of glycogen that the body is forced to reconvert it into fat for storage around the hips and elsewhere.

Fats lubricate the skin, insulate nerve fibres by protecting the delicate filaments and act as a vehicle for distributing vitamins round the body. There are times when the body needs fat for extra energy and to keep out the cold, as in wintertime. Fats are the highest 'octane' fuel you can handle. For instance, 100g (35oz) bread (four or five slices) contain roughly 1,047kg (250 calories) or energy units.

The purest form of fat (margarine, butter and lard) contains – weight for weight – twice as many calories as starch or protein. Especially high in the scale are fried bacon, grilled pork sausages, double cream and Cheddar cheese.

Can the body produce all the fats it needs? Yes, all except one – linoleic acid. This is an essential nutrient, but we need so little of it that 30g (1oz) of oatmeal a day does the trick.

As much as 40% of the average Westerner's calorie intake comes from fatty foods. But researchers now believe that such a high percentage can inflict irreversible damage.

Why is a high percentage of fat to be avoided? Because fats deprive healthy tissue of oxygen. When tissue is denied oxygen for any great length of time, it atrophies and dies. Oxygen is the main necessity of life. It reaches the blood to purify and vitalize it through the process of respiration. Oxygen starvation (anoxia) is where the tissues receive less oxygen than is needful for their work. The blood is not capable of carrying its normal amount of oxygen when it is loaded with lipids and cholesterol after a big fatty meal.

Because an adequate supply of oxygen must be immediately available in the body, any lack of it can prove a threat to cases of heart disease, slow circulation, anaemia and where there are breathing difficulties.

Vitamin E – found in many vegetable foods – is nature's answer to oxygen starvation. Many people augment their body supply by taking supplements of this expensive vitamin. There must be at least fifty million people taking this vitamin in the USA, UK and Europe. It would be interesting to learn how many are heavy consumers of butter and other 'saturates', which rapidly deplete their reserves of this vitamin and render many vitamin E preparations useless.

What are saturated fats?
All fats consist of carbon and hydrogen. Those derived from warm-blooded animals contain a high concentration of hydrogen, so are said to be saturated. They are solid at room temperature and contain a white waxy substance called cholesterol. This occurs naturally in the blood, but tends, over the

years, to build up in the inner lining of the arteries, raising blood pressure and causing blockages that lead to heart attacks and strokes.

Fish are not 'saturated' which makes them preferable to animal meats. The best sources of fish fats are halibut, cod, salmon, sardines and herring – all rich in vitamins A and D.

The rate at which fats are used up in the body is determined by the glands (organs that secrete substances that act elsewhere) such as the adrenals, thyroid and pituitary, whose hormones (chemical messengers) split up fatty acids in the blood. The deposit of cholesterol on artery walls can be accelerated where under stressful conditions a glut of hormones is discharged into the bloodstream. This places heavy fat consumers at risk, the most effective antidote being exercise.

What are unsaturated fats?
Unsaturated fats are those that contain a low concentration of hydrogen. They are liquid at room temperature, and are of two kinds: mono-unsaturated fat (oleic acid) and polyunsaturated fat (linoleic acid). They come largely from the vegetable kingdom. Liquid vegetable fats are said to be polyunsaturated when they contain two or more extra atoms of hydrogen.

Vegetable fats are made up of unsaturated fatty acids and are found in soybean, safflower, corn, cottonseed, sunflower seed, olive oil and other so-called golden oils. This means they are able to take on extra atoms of hydrogen.

More of the younger generation of doctors recommend golden oils to replace butter, lard and the fat of meats. These oils lower cholesterol levels and are therefore a safeguard against high blood pressure and heart disorders.

Dr Nathan Pritikin[1] and other investigators claim that even corn and other vegetable oils may cause temporary clumping of blood cells. 'Clumping' is the sticking together of blood cells, caused by a sticky fatty film forming over each cell. But, by a long way, meat and dairy fats are the worst offenders. First to get plugged up are the tiny capillaries; later the general circulation slows down.

What is meant by cholesterol?

Today, the Western world lays down more fat on the walls of its arteries in a year, than did the Old World in a whole lifetime. A frugal diet knows no cholesterol problem.

The more hard fat we eat, the more difficult it is for our blood to find its way round the kilometres of labyrinthine blood-vessel network of our circulatory system. The more fats we eat from meat and dairy products, the more cholesterol we produce. Any excesses will plug our arteries with its gluey consistency.

Our bodies need cholesterol for vital jobs, such as maintaining the brain and assisting the glandular system. We need it to form bile salts and certain hormones. And since we can manufacture our own fats in the liver, there would appear to be no necessity for any extra intake in the form of animal fats.

As a product of saturated animal fat, cholesterol is found in cream, whole milk, cheese, butter and meat. Skimmed milk products are low in saturated fat and cholesterol. This is one reason why they are recommended for those who may suffer from hardening of the arteries. There are good reasons why we should avoid the kind of fat that causes the blood to sludge and block millions of tiny capillaries.

Carbohydrates – heat and energy creators

Carbohydrates contain carbon, which combines with oxygen and hydrogen, producing energy. They consist mainly of starches and sugars. Starches are present in considerable quantities in potatoes, bread, and also in fruits, green vegetables and nuts.

Nature gives us starch in green plants, then stores it in the roots, stems and seeds. Chief among the seeds are wheat, maize, barley, rye, sago and rice. The presence of starch in roots is best seen in the potato.

The sugar group is also derived from the vegetable kingdom as cane or beet sugar and honey.

Some starches are easier to digest than others. Of these, there are three different kinds.

(1) **Mono-saccharides:** These are the starches that are most easily digested. All starches must be reduced to this elemental state before they can be used in the body. This group contains dextrose, glucose, fructose and galactose.
(2) **Disaccharides:** These starches take the form of cane sugar or sucrose, maltose or malt sugar, lactose or milk sugar.
(3) **Polysaccharides:** These include dextrin, cellulose and glycogen – the latter is referred to as animal starch.

   During digestion sugar and starch must be reduced to a simpler form before they can be burned up in the tissues to produce heat and energy.

As it is soluble in water, sugar cannot be stored in the tissues. So the body converts it into a simpler starch – glycogen – that is stored in the muscles and liver, where it stays until muscular exertion and emotional activity take it out of the body reserves for immediate requirements.

Not all sugars are easily absorbed. Only those that are found in nature, such as those present in fruits and vegetables and in honey, are readily digestible. It is into this kind of sugar that starches are converted in the body, so as to render it easy to digest.

But certain forms of sugar – such as white sugar – in addition to some starches, if taken in excess, are liable to overtax the stomach and cause indigestion. Moreover, they release a substance that activates insulin, which in turn decreases blood sugar and increases appetite. The more sugar you eat, the more you want.

Learned medical societies hear how world experts blame sugar for many problems: tooth decay, heart disease, low blood sugar, obesity, chronic fatigue, sleeplessness and aggression.

'Sugar weakens your body's ability to fight infection.'

B.N. Nalder, Utah State University

Other not so well-known conditions include: hyperactivity in children and adults, depression and mood swings, Crohn's disease and high blood pressure.

Honey is the ideal form of sweetening. There is, however, a digestible form of sugar known as Barbados, a very dark sugar, and rich in impurities. Why are impurities good? They contain a conglomerate of minerals and are a valuable source of nutrients.

'White sugar provides no vitamins, no minerals, no proteins, no dietary fibre – just calories.'

(Sainsbury)

In well-balanced diet the starchy foods should account for 80% of our daily intake. Where they have not been modified by the food chemist, they will contain all the fibre, minerals and vitamins required. In this way we get the maximum from bread, cereals, corn flour, rice, bananas and so on.

Choice of food

Our choice of food is often the result of habit. Most people continue to cook and eat food they've always been used to. This may mean the destruction of essential nutrients.

Happily, more and more people are drawn towards natural foods. All that is needed is the simple good cooking of honest-to-goodness vegetables. It's good to taste the natural food free of seasoning.

Food should taste of what it is. If it's lamb, it's expected to taste like lamb, not mutton. If it's wholewheat bread, not pre-fabricated dough. If bread is beautifully cooked you can smell the goodness in it.

Avoid 'convenience' or fast foods. Go out of your way for natural foods. Make sure all bread flour and cereals arrive at your table 'whole', as they come from the earth – that nothing has been removed, nothing added. Never be tempted to take white sugar – honey will do you twice as much good. Take no sugar with fruit.

Instant potato can lose its vitamin C soon after being opened. Very little butter or soft margarine is recommended. Unsweetened carob powder may be used as a substitute for chocolate. For cooking, sunflower seed oil makes a good alternative to butter.

Keep it simple. Take your time at meals. Don't eat when you are excited or in a hurry. Masticate well before swallowing. Enjoy and savour the flavour of your food. Dry feed, as far as possible. Try not to drink with meals. Drink plenty between meals. Let your credo be: more fibre, less fat; more fresh food, less sugar and salt.

Foods to eat

- **Grains:** All wholegrains. Bread, cereals, rice, pasta.
- **Meat:** Lean beef or lamb, chicken, turkey, venison, poultry, game.
- **Fat:** Margarines with liquid corn or other liquid vegetable oil as the first listed ingredient. Corn oil, safflower seed oil, sesame seed oil, soy-bean oil, cottonseed oil. Fish oils.
- **Dairy products:** Milk. Skim-milk powder (non-fat). Evaporated skim milk. Buttermilk. Low-fat cheese, cottage cheese, skimmed milk cheeses. Yoghurt, eggs in moderation.
- **Fish:** All kinds that have fins and scales (*Leviticus* 11:10).
- **Vegetables:** All vegetables, including potatoes. Beet, sweetcorn, cucumbers, peppers, carrots, cabbage, lettuce, tomatoes, sweet potatoes, beans, peas and legumes generally.
- **Fruits:** All fresh fruits, stewed, cooked or puréed. Dried fruits, raisins, figs, etc. Nuts, seeds.
- **Sugars:** Honey. Demerara (sparingly). Barbados. Condiments: Dressings, sauces, desserts, home-made mayonnaise, salad oil. Powdered herbs and spices, cider vinegar, capers. Wine or cider vinegar. Salt – a bare minimum.
- **Beverages:** Tea (in moderation). Herb teas (vervain, chamomile, hibiscus, lemon balm, parsley, mint, limeflower, ginseng, etc.). Dandelion or other coffee substitutes. Home-made fruit drinks, e.g. barley and lemon. Drink when you are thirsty – water – especially spring water or other mineral waters. Unsweetened fruit and vegetable juices. Use honey for sweetening: never use saccharine or aspartame sugar substitutes.

- **Snacks:** Fresh fruits or raw carrot. Fruit bar. Dates. Nuts and raisins. When engaged on heavy manual work – cheese and onion. Bedtime: oatmeal biscuit, with hot milk well-laced with honey.

Grace Salad

Obtain as many vegetables as available. Line individual plates (or bowls) with lettuce. Cut a tomato into four segments (but do not sever entirely), and place in the middle of the plate (or bowl). Surround by small heaps of grated carrots, beetroot, cabbage, and grated nuts. Add watercress, mustard and cress, cucumber or root vegetables, 2.5-cm (1-in)-long pieces of celery and dates. Add a little cooked brown rice.

Mayonnaise

To 60ml yoghurt, add 15ml olive oil, one egg white, 15ml cider vinegar, and the juice of one lemon. Add chopped garlic or onion, fennel, dill or parsley to taste. Shake well before use. If too thick, it can be diluted with a little concentrated vegetable juice.

Foods not to eat

- **Grains:** Any breads, cereals, rice pastry or bakery goods that have been made with the addition of sugars. All white flour products.
- **Meat:** Frankfurters, hamburgers, organ meats (kidney, brain, sweetbreads). Everything from the pig – bacon, ham, pork, lard. All fat from meat and poultry, sausage, beefburgers, goose, duck, suet.
- **Fat:** Avoid all fat of meat, lard and hydrogenated margarine.
- **Dairy Products:** All cheese containing more than 1% fat. Cream. All substitutes for cream. Whipped cream.
- **Fish:** All canned fish, except that canned in oil. Shellfish; lobster, crab, prawns, shrimps, oysters, whelks (*Leviticus* 11:10).
- **Fruits:** Fruits out of cans, or have been frozen, with sugar added. Commercial fruit juices and soft drinks with added sugar. Blackcurrant syrup with added sugar.
- **Sugars:** All refined sugar, white sugar and confectionery.
- **Oils:** Hydrogenated vegetable oils.
- **Beverages:** Coffee, carbonated drinks.

The law of Moses includes specific instructions regarding foods that may or may not be eaten. Foods which were permitted were 'clean', those prohibited, 'unclean'. Anything declared 'unclean' in the Bible is usually associated with disease. Those who wish to pursue this subject further should look at *Leviticus* 3:17, chapter 11; chapter 19: 19–26.

Acts 15:29 has a special reference to blood taken through the mouth or through the veins, being one and the same thing – to nourish a sickly body or restore to health. In the sight of the Creator there is a special sanctity about human and animal blood, which should not be taken into the body.

A typical week's healthy eating

Monday
BREAKFAST: Muesli with grated apple. Milk or yoghurt – Wholewheat bread, or toast, or rye crispbread. Butter. Honey. LUNCH: Glass tomato juice, or vegetable soup – A raw salad (with or without beansprouts). The ingredients for my recommended salad, which I call Gerard Salad, are given on p.24. Mayonnaise, or lemon and olive oil dressing – Wholewheat bread, butter – Grapes, banana, or apple. DINNER: Melon – Tender chicken or turkey – Cooked vegetables, with jacket potato – Dried fruit.

Tuesday
BREAKFAST: Apple or pear – Blend of grains: rye, oats, wheat-flakes or barley kernels, and milk or yoghurt – Any whole-grain bread. Butter. Honey. LUNCH: Salad, with cottage cheese. Mayonnaise or dressing – Oat cake, yoghurt cocktail (yoghurt, honey and wheat germ). DINNER: Split pea soup – Nut cutlet and cooked vegetables – Fresh fruit salad.

Wednesday
BREAKFAST: Soaked figs, or prunes, muesli consisting of assorted grains, bran, grated nuts, raisins, sunflower seeds, etc. with yoghurt

continued

or top of the milk. LUNCH: Vegetable soup – Salad, with chopped suey, bamboo shoots, etc. – Baked apple stuffed with seedless raisins. DINNER: Poached eggs, on steamed spinach puree – Baked jacket potato, cooked carrots, etc. – Bananas and custard.

Thursday
BREAKFAST: Grapefruit, or apple – Cereal. Few dates or figs. Yoghurt or top of milk – Slice wholewheat bread. Butter. Honey. LUNCH: Salad, with chicken. With or without dressing – Baked apple, stuffed with seedless raisins. DINNER: Bean soup – Poultry or fish, with creamed potato, broccoli, and a pinch of curry powder (if desired) – Peach Melba.

Friday
BREAKFAST: Apple – Shredded wheat or buckwheat (kasha), Yoghurt or top of milk – Toast. Butter. Honey. LUNCH: Vegetable soup with noodles – Salad, with cottage cheese – Oatmeal biscuit. DINNER: Cooked sweetcorn on lettuce leaf or, lamb with mint sauce. Cooked potatoes and vegetables – Fresh fruit salad made from available fruits. Yoghurt or top of milk.

Saturday
BREAKFAST: Fruit. Grapes – A blend of grains: oats, rye and barley. Yoghurt or top of milk – Wholewheat bread. Butter or margarine. Honey, or homemade preserve. LUNCH: Lentil soup – Salad, with eggplant. Chopped chives – Fresh fruit, with spoonful of wheat germ. DINNER: Melon, with ginger – Fillets of sole, haddock, trout or other fish. Cooked brown rice – Stewed apples or pears, dried or fresh fruits as available.

Sunday
BREAKFAST: Fruit – A nut crunch, with yoghurt or top of milk – Wholewheat bread. Butter or margarine. Honey, or homemade preserve. LUNCH: Barley and vegetable soup – Onion cheese omelet – Oatmeal biscuit, with butter. DINNER: Fish with chopped parsley. Or nut cutlets. Cooked vegetables. Potatoes – Rice pudding or fresh fruit salad.

Note: Menus for lunch and dinner are reversible.

High-fibre diet

Something might be missing from your diet – insufficient roughage, or fibre.

Dietary fibre is the supporting structure of plants that forms the cell walls – the outside envelope for the plant's nutrients. For decades we discarded roughage in the belief that it had nothing to offer human nutrition. Now, scientists see how necessary it is to keep us healthy.

The role of fibre is partly mechanical, partly to increase the population of beneficial bacteria, and to hold sufficient water in the faeces to ensure easy evacuation. This latter factor is important, the stool becoming softer, bulkier, and easier to pass. It also causes the person to lose weight, if too fat. It is in the fibre that many vital minerals are contained.

The most fibre-containing substance is bran. An increasing number of doctors believe that were we all to add bran to our diets, bowel troubles, gallstones, piles and varicose veins would gradually disappear. A diet low in fibre also seems to be a contributory cause of coronary heart disease.

One great advantage of roughage is that a high fibre diet is at the same time a low fat diet, and vice versa. This is important to those with obesity.

People in the West are beginning to reap the benefits of health education about the value of a high fibre diet. Bakers report a greater demand for wholemeal bread, greengrocers report increased sales of fresh fruits and vegetables. Appendicitis is one of the many conditions resulting from a low-fibre diet. Surgical wards of our hospitals now receive fewer cases of appendicitis than in previous decades because people make more specific demands upon their baker and greengrocer.

A simple and cheap insurance against many diseases is to add one heaped dessertspoonful of bran or flaxseed to our daily diet. How much fibre should we eat daily? Vegetarians take about 40g (1.4oz) a day, and this is regarded as a good average. Not all need this amount but by starting with it, they can adapt to individual requirements.

Three or four slices of wholemeal bread and a good plateful of bran- or flaxseed-enriched muesli will supply at least 20g (¾oz). Fresh fruit, vegetables, dried fruits and nuts can make up another 20g (¾oz). The proof is in the eating.

Gluten-free diet

Untold millions of Asians (especially Chinese) have, since the beginning of their race, lived vigorous healthy lives on millet, rice or soya. These three have no gluten in the grain.

Gluten is the gluey incomplete protein part of some grains: wheat, oats, rye and barley. It is present in ordinary flour, bread, biscuits and cakes.

The gluten-free diet has become very popular among people with allergies. Nutritionists have discovered that this sticky substance can be the unsuspected cause of a number of disorders, ranging from coeliac disease (nervous colitis – an allergy) to rheumatoid arthritis, in those who cannot absorb gluten.

It has come to light that some people cannot take for granted bread, cereals, pastas and cakes that may contain wheat gluten. It is now a common experience among some children who have never been robust, but never really ill, to gain unbelievable vitality and freedom from certain allergies when put on a gluten-free diet.

A number of books on the subject have been published, including *Easy Gluten-Free Cooking*,[2] by Rita Greer. Bread is the real problem, an all-gluten loaf being unsatisfactory. A more acceptable loaf can be made by using equal parts of wheaten flour and soya flour.

The humble potato comes into its own in the gluten-free world, especially for thickening soups and casseroles.

In her book we learn how Rita Greer, already well-known as a gifted painter, achieved the seemingly impossible task of improving her husband's 'hopeless' chronic limitations from multiple sclerosis by putting him, literally, back on his feet again. She did this after years of experimentation in her kitchen where she found that her husband's condition really improved when gluten was excluded from his diet.

One does not have to suffer from allergies to enjoy some of the attractions of the gluten-free diet which many people find surprisingly agreeable.

Natural waters

Almost the whole of Europe is going 'natural' in its consumption of drinking water. Bottled mineral water from European springs is literally bubbling its way into our homes. Even in rainy Britain, sales of natural waters (not gaseous or aerated waters) have spurted significantly in recent years.

Why this sudden upsurge?

A lot of people are no longer happy about their public supplies of drinking water. While Britain lags behind some other countries, bottled waters from pure natural springs in Scandinavia, Germany and France are the 'in' thing. They contain no sugar, no artificial preserves or flavourings, no fluorides or chlorine, no calories. Most are bursting with valuable mineral salts.

The French Government has a special authorization for its natural spring waters. Deep in the mountains, its Evian waters are filtered as they flow through glacial sand. This impregnates them with mineral salts – 'sufficient to be of value, but low enough not to have any contra-indication for young and old'.

These waters are available widely and are ideal for those on a salt-free diet. It is not necessary to boil for purity – either when babies and young children require a base for dissolving powdered milk and foods or for between-feed drinks.

What your body needs is not so much tea, coffee and soft drinks, but just plain water. Our bodies call out for elemental 'aqua pura' which we tend to stifle with soft drinks and anything else that's going. We should all drink more water!

'Nothing can be more important or necessary to know than the science of nutrition, so let your medicine be your food and your food your medicine.'

Hippocrates

2

Vitamins

The remarkable fitness of the Hunzas, Maoris and inhabitants of Fiji, Tonga, Samoa, Hawaii, East Island, etc., is due to food loaded with vitamins. Vitamins have, of course, always been with us, although vitamin A, the first to be discovered, was not recognised until 1913.

It all started when Sir Richard Hawkins (1562–1622) and Captain Cook (1728–79) mentioned in their log books the cure of scurvy with lemon juice. The advent of the humble potato made a powerful impact upon European health in the sixteenth century. Vitamins increase our ability to resist disease.

When we eat a well balanced diet, Nature ensures us a plentiful supply of vitamins. But these can be vitiated by processed foods containing chemical additives for colouring and so on. Processed foods lack the vitality of raw foods.

How can we make up vitamin deficiencies? Each food contains many different vitamins. Food should be eaten raw and fresh when possible, with little cooking. Supplementation by natural vitamins may make all the difference between glowing health and a life without fun.

Women lose their mobility through lack of vitamins. Men lack potency and fertility because of a lack of vitamin A. Mental confusion in elderly people may sometimes be caused by lack of enough B vitamins.

Get to know your vitamins for what they are – invisible workers laying down sound bricks and mortar in the building of a durable constitution. They are not a substitute for honest-to-goodness food. Stress makes such heavy demands upon our vitamin resources that we cannot afford to gloss over this important nutritional factor.

Vitamin A (*retinol*)

There are folk alive today who may remember the discovery of this vitamin in 1913, but thousands felt the benefits of cod liver oil years before that.

Apart from fish oils, other sources are eggs, cheese, margarine, dairy products, liver, apricots, alfalfa leaves, spinach, broccoli, sweet potatoes, deep green leafy vegetables and, of course, carrots.

Vitamin A keeps the shiny surface of the eyeball moist and transparent. When it is short in the diet, these cells stop secreting mucus and produce keratin, which pits and beclouds those delicate structures. This occurs chiefly in rice-eating countries where vitamin A is scarce.

Eye troubles were once India's top medical problem. Thanks to vitamin A, one of the simplest and cheapest of remedies available in green vegetables, these are now much less severe.

Combined with vitamin D, it maintains sound bones and teeth and helps build up resistance against winter's colds. Vitamin A is also useful for people with rheumatoid-arthritis, and there is some evidence that a deficiency of this vitamin may be related to lung cancer.

Give yourself a simple test.

Vitamin A is stored as yellow carotene just under the skin. So clench your hand tightly. Open out quickly. Before blood has suffused back into the tissues, you should see a yellow pigment under the skin. If this temporary yellow hue is absent, you're not getting enough vitamin A.

Vitamin B1 (*aneurine or thiamine*)

Vitamin B1 is found in brewer's yeast, wheat germ, nuts, vegetables, beans, organ meats, sunflower seeds and wholegrain products.

All vitamins of the B group are closely related to mental health and the well-being of the nervous system. If we are short of any one of the group, we are likely to be short of others. It is wise not to take one single kind of vitamin without also taking a supplement of the whole group.

When appetite is poor, it is likely your vitamin B1 is in short supply. If it is accompanied by low physical endurance, muscle weakness and flitting pains in the limbs, you can be almost certain B1 is what you need. Take it also for nervous disorders, low blood pressure and a decline in well-being.

Vitamin B2 (*riboflavine*)

Vitamin B2 is found in brewer's yeast, asparagus, cheese, almonds, milk, liver, green leafy vegetables, broccoli, organ meats, brown rice, wheat germ, wholewheat bread and chicken.

A watery or bloodshot itching eye and undue sensitivity to light may be caused by a deficiency of vitamin B2. If we don't take enough B2 we are likely to get influenza germs more easily. Dryness of hair and skin are possible, as well as a sore tongue and a rash at the corners of the mouth.

Vitamin B3 (*nicotinic acid*) (*niacin*)

Vitamin B3 is found in brewer's yeast, game, poultry, fish and seafoods, organ meats (liver, kidneys, etc.), beans, wholegrain cereals and wholewheat bread.

We must renew supplies daily if we are to avoid undue nervous tension and instability. End results of a diet weak in this nutrient can be unpleasant, what doctors call the 'three Ds' – dermatitis, diarrhoea and dementia. Where deficiency is not corrected it may lead to a deterioration of the nervous system.

Headache and depression have been known to follow a reduced intake. Prolonged shortage throws up an uncomfortable set of symptoms known as pellagra, which develops with a rough skin, neuritis and digestive troubles. It starts with depression and confusion.

Schizophrenics (literally 'split minds') and alcoholics are known to have low blood sugar, which can be corrected by this vitamin. Hyperactive mentally disturbed children can also benefit. An encouraging development has been an ability of this vitamin to improve school performance and straighten out social maladjustments in young children. B3 deficiency symptoms cannot appear in those who enjoy a varied diet including ample protein.

B3 is associated with the body's utilization of sugar. Excessive use of white sugar has been found to be intimately connected with mental symptoms where heavy demands are made upon the body's reserves of vitamin B3. Penicillin and the other antibiotics destroy this important vitamin.

Vitamin B6 (*pyridoxine*)

If we took advantage of our accumulated knowledge of vitamins, practically all common complaints and dental problems could be eliminated in one generation. On the strength of vitamin B6 alone, this might well be true.

It is present in sunflower seeds, bananas, brewer's yeast, peanuts, wholegrain cereals, wholewheat bread, brown rice, buckwheat products, chicken, poultry, organ meats and fish.

Adelle Davis, noted nutritionist, writes: 'The intense pain of so-called arthritics could be largely alleviated. Deficiencies induced by dangerous and often needless diuretics could be avoided. Not only could pregnancy become relatively free from sickness, but more intelligent healthy children could be produced with the aid of vitamin B6.'

Vitamin B12 (*cyanocobalamine*)

This vitamin is present in liver, beef, eggs, milk, cheese, organ meats, fish and seafoods.

When we do not get a sufficiency of this vitamin our blood cells suffer. Vegetarians are at risk as it is usually found in meats, especially liver. Vitamin B12 foods are essential for sufferers of polyneuritis, diabetes and pernicious anaemia.

Vitamin B15 (*Pangamic acid*)

What is so special about this vitamin? It was the secret that enabled Soviet athletes to startle the world with such extraordinary performances at the 1968 Olympics. If, at first, it was believed that the Russian women were training on male hormones, it soon became apparent that a new vitamin had been discovered. Since then, claims made for its life-saving and life-rejuvenating properties have caught the public imagination.

How does it work? It increases the volume of oxygen in the bloodstream, thereby promoting more efficient expulsion of body wastes and by-products of combustion. In this way it is able to delay ageing of body cells.

Dr Shpirt of the Academy of Sciences said: 'I believe the time will come when supplements of the vitamin will be on the table of every family with people past forty.'

Every time a muscle contracts it expends energy. This energy is provided by fresh oxygen, which cells select from the bloodstream. When oxygen is in action, it leaves behind a chemical waste – lactic acid – the build-up of which is retarded by this 'stamina' vitamin.

B15 puts a heavy brake on the pathological craving for drink. The Russians use it for drink and drug abuse, and find that it gives a boost to low blood sugar.

'You seldom see high energy people who are shrinking violets or who suffer from certain self-images,' writes Brenda Forman, medical journalist.[3] 'High energy folks take more risks and are less prone to negative psychological ramifications of rejection and failure. Low energy people are those you often see who have psychological problems – who suffer from depression and psychological blockages.'

Vitamin B17 (*amygdalin*)

Fruit stones and certain berries contain vitamin B17, claimed to be an anti-cancer vitamin. Some investigators believe it will be to cancer what vitamin C is to scurvy, and vitamin B12 to pernicious anaemia.

Few sources are as rich as apricot kernels. Reduced quantities are found in apples, cherries, currants, nectarines, plums, prunes and pears. Green vegetables contain scarcely any at all. It is to the Chinese restaurants that we owe chop suey made from bamboo shoots, which is one of the pleasantest ways of eating B17. Sprouted bamboo shoots, alfalfa seeds, mung beans and wheat grains are all over twenty times richer than the unsprouted.

Parts of the world where kernels of fruit stones are eaten in the diet have thrown up evidence to suggest that they afford the body some protection against cancer, which some investigators believe to be a deficiency disease.

Until science comes up with all the answers, we shall not know the truth. In the meantime, maybe there is something to be gained from a sprinkle of ground roasted apricot kernels – or would you prefer the potential pip-power of Cox's Orange Pippins?

Vitamin C

This is a vital nutrient, though most people consume too little. Most unstable of all the vitamins, it is easily lost by heat, water, oxygen in the air, drugs and smoking. The most important causes of loss are stress and emotional exhaustion. Vitamin C is known to many as the 'stress' vitamin.

While few things compare with a strong spiritual background and positive thought for dealing with stress, vitamin C is known to have a steadying effect on the psyche in highly charged emotional situations when the vitamin is used up rapidly. Sources include citrus fruits, leafy green vegetables, green peppers, cabbages, potatoes, acerola, rose-hips, broccoli, cauliflower, Brussels sprouts, tomatoes, cantaloupe, blackcurrants, papaya, guava, strawberry, persimmon, spinach, lemon juice, orange juice, fresh pineapple, grapefruit and grapes.

Allergy is one of the common causes of minor ailments. This is a field in which vitamin C supplementation excels.

Enormous interest was evinced in this vitamin when the Nobel Prize-winner, Dr Linus Pauling, Professor of Chemistry, published his book *Vitamin C and the Common Cold*.[4]

Vitamin D

It is an interesting fact that practically all vitamins are made by plants. An exception is vitamin D, for which direct sunlight is responsible. The 'sunshine' vitamin regulates the degree in which calcium and phosphorus are laid down in our bodies. It is essential for the proper formation of bones and teeth.

A deficiency can cause rickets, retarded growth, tooth decay and other weaknesses. Bone malformation was once believed to be a disease of poverty and ill-ventilated dwellings, until a Far Eastern missionary remarked that these did not cause rickets where there was strong sunshine. Actually, we synthesize most of our requirements of this vitamin when our skin is exposed to sunshine.

Foods that contain vitamin D include fish liver oils (cod, halibut, etc.), sardines, salmon, herring and mackerel.

Our bodies can manufacture vitamin D from sunlight. The more clothes we wear, the less our bodies are exposed to the sun, and the more likely we are to sustain loss of this vitamin. Black children living in northern Europe require more protection against rickets than whites living under similar conditions. A dark skin offers protection against excessive sunlight.

Glass windows and normal clothing are barriers to your intake of this vitamin, so you can see there is much to be said for out-of-doors exercises with a minimum of clothing. We all need summer's sunlight to lay down adequate stores of vitamin D for the winter, to give added strength to our body's defence system. How we all need the sun!

Vitamin E (*alpha-tocopherol*)

'Life is a constant struggle against oxygen deficiency,' wrote the Russian physiologist Ivan Pavlov (1849–1936). Of all vitamins, vitamin E rouses most controversy. It is a vital nutrient which keeps our cells healthy by ensuring they have a good blood supply.

In the early eighties, there came from Doctors Wilfred and Evan Shute, Canadian physicians, a success story which thrilled world medicine.[5] It all started when they treated their mother who had angina and swelling of the legs. When she took this vitamin her anginal pains vanished and dropsy dispersed within one week. Heart disease was their speciality. They were regarded as experts in the use of vitamin E for heart disease, thrombosis, serious burns, varicose veins and certain menopausal symptoms.

The vitamin comes to us in many forms; chiefly in freshly ground whole-wheat flour, wheat germ, vegetable oils, green leaves, meat, margarine, wholegrain cereals, olive oil, safflower oil, soy-bean oil, peanut oil, sesame oil, sunflower seed oil, wheat germ oil, corn oil, almonds and sprouted seeds.

This 'life of the wheat' is found in the germ, which is a powerful anti-coagulant. Its most useful property is that of an antioxidant. As an anti-coagulant, it has an ability to remove deposits of cholesterol from arteries caused by saturated fats and calcium. The Shutes regarded it as the key both to prevention and treatment of conditions arising from a lack of blood supply due to thickened or blocked blood vessels.

Its use in the healing of wounds has shown how it can heal by leaving the smallest of scars. A growing number of practitioners regard it as one of the few safe substances that can be added to the list of so-called 'wonder-drugs'.

Vitamin K (*phytomenadione*)

Discovered by a Danish scientist, Henrik Dam, in 1935, vitamin K, the anti-haemorrhage vitamin, opened up a new horizon in surgery. Patients who previously died from loss of blood were saved. When vitamin K is scarce, clotting time will be so prolonged that it is unlikely we would recover from the slightest wound.

There must be adequate calcium in the blood if vitamin K – which is produced by bacteria in the intestines – is to do its work properly. Aspirin, often used in the treatment of the elderly, destroys this vitamin and prolongs clotting time.

Bio-flavonoids

These assist the action of vitamin C in the body. They are protective against allergies and play a part in the body's defence system. By strengthening walls of the capillaries, they help prevent strokes in cases of high blood pressure.

They are present in the pulp and peel of citrus fruits, grapes, rosehips, buckwheat and blackcurrant.

It takes about three or four oranges to supply the normal daily requirements. Green peppers are another popular way of obtaining this useful factor.

Biotin

This is a member of the B group – a co-enzyme assisting others in their function. It is present in all animal tissues and, like vitamin K, is produced in the intestines by bacteria.

It is present in milk, liver, eggs, nuts, brewer's yeast, yeast, beans, lamb, veal, beef, molasses, fish, cheese and whole grains.

Deficiencies are rare as it is so widely distributed among the foods we eat. It forms part of enzyme systems related to the metabolism of proteins, fatty acids and glucose. But where deficiencies do occur, they spell lack of energy, dry skin, muscular pain and hair troubles.

Choline

Essential for metabolism of fats. It is required by the kidneys, for milk production in lactation, for the spleen and thymus gland. Choline and inositol are more effective when taken together than separately. A liberal intake is helpful for nerve troubles.

Deficiencies may give rise to high blood pressure with symptoms of headache, dizziness, ear noises, palpitation and constipation, all of which have almost disappeared after supplementing the diet with choline.

Folic acid

Also a member of the B group, folic acid was first isolated in spinach. The name 'folic' comes from the word 'foliage' – being found in leafy green vegetables. Other sources are cheese, milk, corn, wheat germ, beef, asparagus, beet green, endive, potatoes, lima beans and kidneys.

It is a substance that enriches the blood, restoring vitality to body cells. By its stimulating action on the bone marrow, it is essential to form red blood cells. We have seen how a deficiency of B12 can cause pernicious anaemia. There is another kind of anaemia (macrocytic, or giant cell) which is caused by a shortage of folic acid. Both B12 and folic acid are found in liver and yeast.

Where an insufficiency exists, the person becomes susceptible to fungus infections. Onset of early senility in the elderly may be the result of too few green salads, with inadequate folic acid.

Inositol

Inositol is an essential B group nutrient for all organs. High deposits in the lens of the eye imply that clarity of vision is partly dependent upon it. This member of the B group has been used with success in cases of psoriasis (a chronic skin condition) and is said to assist hair growth. Deficiencies lead to premature ageing.

Natural sources are fruits, nuts, yeast, milk, liver, brewer's yeast, wheat germ, yoghurt, beef heart and brown rice. Caffeine in tea and coffee counteracts its beneficial effects.

Nicotinamide

A form of vitamin B3 which dilates the blood vessels, being helpful for ringing in the ears (tinnitus) and dizziness. Maintains normal function of the skin, nerves and digestive system. Helpful for prevention of premenstrual headache.

Pantothenic acid (*also known as vitamin B5*)

Little is known of this important food factor apart from the fact that its absence in the diet favours the onset of neuritis and rheumatic aches and pains. A deficiency in animals causes inability to walk straight and weakness of the hindquarters.

Thinning and greying of the hair has responded to supplementation. Some claim it is helpful for allergies. A member of the B group, its richest source is 'royal jelly', as fed to bee larvae by worker bees to rear the queen. The prodigious effort required of these marvellous creatures in propagating the hive population demands nutrients of great power and sustenance.

As our bodies cannot synthesize this acid, daily supply must be made up through food or supplements, usually in the form of calcium pantothenate.

Para (*para-aminobenzoic acid*)

This component of folic acid helps protect the skin against sunburn. If it is omitted from the food of animals, their hair turns white; but colour can be restored on resumption in the diet. Like other vitamin B deficiencies, attendant symptoms are depression, digestive upsets and nervousness.

'The science of medicine will some time resolve itself into a science of prevention rather than a matter of cure. The best medicine I know of is an active and intelligent interest in the world of nature.'
Dr Erasmus Darwin Grandfather of, Charles Darwin

'Vitamin E is the most valuable ally the cardiologist has yet found in the treatment of heart disease. It has no rivals.

Vitamin E replaces "rest and reassurance" – which have no authentic basis – with real help to the damaged labouring heart itself.'
Dr Evan Shute

3

The Master Minerals

Our bodies are made up of a wide range of minerals. They regulate body fluids and the balance of chemicals. The role they play is little appreciated. In water and soil, they have a greater effect upon our health than climate.

Without the basic minerals life is impossible. It takes a mineral-rich soil to produce healthy food.

For the classic effects of a mineral-rich diet we return to the Hunza of Pakistan. It would be difficult to find women more energetic, men more virile. The secret of their superiority has been proved to be due to their raw diet. This is not because of any special custom, but because there is so little fuel in their country. No wood or coal is available for cooking. What precious fuel they have is stored for use against the long harsh winter.

Almost everything eaten is high in calcium, magnesium, iron and numerous valuable salts taken up from the soil by their fruits and vegetables. An interesting picture of their feeding habits appears in John Tobe's *Guideposts to Health*.[6] Their breakfast consists almost entirely of a mixture of dried apricots, grain meal and glacial water. They rub the wet apricots in the water between their hands and make a sort of gruel. To this they add freshly ground wholewheat, buckwheat, oats and barley meal. This is drunk like soup.

Apricots, both fresh and dried, form a vital part of their food supply and the kernels are stored until utilized. They are used as nuts or for the making of oil.

The oil is made by each individual householder, as and when required. This permits no rancidity. None of the important nutritive properties are removed.

Hunzas consume many varieties of raw vegetables: onions, potatoes, peas, beans, carrots, turnips, lettuce, radishes and others. English walnut trees are scattered throughout the country, but the apricot is the mainstay. Also eaten are wheat, buckwheat, millet, rye, barley and some rice.

Few can afford to raise cattle for food since pasturelands are extremely scarce. They drink some wine and practically every home has its own little vineyard; that is, a few grape vines strung along a wall against the house.

Every year thousands of pilgrims travel from all parts of India in order to bathe in and imbibe the water of the River Ganges, at the holy city of Benares. This must be the most heavily polluted river in the world. All kinds of germs from noxious diseases have been identified in it. Strangely enough, not many cases of infection are recorded. Why this strange phenomenon?

Local people will tell you that the upper reaches of the Ganges flow through soil containing a wealth of different kinds of minerals that render germs and bacteria inactive.

Does this mean that an adequate intake of various minerals in our food will heighten our resistance to infection? Scientists think it does.

Boron

An important mineral indicated for osteoporosis and arthritis, for its ability to repair magnesium and calcium losses from the bones. It also reduces risk of loss of these elements through expulsion through the kidneys.

Boron is used increasingly for the menopause. Sources include green vegetables, dried fruit and nuts.

Calcium

Minerals calcium and phosphorus are the main constituents of the bones and teeth. They are necessary for normal functioning of muscles and nerves, for clotting of blood, to regulate heart rhythm, and to sustain vitality and endurance.

Calcium is present in dried milk, cheese, green vegetables, wholewheat products, soy-beans, sesame seeds, brewer's yeast, almonds, figs, molasses, beans, broccoli, sardines, salmon, mackerel and herring.

Deficiencies bring on cramp, nervous tension, bad teeth and rickets. Some nutritionists believe it guards against radioactivity; others think it counteracts lead toxicity. A deficiency may be indicated by rheumatic and arthritic disturbances, sinus troubles and low back pain.

Hard water means a high calcium (lime) content, which is essential for keeping the central nervous system resilient. The softer the water, the higher the number of newborn infants with deficient brain power.

Loss of lime salts in the body may lead to softening of the bones, as in the elderly whose femurs are liable to fracture. Adequate calcium keeps hearts robust, capable of taking all the stresses imposed by such active exercises as cycling, mowing the lawn and jogging.

Chlorine

Present in sodium chloride (salt). Regulates the acid–alkali balance of the blood. It is a non-metallic essential mineral maintaining the body's water balance. Salt is necessary for efficient function of the adrenal glands. Loss of teeth and hair may follow deficiency.

Natural sources of chlorine are common table salt, olives and seaweeds.

Those who overdo the salt-shaker are at risk of developing strokes or cancer of the stomach. Try to keep daily intake to not more than 10mg daily.

Chromium

Chromium is in some ways essential to the body. Hypoglycaemia is a deficiency in chromium, and causes low blood sugar responsible for weakness, breathlessness and nervousness.

A superb piece of medical detection was carried out in Israel when experts could not understand why a group of children in the Jordan River Valley and another group in Jerusalem, fed on the same diet, should differ so much in health.

The Jerusalem children suffered from very low blood sugar alternating with high blood pressure levels. The Jordan River Valley children were quite free from these disturbances. Hospital staff were baffled, until someone hit on the idea of testing the water supply of each district. Drinking water from wells in the Jordan Valley contained much higher levels of chromium than those in Jerusalem. One single minute dose of chromium to each child wrought a miracle within 24 hours.

In the West, over-consumption of sugar makes serious inroads into our chromium levels, which are quickly affected every time the pancreas releases insulin. The more sugar we eat, the more chromium we use.

Those troubled with diabetic symptoms have a ready 'chromium' food in the form of brewer's yeast.

Cobalt

Cobalt (cobalamin) is the part of the molecule of vitamin B12 used in radio-therapy, and is essential for the production of red cells. Vegetarians may find supplementation necessary.

Sheep and farmyard cattle synthesize their own vitamin B12 requirements, but the human body lacks this ability, supplies being available from meat, liver, kidneys, milk and oysters.

Copper

Without copper, our bodies cannot form red blood cells. Deficiencies in human diet are practically unknown, being readily available in most foods.

Copper is present in all kinds of meat and fish, including shellfish, liver, brazil nuts, wholewheat products, brewer's yeast, curry powder, mushrooms, parsley, honey and red wine.

Women who take oral contraceptives tend to a low copper level and some antibiotics destroy its efficacy.

Fluorine

Fluorides help prevent dental decay by strengthening the enamel and preventing formation of plaque. Fluorine can be found in seafood, fish and seaweeds.

Iodine

Iodine is essential for the secretion of thyroxin, a hormone for the metabolism of fats. When depleted, it causes a swelling of the thyroid gland known as goitre. Good sources of iodine can be found in seafoods, fish, kelp, meat, onions and cereals.

Iron

Without iron, life cannot go on. When low in this mineral, bone marrow fails to produce healthy red blood cells. Cells will be malformed and pale in colour – the result of oxygen-starvation. It is the important constituent of haemoglobin – known as the oxygen-carrier of the blood.

Sources of iron foods are liver, kidneys, meat, eggs, wheat germ, wholewheat bread, wholegrain products, potatoes, green vegetables, beans, peas, lentils, parsley, spinach, sunflower seeds, rye crispbread, figs, brazil nuts, brewer's yeast, fish, crude black molasses and apricots.

Your body should hold five grams of iron, but its daily need is about 12 milligrams because it is poorly absorbed. Daily losses of iron are considerable, in the form of sweat, urine and worn-out cells, in spite of much being recycled in the liver.

When we reflect that only 10% of all the iron we eat is used, we see how necessary it is to eat from as many varied sources as possible. The more we examine each separate element, the deeper grows our understanding that all minerals, as well as proteins, vitamins and so on, work together for our good.

Acid is required to dissolve iron from the stomach and if you have any doubts about your body's ability to cope, two teaspoonfuls of apple cider vinegar in half a tumbler of water taken at meals will create the right environment for your intake of iron to be well broken down.

If we could convince children how vitamin C (in fresh fruits and vegetables) assists in the assimilation of iron, we would make a lasting impression upon the future health of nations. A little learning is no longer a dangerous thing.

Girls who eat no breakfast in the mistaken belief that they will avoid putting on weight produce too little oestrogen, which results in an iron shortage. Ovaries get lazy, and every cell in the body reacts by pillaging iron from its neighbour; complexion pales, hair becomes lifeless, nails get brittle, before emotional instability sets in with rapid tiredness from little effort.

This loss of iron must be made up if good health is to return. One of the fastest iron-rescue substances we know is crude black molasses (black-strap molasses), containing ten times more iron than ordinary sugar. When we consider that this is an ideal cattle food, we know we must be on the right lines – Europe has a habit of feeding its animals better than its children.

Magnesium

Magnesium is important for the metabolism of calcium and vitamin C, and essential for the functioning of the nervous system. It protects the myelin sheath, which encloses many nerves in the brain and spinal cord, and activates some enzymes in the body.

Enzymes are proteins that speed up chemical reactions. All foods we eat are totally indigestible until enzymes break them down into simpler substances before they are absorbed into the bloodstream. None of this would be possible without magnesium.

Magnesium has a relaxing effect upon irritable muscles and nerves, helps allay the onset of kidney stones, strengthens a weak heartbeat, safeguards blood vessels, and is important to bones and teeth.

Do alternatives to the controversial fluorides exist? A strong case has been put up for the use of magnesium for dental decay. Were water and soil treated with this mineral, the toxic effects of fluoride might be avoided. Our teeth are made up largely of calcium and magnesium, so what better protection could be offered than dolomite limestone, a naturally occurring combination of calcium and magnesium, which many dentists recommend?

Soft drinking water is low in calcium and magnesium, and is believed to carry the risk of heart disease. People living in soft water areas are encouraged to take a calcium and magnesium supplement.

To jog our memory from time to time is to make sure we do not overlook mineral-rich foods. When did you last eat almonds, cashews, peanuts, brazil nuts, walnuts and dried apricots – all prime sources of magnesium?

When we use them in salads, we have the satisfaction of knowing we are injecting precious chlorophyll as well as magnesium into our bodies. Chlorophyll is that mysterious colouring matter in plants about which so much is written, but so little known.

Magnesium is required to keep your heart strong and resilient, and to trigger electrical stimuli to keep it ticking over. Without magnesium there would be no heartbeat.

In any serious drop in energy levels, the heart is certain to be involved. You may not have heart trouble but can be scared out of your wits if a bout of palpitation overtakes you in the night. If your doctor gives you anticoagulants because he suspects thrombosis, it is a good thing to consider if your diet is falling down on magnesium.

Magnesium is a first-class vasodilator. It opens vessels wide, thus helping blood along its route through the body. We see the advantages of this in poor circulation. On stepping up her intake of magnesium levels by taking five almonds daily, a woman said her feet and hands were no longer cold in winter.

She said: 'Now, I don't have to place my feet on my warm husband at nights to keep my feet warm. He's no longer irritable and my feet don't wake him up any more.' Little did she realize that her almond supplement could delay hardening of the arteries.

Foods containing magnesium include nuts, peas, beans, crude black molasses, Brussels sprouts, bran, chard, corn, oatmeal, whole grain products, green vegetables, brown rice, prunes, raisins, honey and – one of the richest of them all – spinach.

Manganese

Nothing can happen in our bodies without enzymes. They really run the organism. Manganese is a powerful activator of enzymes, especially those present in the blood, which affect the heart and vessels.

When manganese is scarce, the reproductive organs are the first to suffer. Feeble sexual function sets in, and there is a possibility of stillbirths and infertility.

Surprisingly, one of the best sources is tea. A single cup of tea produces one milligram, so there is little likelihood tea drinker will be light on manganese. Average daily requirements are three to four milligrams. Buckwheat is also rich in this mineral.

It can also be found in bananas, wheat germ, wholegrain products, bran, oatmeal, brown rice, corn, rye crispbread, sweet potatoes, chestnuts, hazelnuts, walnuts, peas and beans, spices, prunes, spinach and celery.

A deficiency of this mineral is said to reduce a woman's concern for her young. We know that in animals a deficiency causes rat mothers to be lacking in the maternal instinct. It is certain that it is required somewhere along the line in the transmission of hereditary factors via the genes.

Molybdenum

This is a trace mineral present in dark green leafy vegetables (cabbage family), peas, beans and wholegrains. Is necessary for conversion of iron into haemoglobin (the red colouring matter in the blood).

Phosphorus

Phosphorus plays an essential part in releasing energy from food. It is present in all body cells. Together with calcium, it is highest in quantity of all minerals in our body. Composition of body fluids is in a large measure kept in balance by this mineral. Cavities in teeth are believed to be due to a deficiency of phosphorus. It is vital to growing infants.

So close is the action and interaction of calcium and phosphorus that a disturbance in one is immediately reflected in the other through what is known as the calcium-phosphorus balance. This balance has to be maintained at all costs, but is easily upset by the disastrous effects of white sugar.

Our phosphorus levels can fall dramatically two hours after eating confectionery or chocolate. Sufficient evidence now exists to show that tooth decay, arthritis and some other chronic diseases are often self-produced by eating substances that disturb the calcium-phosphorus balance.

Phosphorus is found in brewer's yeast, wheat germ, wholewheat bread, cereals and other products; eggs, cheese, liver, lecithin, yoghurt, sweetbreads, sardines, salmon, halibut, cod, milk, sunflower seeds, peas, peanuts, walnuts and brazil nuts.

Potassium

Potassium is one of our body's most needed elements. One of its restorative properties is to take the weariness out of heavy eyelids. In later life, when resistance and muscular strength are low, people respond positively to potassium.

Potassium foods are brewer's yeast, seeds (sprouted and unsprouted), sesame, sunflower and other seeds, tomatoes, wheat germ, apples, oranges, bananas, apricots, meats, broccoli, carrots, molasses and potatoes.

When we have periods of excessive tiredness, it can be helpful to turn to potassium-rich foods, such as tomatoes.

Selenium

At the end of the seventies, inhabitants of Rapid City, South Dakota, showed the highest selenium blood levels of any state in the USA. They also had the lowest cancer rate. Soil rich in this element produces selenium-rich green vegetables for strengthening our body's defences.

At Lima, Ohio, the mineral is scarce. This is reflected in people's low selenium levels – and twice the cancer rate of the South Dakotans.

Selenium works together with vitamin E, their combined effect being greater than the sum of their action apart. Together, they protect our bodies from early physical and mental degeneration.

Selenium foods: spinach, brewer's yeast, milk, liver, kidneys, sweetbreads, soy-beans, corn (maize) and fish.

Deficiency symptoms include hair loss, cataracts and reproductive difficulties.

Modern methods of production include growing the mineral in brewer's yeast, which results in a natural product containing the mineral in an identical form in which it has always been eaten by humans. Finland has made an impressive contribution by supplying a selenium preparation from enriched barley.

Recommended daily allowance: Supplements – 75mcg for men; 60mcg for women. *See*: Brazil nuts p. 57.

Sodium Chloride

Sodium chloride (common table salt) is necessary to hold water in the body, thus preventing dehydration. One effect of stress is to so interfere with the behaviour of salt in our bodies that water may be retained, eyes and ankles becoming puffy.

When the adrenal glands are exhausted, too much water and salt may be lost from the body, resulting in dehydration and low blood pressure. At such times extra salt may be necessary.

But it has been said that the average diner consumes ten times more salt than needed. What happens to any excess? The burden of its elimination falls on the over-worked kidneys. Few people ever give a thought to conserving the efforts and energies of their kidneys.

This salt is readily available in most foods and does not need supplementation at the table. It is found in all seafoods, kelp and sea salt.

Common salt produces acid. Excess can result in over-acidity. It also inhibits the elimination of uric acid, which paves the way to rheumatism and gout. It also creates abnormal thirst which, if satisfied, makes watery blood. Watery blood makes fat. In this way, salt is converted into fat.

Scientists warn of 'the salt menace', the largest contributory cause of death from high blood pressure, heart disease and other serious health conditions. The US Department of Agriculture are aware of the overloading of processed foods with a high level of salt. They believe that if the food industry fails to reduce the amount of sodium in foods, the health of millions will continue to be at risk.

Refined salt is pure sodium chloride from which all the valuable trace minerals have been removed. It can cause a strong thirst and the temptation is for it to be satisfied with alcoholic drinks. It destroys protein compounds, causing their excessive excretion as albumin in the urine.

Excessive salt 'pickles' the tissues, interfering with the absorption of food and deranges osmosis (the interchange of fluids through tissue membranes). It lies hidden in the background of a number of skin diseases.

Salt weakens the relish for natural flavours and dulls your sense of taste so that it is not able to detect the subtle delicate flavours of natural foods.

Reducing your salt intake is a wise step to take before you get high blood pressure or any other threat of the sodium menace.

Sulphur

Only sulphur-containing protein foods can be utilized as a source of sulphur. These include lentils, wheat germ, cheese, peanuts (peanut butter), eggs, onions and meats. It is present in cabbage in small quantities.

It is also present in the B vitamins (B1 and biotin). The element is vital to healthy hair, nails and skin. It has powerful blood purifying properties. We do not know why it concentrates in hair and nails, but we do know that brittle nails and hair can improve through a wider selection of the sulphur foods and other essential minerals.

Zinc[7]

Have you ever looked at your nails and pondered the cause of those white flecks? They are most likely to be due to a shortage of zinc. Have you ever lost your sense of taste and smell? If so, zinc may be the culprit.

Rudy Coniglio, proprietor of a restaurant bar in Texas lost his sense of taste and smell. He didn't notice anything wrong until he thought tomatoes smelt funny. They tasted awful. Antibiotics failed to bring relief. Loss of weight followed. He felt sure he was going to be really ill.

He had all sorts of elaborate tests including a brain scan, eye and nerve examinations, and others. Even a tiny segment of his tongue was sliced off for laboratory analysis. His records were passed on to Coniglio's specialist, who was in for a surprise. The biopsy revealed gross abnormalities of taste buds, which were described as frayed, worn down and moth eaten.

Rudy's morale was never so low. Then his specialist put him on a supplement of zinc. The effect was dramatic. Appetite bounced back and he no longer felt he was going out of his mind. His sense of taste and smell returned.

If you happen to be a diabetic you will probably know that your zinc levels are lower than average. This is where the practice of prescribing chelated zinc equivalent to 10 milligrams daily has something to commend it.

A child had body odour all the time; nothing could touch it. Somebody recommended 30 milligrams of zinc supplement twice daily. A week later the offensive smell was gone.

Foods containing zinc are all foods from the sea, meat, lamb, eggs, cheese, wheat germ, wholegrain foods, nuts, pumpkin seeds, brewer's yeast, lima beans and green beans. It is also richly present in sunflower seeds. Sunflower seeds and pumpkin seeds are a popular way of taking the mineral to preserve health of the prostate gland.

Be convinced that a high level of health is not beyond your reach. You can be the man or woman you want to be. Health and happiness are waiting for all who are determined to have them.

We cannot all enjoy the natural mineral–rich foods of Hunzaland, as eaten in a beautiful valley under blue skies, flanked by tall snow–capped mountains. However, we can live to the best of our ability in the society in which we find ourselves.

You have so much to gain. Learn to move with the easy grace of a spine firmly sustained by a galaxy of master minerals. Feel your bloodstream purer, your heart stronger, and your eyes clearer. Be determined no longer to be at the mercy of a minor-key metabolism but majoring from *adagio lethargica* to *animato con spirito.*

4

Super Foods and Super Diets – Our Daily Bread

'Be gentle when you touch bread,
Let it not go uncared for . . . or unwanted.
Too often bread is taken for granted.
There is much beauty in bread; beauty of sun and soil: beauty of
patient toil.
Wind and rain have caressed it: Christ often blessed it.
Be gentle when you touch bread.'

Women's Land Army Christmas card

Brown is beautiful

Your newly discovered well-being is part of the good life you don't get when following mass eating habits. We cannot look to government food regulations for sound nutrition, but to ourselves.

The challenge of baking your own bread will be worth all the sophisticated whiter-than-white loaves of the public marketplace. You will be like those lucky animals for whom the millers reserve the germ, and whose alimentary canal is not irritated by ammonium persulphate, potassium bromate, glycerol monostearate – to say nothing of the added chalk.

Once you form the habit of home-baking you are not likely to go back to that which masquerades as the staff of life.

Hippocrates, the physician who died about 370 BC, couldn't have known anything about calories, but he knew bread to be an energy food. Neither had he any knowledge of those indispensable B vitamins and trace elements. But he trusted Nature to provide all the nutrients our bodies needed. She worked it out for us so many years ago.

The only thing Nature didn't work out was the blindness of man, who think they can pillage vital elements from our daily bread, and remain healthy.

Doris Grant took all the hard work out of bread-making years ago when she conceived her famous Grant Loaf.[8] What utensils do you need? Apart from a large basin, you need a wooden spoon, a set of scales, baking tins – and a pair of hands. Tins should be well-greased and sprinkled lightly with flour. When you enlist the help of an electric mixer you slightly shorten the process, but if you are a self-sufficiency expert you will want to do the job with your hands.

Many people have found bread-making to be a simple yet rewarding occupation. Its fragrance is intoxicating. No heart warms as much as that of the mother sitting down with her family with fresh homemade bread. If you have been ill, or just down-hearted, its therapeutic value will make you feel better.

Beside a roaring coal fire on a cold winter's day, our friend Doris described her famous loaf.

Experienced bread-makers always pre-heat their ovens to the right temperature before inserting the tins of dough. As baking arrests fermentation of the yeast, they make sure the dough has risen sufficiently before baking.

Warm your flour if your kitchen is cold. Organically-grown wheat is heavier on the hands and produces a loaf with a tendency to crumble easily. To bind the mixture and make a more manageable loaf, add one beaten egg to every 1.5kg (3lbs) flour.

Sugar

Bread-making is one of the few exceptions when we use sugar. Its presence encourages the dough to rise adequately. It gives yeast 'something to feed on'. Barbados sugar helps the flavour and produces an attractive browning of the crust. However, too much sugar hinders the rising of the dough and dampens down activity of the yeast.

All kinds of exciting flavours can be obtained by the use of honey, crude black molasses and Barbados sugar. Our Canadian and American friends impart a unique and persuasive flavour by their use of maple syrup.

Fat

Maybe you wish to bake a softer loaf, with more flavour? If so, add a little melted butter, or a teaspoon or two of any one of the golden oils: safflower, sunflower or corn.

Water

Most recipes specify the quantity of water to be used. There is no reason why you should not use milk as part of the quantity of water.

The Grant Loaf

Here is the original recipe of the famous loaf which home cooks make all around the world. There isn't an easier loaf you can make. You could substitute 40g (1½oz) of medium cut oatmeal for the same amount of the wholemeal flour for a different texture and flavour.

Pre-heat oven to 200°C/400°F/gas 6.
Bake for 35 to 40 minutes.
Makes 3 loaves

25g (1oz) fresh yeast or 3 level teaspoons dried yeast.
2–3 rounded teaspoons honey or black molasses.
1.25l (2 pints) lukewarm water.
2 scant teaspoons salt.
5kg (3lb) stoneground wholemeal xour.

Cream the fresh yeast in a small bowl with the honey or black molasses. Add 150ml (5fl oz) of the water at 35–38°C (95–100°F). The temperature is important; it is best to check with a cooking thermometer. Leave for 10 minutes to froth up. If using dried yeast, mix with 3 tablespoons of the water and then add 3 teaspoons honey or black molasses.

Put the flour into a large bowl and add the salt. In very cold weather warm the flour slightly, just enough to take off the chill. Pour the yeast mixture into the flour and add the rest of the water. Mix well – by hand is best – working from the sides of the bowl to the middle till the dough feels elastic and leaves the sides of the bowl clean. Divide the dough, which should be slippery but not wet, between three 1.25l (2 pints) bread tins, warmed and greased.

Cover the tins with a cloth and put in a warm place for about 20 minutes, or until the dough is within 15mm (½ in) from the top of the tins.

Milk gives a smoother texture and, of course, provides more nourishment. But water leaves you with a crisper crust and is the best solvent for yeast.

Other ingredients

Nothing brought more pride of achievement to a brigadier patient and friend than the quality of his homemade loaf. His wife never knew what to expect next. He rang the changes with the addition of grated nuts, molasses, wheat germ, herbs and spices with the panache of a chef at the Ritz.

Salt

Salt slows down the fermentation process and should be mixed separated from the yeast.

Kneading

Some people cannot believe you can produce a good bread without kneading. 'Try and experiment yourself,' said Doris Grant. 'Make two identical loaves, as I have done, kneading one and leaving the other, baking them together. The one you haven't kneaded has goodness and flavour. The other one – few bother to have a second slice.

'I only discovered the method by accident. I had been put on to a wholemeal bread by a doctor – to help solve a fifteen-year problem of indigestion, which it did. As I couldn't buy any good wholemeal bread, I had to make my own. One day I was making it, and simply forgot to knead it. In spite of this, the bread was delicious.

'I began to think then that it was because of not kneading it. I was later told by an old and experienced baker that kneading breaks down the air spaces caused by the yeast, letting some of the pleasant flavours and goodness of the grain escape. It doesn't matter two hoots if you knead white flour because it has already lost most of its goodness in the milling process.'

Baker John Reynolds says: 'Bread reflects your state of mind when you bake it.' The moral is, never to bake when you're in a bad mood. Positive thinking is your first requirement for successful home-baking. You naturally expect everything to turn out right.

Breakfast

We believe in a good breakfast. This could be the most important meal of the day. Why? Because the way you feel in the mid-afternoon depends very much upon the nutrition it provides.

When we skimp this meal we are likely to droop into that mid-morning sinking feeling with the temptation to boost our flagging energies with nutrient-deficient high-calorie snacks.

Some people prefer a light breakfast. Many now turn to a bowl of whole-grain cereals including rice, barley, rye and oats. All these provide an abundance of vitamins, minerals and antioxidants in addition to the fibre which we are constantly reminded is necessary for intestinal health.

Whole cereals can be delicious, including muesli, porridge or flakes with milk (or nut milk), and have much to offer. One or two dried fruits – dates, raisins, prunes, dried apricots, dried bananas, figs, peaches or pears – followed by toast, marmalade or honey, help to add to our vitality.

Others prefer a breakfast starting with fresh fruit, followed by nut rissole, sweetcorn, eggs or tomatoes on toast and dried fruits.

Scientists are discovering more and more on delaying the onset of old age. They tell us wholegrain products make a vital contribution to the quality of life in our retirement years and how they can reduce the risk of chronic disease.

Muesli

100g (4oz) coarse oatmeal
25g (1oz) flaked almonds
50g (2oz) apricots, dried
25g (1oz) sultanas
250ml (8 fl oz) milk or yoghurt
150g (6oz) fresh fruit (bananas, oranges, grapes, apples, or whatever is in season)
1 tablespoon honey

Method: Mix together the oatmeal, almonds, apricots and sultanas. Soak in the milk overnight in the fridge. Add fresh fruit and honey when serving.

Serves 4

Grains are a great source of B vitamins and provide a healthy energy-giving breakfast to start off your day of well-being.

Alternatives
- Wholegrain cereals with fruit toppings such as canned or fresh peaches, bananas or apples.
- Hot wholegrain cereal or porridge (oatmeal) with added wheat germ and raisins or chopped dates.

- Dried fruit salad.
- Cooked brown rice as a cereal with raisins, bananas or dates.

Almonds (*Prunus dulcis*)

We think of almonds in the spring when, in the country of their production, the tree bursts out into magnificent pink and white blossoms. It is a cheerful sight after winter. They are now regarded as one of the super foods, including olive oil, garlic and watercress. All contain high levels of vitamin E, zinc, calcium and iron. Their essential fatty acids Omega-3 and Omega-6 burn up excessive fat and raise the metabolic rate. All have the property of reducing cholesterol deposits.

The nuts have no animal fat to clog the arteries and have as much protein as prime steak.

Almonds make an excellent ingredient in weight-loss diets and are completely alkaline, hence a major factor in maintaining the body's alkaline balance.

Almonds are also rich in phosphorus, potassium, lecithin, niacin and folic acid. The effect of five to ten per day may first be apparent in a firming-up of brittle or diseased fingernails.

Being rich in vitamin B1 they are excellent for the nervous system. Almonds have a traditional reputation in preventing formation of tumours, for which they should be eaten raw and uncooked.

Eat almonds chopped up in salads. Or you may take them whole, but be sure to discard the outer skins, which are indigestible. Whatever is indigestible is usually constipative. Place in boiling water for a minute, after which the skins may easily be rubbed off. They may be used as a sauce for fish or chicken.

Try to avoid ground almonds, unless you grind them yourself. On exposure to air for a few hours they may go rancid.

Almond oil has great cosmetic value when massaged into the skin, feeding and softening it to make your body supple. Used on hair it is a fine conditioner.

Apples

An apple a day is said to 'keep the doctor away'. From recent research it appears an apple can also keep the dentist away. It is said they are about 30% more effective than brushing teeth. Dentists call it 'the detergent effect'. One of the most maddening sights is the neglected tree where no one picks the fruit. We should make the most of Nature's bounty while we may.

Dr Eugene H. Lucas, of Michigan University tested apples in an experiment in which 1,300 students ate one or more apples a day. After a period of three years, it was found that those who ate apples regularly had 33% fewer colds and flu. An unexpected and welcome discovery emerged: there was much less nervousness, sense of insecurity, anxiety and pressure headaches. Do apples contain some kind of natural tranquillizer?

Dr Healer of the USA reported the cure of a patient of long-standing mucous colitis and chronic catarrh by a diet of grated raw apples.

Apples contain pectin, a polysaccharide detoxifier which lowers the level of cholesterol in the blood, thus reducing the risk of hardening of the arteries. It also reduces blood glucose as in diabetes.

What is not generally known, is that apples are an excellent brain food for a clear head. Their pectin promotes elimination of toxic metals cadmium, lead and mercury from the body.

Their phosphorus feeds the brain, strengthens the nerves, and may reduce the risk of such degenerative disorders as Parkinson's and Alzheimer's disease.

Apples contain flavonoids that protect mucous and airway surfaces – of some value for asthma. Today's studies show how they cut the risk of heart disease, osteoporosis, high blood pressure and strokes, and it is also believed they can reduce the risk of breast cancers.

In your kitchen, apples are invaluable eaten raw or as apple strudel.

Apricots

The apricot is a powerhouse of nutrition. It is one of the richest sources of iron, correcting simple anaemia due to shortage of iron in the red blood cells.

Apricots are a valuable source of vitamin A for bright eyes, resistance to disease, and the health of the mucous membranes especially of the nose and throat. They are equally valuable dried, and should be eaten in that form in winter when the fresh fruit is not obtainable. They are excellent for those who do not have to count their calories because of a weight problem.

This versatile fruit adds a piquant flavour to most dishes and may be brimming with golden juice where ripened naturally in the sun. Try to avoid the sulphur-dioxide variety for optimum health. Rich in beta-carotene (revealed by their colour), they are good for the skin and for general condition.

Avocado

Avocado has outstanding nutritional values, being high in potassium for clear thinking, manganese for healthy blood cells, and phosphorus for bone and dental health.

Avocado also contains an impressive selection of vitamins: vitamin E to keep our arterial walls and heart resilient, and vitamins B1, B2 and niacin for mental alertness. They are a rich source of folic acid for pregnancy, and contain no less than eleven vitamins and fourteen minerals. All these make for healthy brain cells, improving memory loss and concentration. It is said to be rich in tyrosine, which is good for depression.

You can enjoy eating avocado with citrus fruits or tomatoes.

Bananas

A banana is so easy, quick and yummy!

Ripe and ready to eat, a golden banana makes the ideal snack at any time of the day.

The greatest assistance you can give your heart is an adequate supply of potassium. We really can never take too much. This mineral can rectify an excessive salt intake, which means it is of value for high blood pressure and high cholesterol levels.

Did you know that bananas offer a harmless alternative to chemical antacids for acidity and some stomach troubles? Some diners claim it to be a mood-lifter.

Green bananas are now known to help cure stomach ulcers, though they do tend to constipate. In the 1920s a patient was diagnosed suffering from gastric ulcers. A Manchester general practitioner informed him that if he wished to avoid surgery he should try dieting on green bananas and cheese for a month or two. It proved successful. For the next twenty years, until he died in his early eighties, there was no apparent relapse.

Eat a banana when anything gets stuck in your throat, to carry it down to the stomach. To assist the passage of medicinal tablets to the stomach of a patient in a recumbent position, let them swallow a few bites immediately after.

The Zulus used to apply banana skins to the skin for irritative rashes. A study discovered that about 50% went into remission.

Not-too-sweet dried bananas are soft and chewy, but make sure you buy the non-sulphured dried fruit from your health store. Banana chips, which are made from banana slices partially fried in coconut oil, then dipped in honey or glucose, are popular snacks with children.

From the dawn of civilization the banana has not lost its popularity. What is yummier than a plate of cereal and bananas? Or a banana split? Or just a plain banana?

Beetroot

Beetroot is a popular vegetable for enriching the blood. The vivid red juice of the fresh root discolours everything in which it comes into contact. It is at its best and most delicious when eaten raw, grated in salads. Beets and carrots go well together.

Like carrots and almonds, beetroot is rich in minerals. Its leaves are a source of potassium and vitamin A. Grown on organic-enriched soil, it will be rich in zinc and iron that enhance its effect upon the haemoglobin in the blood, enabling it to take up more oxygen.

It is indicated in simple iron-deficiency anaemia.

A diet of calcium and magnesium-rich foods should be eaten regularly. Such foods are green leafy vegetables, including beetroot green tops. The palatability of beets is improved by a sprinkling of thyme.

Brazil nuts

Brazils contain a mineral essential for an efficient immune system. Not only are they a good source of protein, they are endowed with a whole galaxy of 'goodies'. Such include: vitamin E, mono-unsaturated fatty acids, calcium, magnesium, iron, zinc and – what appears to be the most important of all – selenium. *See* Selenium p. 46.

Brazil nuts provide from 230mcg and 5,300mcg selenium per 100g. For those trying to overcome the ravages of heavy drinking and smoking, they are a must. They are of help for the prevention of a whole range of ailments. The elderly, vegetarians and pregnant and breast-feeding women do well on two to three nuts per day.

For the sake of your liver two to three nuts per day should keep it sweet and clean.

Brewer's yeast

With the rapidly developing market of health foods all over the world exceeding expectations, it is understandable that brewer's yeast comes into its own.

Sweden's increased sales reflect growing interest. It could be that harsh winters are responsible, when people are subject to unequal stresses from rapid temperature changes.

Brewer's yeast is a biological force of considerable power. Its cells actively influence what goes on in our bodies. Have you ever thought what a mighty reserve of energy is needed by your body to meet the basic requirements for the action of the heart, lungs and other organs? To liberate this prodigious energy we must have the B vitamins to form the different enzymes.

So you see, there is a relationship between our output of energy and the B vitamins. If we eat food which is lacking in these – such as processed cereals – we need to eat some other food rich in them, to make good the loss.

What are the B vitamins? They are matches which burn up the starches in our body. Calories from sugar and starch cannot be released without them.

In their natural state, wholewheat, brown rice, whole corn, whole barley and rye all contain the necessary B vitamins for unlocking their latent energy. When these grains are factory-processed, white sugar, white rice and white flour will not contain any vitamins at all, except those purposefully restored in order to measure up to acceptable standards of sale.

One great advantage of the amazing fungal phenomenon of brewer's yeast is that it brings to our table a high quality protein. Would you believe it carries, gram for gram, more than four times the protein of an egg, and even more than sirloin steak!

In what other form of nourishment would you find as many as seventeen vitamins (including the whole of the B group, except B12 present in liver), sixteen amino acids and fourteen essential minerals? One tablespoonful of brewer's yeast contains 1.25 milligrams of thiamin (vitamin B1), absolutely necessary for appetite and digestion.

Those looking for a no-starch, no-sugar and non-fat diet need fix their eye no further than brewer's yeast. Do you wonder why vegetarians attach so much importance to it? Not so many years ago it was called 'the vegetarian's protein'. It is easily metabolized. It leaves no toxic wastes to overtax the liver and kidneys.

Japan has recently become more interested in brewer's yeast. This is understandable because of an unexpected return of cardiac beriberi (neuritis of the heart) in teenagers eating too many refined starchy foods, which lack vitamin B (thiamine). Such weakness becomes apparent during the holiday season when young people are likely to exert themselves more physically outdoors.

The disorder was tracked down to powermill polished rice, sweet soft drinks and instant noodles. Boys were easily fatigued, short of breath and harassed by a persistent aching neuritis. Dramatic results followed the use of vitamin B, which abounds in brewer's yeast.

Close involvement with Japan's urgent economic drive, finely geared for international competition, makes heavy demands upon its population. People work hard. They are well looked after socially and medically. Their scientists, too, recognize the benefits of the B vitamins in yeast and the material role they play in the life of modern industrial communities.

It is no longer an act of professional courage for a doctor to prescribe brewer's yeast for certain skin conditions – boils and acne, for example. Some practitioners are impressed by its growing reputation as a 'blood purifier' though those two words have been purged from official medicine.

Pale, emaciated patients may lie in hospital a long time before generating sufficient vitality to spring back into top gear. In itself, brewer's yeast is a living sustaining food, building up post-operative cases and accelerating recovery.

A Gloucester woman took brewer's yeast for her nerves. Her hair had started to 'go white' at an early age due to shock, but, much to her delight and surprise, it started growing dark again, especially underneath and at the back. Now, she finds life rewarding.

Is it all in the mind? Evidence mounts to show how delinquency and even low scholastic performance can be affected by an absence of the B vitamins. When our diet is deficient, especially where accompanied by some of the 2,000 odd additives and colourings in our food, the most extraordinary things happen.

Does food affect our emotional life? Dr Russell Wilder, Chairman of the Nutrition Committee of the National Research Council of the Mayo Clinic thinks it does: 'I am personally convinced that insufficiency of vitamin B is the principal cause of the psychological state known as loss of morale. I suspect that many industrial workers are led to make unreasonable demands because of inadequacy of this vitamin in their diet. Consequently, they become hypersensitive and unwilling to co-operate.'

A hyperactive child, screaming the whole time, who would be awake for over thirty hours with severe colic and sickness, caused the doctor and her mother to wring their hands. Her tantrums were frightening. Exhaustive tests proved of no avail. The breakthrough came when the child was put on a natural diet, including brewer's yeast. What was once a restive menace now plays happily with her friends.

The riboflavin (vitamin B2) of this extraordinary food is found to be intimately related to our emotional balance.

When our diets are deficient in this group of vitamins, we are likely to feel highly-strung. Such diets induce nervous tension. Like loosening screws on an over-strung musical instrument brewer's yeast reduces tension on the strings.

Are you bothered with lapse of memory and forgetfulness? It can be a problem when trying to hold down an exacting job. Researchers claim it is related to the kind of food we eat. Conducting tests for speed of thought and memory, it was found that marked improvement followed brewer's yeast because of the enlivening vitamins it contained. If your memory is not what it used to be, yet you are far from being doddery, don't hesitate to add it to your diet.

How can you take brewer's yeast? All calorie-conscious people will be delighted to learn that they can enjoy all the rich nutrition of brewer's yeast at very low calorie cost. One tablespoonful offers only twenty-two calories – about one hundredth of the recommended daily intake. Whatever other form of protein is taken, you have everything to gain from the addition of one tablespoonful daily on your salad, soup or cereal.

You're not likely to mistake brewer's yeast for fresh yeast, which is used in baking and which can be very bitter.

Powdered brewer's yeast blends happily with fruit juices, water and even milk. To make your vitamin B drink, pour 300ml (10fl oz) of liquid into a 600ml (1 pint) jug; add one or two tablespoonfuls, and stir. Store in a cool place. Drink it when you get that sinking feeling.

That tangy taste may be a welcome change from sugar's sweetness. If your taste buds do not take to it kindly, there are palatable preparations on the market as well as tablets.

Why not thicken-up soups and sauces with it? Your 'iron-ration' protein could take the form of brewer's yeast; it contains that metal and is a splendid fortifier in place of meat and it's very inexpensive. Its vitamins and minerals are more easily absorbed in the presence of food.

If you feel it's the stuff for you, but really can't take it, B-complex supplements offer an alternative. These will contain B12, the only member of the B group missing in yeast. When your country-fresh health begins to fade, think of this enigmatical food, which will not only stimulate your vitality but also keep you pulsing with energy.

Broccoli

Broccoli is one of today's top phyto-nutrients as an anti-cancer vegetable. It is now being prescribed for cases of cancer of the lung, larynx, oesophagus, colon, throat and prostate. American research asserts it is particularly effective in inhibiting tumours of the ovaries and breast.

Broccoli is high in magnesium, calcium, iron, vitamins A, B (especially B2, B5 and B6), beta-carotene, C, K and folic acid. But it is the anti-cancer substances of genistein and sulphoraphone, which attract medical attention. Tests suggest that it can help fight cancer of the womb.

Yet broccoli has another important property. It assists the production of dopamine, mood-lifter and antidepressant, which is almost always in deficit in brain disorders. It is particularly relevant to those with Parkinson's and Alzheimer's disease.

Broccoli sprouts, from the seeds, contain live detoxification enzymes and valuable immune nutrients.

The vegetable is best eaten raw or lightly cooked. Grated raw on salads or lightly steamed (no more than five minutes) can be a gourmet treat.

How frequently should we eat this attractive vegetable? Scientists advise two or three times a week for health and well-being.

Carrots

Carrots are one of today's top phyto-nutrients with a rich source of beta-carotene and as many as seven anti-cancer substances.

Carrots should be used in the kitchen every day of the year. Eaten in salads, they offer a wide spectrum of nutrition. For many years a health farm in the south of England gave a glass of carrot juice to its patients as part of its treatment. It carried with it a bonus: a protection of the lens of the eye from damage by ultra-violet light, and the health farm was convinced it also protected against cataracts.

Carrots produce an alkaline drink for an over-acid condition, especially where there's a weight problem. We have known cases where pounds have just 'peeled off'.

It is a splendid blood purifier. Also, cases of appendicitis, acidosis and colon disorders are known to benefit.

Much can be said for fruit and vegetable juice cocktails. Many people are allergic to fresh milk. They may find juices of apple, apricot, carrots, grape, loganberry, orange and pineapple are alternatives to be relished.

Small segments of raw carrots may be nibbled when entertaining the Jones'.

Carrots and fruits will delay or prevent cataracts. Tufts University (USA) has researched the use of fruits by people aged forty to seventy years. Those who ate less than 1.5 servings of fruit, or less than two servings of vegetables per day were three times as likely to develop cataracts.

Celery (*Apium graveolens*)

Celery was introduced into Britain by the Romans, who used it in the kitchen and as a medicine. It was taken as a tonic for stiff joints.

For many years Europeans recognized its virtues for reducing high blood pressure. Being a vasodilator it opens up blood vessels thus allowing that vital fluid a freer circulation.

This versatile food is rich in iron, sodium, vitamin B3, folic acid and no less than eight anti-cancer chemicals!

It has been found to contain magnesium also, a deficiency of which is known to cause muscular aches and pains. Few people are aware that fresh stalks eaten as a vegetable assist sound sleep, seeping the tension from overwrought nerves.

Herbalists of Britain have been advising celery seeds for rheumatism for the past 300 years. Today they may be made into a tea (simple infusion) by placing one heaped teaspoon into a teacupful of water and bringing it to boiling point. Simmer for half minute and drink cold throughout the day.

At the end of a meal, what could be better than a stick of celery? A crunchy companion to cheese for a healthy digestion!

Cider vinegar

The health-giving power of cider vinegar has been recognized since time immemorial. But it was left to Dr D. C. Jarvis in Vermont, USA, to 'rediscover' its extraordinary possibilities in nourishing the body and curing disease. Cider vinegar is rich in potassium, and this is what he says: 'Folk medicine holds potassium to be the most important mineral – in fact, the key mineral in a constellation of minerals. It is so essential to the life of everything that without it there would be no life.'[9]

What calcium is to the bones, so potassium is to the soft body tissues. When short of this mineral, cells shrink in size and lose their fluid; their normal activity becomes exaggerated. This makes our nerves 'all on edge' and we become over-excitable.

Our bloodstream is our river of life sending nourishment all over the body, circulating every twenty-three seconds. Sickly blood passes through the capillaries more slowly and wastes tend to accumulate. It is a surprise to discover the relationship between stomach acid and a healthy bloodstream.

A man suffering from achlorhydria (absence of hydrochloric acid from the gastric juices), for whom a number of different treatments proved unsuccessful, was advised to try cider vinegar in water. After two days he was beside himself with enthusiasm – pain, flatulence and bloated sensations were gone. He thought it was a fluke.

Not everybody needs vinegar, but often it can be the natural answer to under-acidity. Digestive-acid levels of people get lower with age, unless they are stoked up with excessive protein and other acid-promoters. Alkaline stomachs make their hosts lethargic, easily tired, always sighing and yawning.

We can spend large sums of money on the best food, but if we lack this vital acid our digestion will be imperfect. A weak digestion means less than adequate nourishment – general health suffers.

Hydrochloric acid (HCl), so necessary for breaking down proteins, also serves the valuable purpose taken with fluid of destroying harmful bacteria, although there are times when its defence is weak. Its action is assisted by cider vinegar.

The vinegar contains oxygen and hydrogen among other elements. Metabolism in the body releases the hydrogen ions, which themselves are powerful antiseptics and destructive to germs. They have a purifying effect, assisting elimination of accumulated toxins.

When you have no digestive-acid, calcium cannot be absorbed. Absorption of this important salt is dependent upon the presence of HCl. When this salt cannot be utilized, it is dumped on some off-the-beaten track where it consolidates. In the course of time it forms deposits in the collagen around the joints to create a focus for arthritis.

For a feeble secretion of digestive-acid some authorities recommend glutamic-acid hydrochloride after meals. Others favour drugs of modern pharmacy. Some advise yoghurt. The acids of yoghurt may not be strong enough to cope with achlorhydria, in which the stomach loses its ability to secrete acid, and this is where cider vinegar may step in and fill the breach. I would recommend two teaspoonfuls to a tumbler of water with meals, three times daily, and on rising first thing in the morning.

We have referred to the acid/alkaline balance. Researchers have shown how a persistent excess-alkalinity of the stomach juices is invariably found in cancer patients. Some suspect that a tilting of the balance towards an excess alkalinity can create the environment in which the disease takes root. They support the theory with evidence that hyper-acid stomachs seldom succumb to malignant disease.

What else can be said for this unique drink? It enables us to get more benefit from our food, helping us to assimilate calcium and iron. When a sluggish circulation slows down, hands and feet get icy cold. Cider vinegar is an inexpensive stimulant – cheaper than brandy!

Some people will frighten you by saying that vinegar is harmful. They say it is too acidic. That may be so to a few. It is understandable if some people cannot take it: they cannot tolerate any vinegars at all. After all – cider vinegar is just vinegar made from cider.

Dr Jarvis has a word to say on this: 'I have heard it said that acid harms the body, but if an acid derived from fruit like the apple is harmful why has Nature spread acid about with a lavish hand in fruits, berries, edible leaves and roots? I have offered vinegar mixed with drinking water or ration to chickens, hens, minks, cats, dogs, goats, dairy cows, calves, bulls, farm-horses and racehorses. Always an improvement in health resulted. If the vinegar was harmful in any way I would certainly have observed some adverse reactions.'

Though cider vinegar is an acid, it has an alkaline effect on the blood.

There are times when our energy levels are at a low ebb. Do you some-times feel like that? We need just that little extra zip to enable us to finish off some important job such as tackling the week's washing, or raking the leaves in the garden.

I once knew a busy executive who said he always took a drink of cider vinegar following an afternoon's boardroom stress. He said it always calmed him down.

That set me thinking. That was the first I'd heard of it used as a relaxant. Then it occurred to me that stress arrests the flow of hydrochloric acid in the stomach almost immediately. The vinegar had the effect of stimulating the body's production of hydrochloric acid.

So, when you find yourself under stress at work, in a broken home, or wrestling with money worries, lessen their physical impact with a tangy draught of cider vinegar: two teaspoonfuls to a tumbler of water.

As an instant reviver there can be many variations on this theme. When hard put to it, don't reach for pep pills. Do yourself a favour. Take one calcium tablet, dissolved in two teaspoonfuls of cider vinegar, add one tea-spoonful of honey and stir together in juice or water. Try it as an alternative to those interminable cups of coffee you are tempted to take when you feel exhausted from under-resting and overworking. Nature's lesser-known revitalizers can help you.

When is cider vinegar helpful? Dizziness was a troublesome symptom for which the Vermonters reckoned the vinegar was a reliable remedy. Tinnitus (noises in the ears) is in many cases a potassium disturbance; it can be a wearying experience. The vinegar has a number of successes to its credit and offers a harmless alternative to drugs. It may be reduced from two to one teaspoonful after one month.

It is difficult to believe that one single remedy can exert a favourable action on two opposite clinical conditions such as low blood pressure and high blood pressure. Yet cases exist where one person's low blood pressure from anaemia has improved and another man's high blood pressure has been reduced.

Although there is no such thing as a panacea, other complaints known to react favourably include: hiccups, eneuresis (bed wetting), hay fever, migraine, insomnia, brittle finger nails, falling hair, hard callouses on feet, watery eyes, runny noses and catarrh.

One small warning – all acids, including those from fruits and sugar con-fectionery may attack enamel on the teeth. This includes cider vinegar. The secret of drinking it is to bypass the teeth.

By stimulating metabolism, cider vinegar has become a popular slimming aid. As a lotion, applied neat, for that terribly irritative skin condition, shingles, it can often take away the pain within minutes. As a gargle for sore throats it has something to commend itself.

Little wonder Dr Jarvis can write so convincingly: 'My wife and I have taken vinegar and water every day for thirty years, as nearly as I can remember. Most of the time we have added two teaspoonfuls of honey. The results have been excellent in every way. For example, as conductor of the Barre Junior Symphony Orchestra for twenty-one years, I have missed only one weekly rehearsal and never missed a concert, which shows what it did for me. My daughter has taken vinegar for eighteen years. The three of us as a family are resistant to disease, free from colds, and rarely ill'.

Where there is life and activity, there is acid.

Cod-liver oil

This is perhaps one of the richest natural sources of the protective vitamins A and D, essential for good health, durable teeth and strong bones.

Research confirms its value for certain skin conditions, sores and ulcers. It is rapidly becoming an official medical treatment for high cholesterol levels and coronary heart disease, arthritis and diabetes, known to have high cholesterol levels.

It is increasingly advised for pains of rheumatism in the joints and protection against winter coughs, colds and flu. At one time it was regarded as a preventative of tuberculosis, building up resistance against the disease.

Did you know it could keep your nails in good condition? An early sign of improvement being an absence of dryness and brittleness.

Cod liver oil helps you maintain a healthy heart, joints and immune system. If you feel you cannot stomach the oil, capsules are available from your health store.

The synthesis of prostaglandins is said to be enhanced by the special polyunsaturates found in the oil.

A well-known typically English beauty takes at least a tablespoon every day: 'It's good for my hair, skin, eyes and nails . . . really wonderful stuff!' she says.

Curry

Kari is a Tamil word meaning 'sauce'. It is one of the oldest recipes in the world, being a combination of pungent aromatic spices, sometimes fiery, to go with cooked vegetables, meat or fish.

The best curries seem to come out of Madras, blended by masters of the craft. They contain a mixture of precious spices which can prove useful in the treatment of certain digestive disorders and to provide a wide selection of antioxidants: chillies, cinnamon, cloves, coriander, cumin, mustard, pepper, saffron and turmeric.

An Indian housewife buys her curry spices in the market and roasts them herself. This requires skill – every spice needs a different roasting time and too much heat can destroy the subtle aromas. Then she blends the spices. Finally, she pounds them to a fine powder, painstakingly using a pestle and mortar.

You, too, could roast, mix and grind your own curry powder. Or you can buy one already blended. Sharwood's authentic curry powders are imported from India and have a long traditional reputation in the field.

Dates: Allah's greatest gift

From a land of mosques, mosaics and minarets comes to us fruit of the date palm – Allah's great gift to dwellers of the desert. One of the sweetest and most nourishing of fruits, dates are the staff of life to millions in the Arab world.

Dates mature in a wonderland of perfumes under azure skies. Little wonder they are rich in vitamins A and D. The sun is the giver of life and closely related to the presence of these vitamins. The date is almost a complete food in itself. Bedouin have been known to survive for weeks on little else. Dates and camel's milk are still a staple diet for many.

The world market is supplied chiefly by Iraq, Tunisia, Iran and Egypt. India receives an enormous importation of dates every year. France, Syria, Britain and the Scandinavian countries import heavily. Since the introduction in 1890 of rooted suckers from Arabia, America now has a thriving date industry in the Coachella Valley, Arizona, and New Mexico.

The Arab believes that the date palm should have 'its feet in running water, and its head in the fire of the sky.' Wherever they grow, they flourish in an abundance of water, plenty of sunshine and a hot dry climate. Where these conditions are met, they develop huge root systems in which there is almost as much under as above the ground.

These roots are important. Their penetration is deep. They ramify through soil and rocks, extracting from the lower-most depths vital minerals that can offer our bodies precious nutrients: sodium, potassium (very high), calcium, magnesium, iron, copper, phosphorus, sulphur, and chloride.

When ripe, dates contain proteins, fats, carbohydrates, vitamins and minerals – all in easily assimilable form. The fleshy part may contain as much as 60% sugar.

Dates are high in potassium and therefore help to preserve the acid/alkaline balance of the body. Besides vitamin A, they contain vitamin B1 (improves general metabolism); vitamin B2 (promotes healthy nerves, eyes and skin); and B3 (allays digestive, nervous and mental unrest).

Date starch is readily convertible into sucrose through the action of enzymes present in the fruit. It also has something small to offer by way of protein (cell-replacement material). Few fruits contain protein as well as sugar and fat.

Strange as it may seem, dates have to be pollinated by hand – bees and insects take no part in it. In spite of their long history, pollination has always been carried out by the hand of man. It seems it was the Creator's intention for men to shin up to the dizzy heights of trees sometimes reaching over 24m (80 ft). Fertilization is artificially aided by cutting off the male flower clusters from another tree just before the stamens ripen, and for them to be suspended among those of the female trees.

A single bunch of dates may contain over 1,000 individual fruits and weigh 9–18kg (20–40lb).

Bunches of male date blossoms can be seen in the Arab marketplace, a sprig of which is placed near female flowers. Also, can be seen piles of date stones, so huge that one wonders at all the labour, sun and water that will be needed before mature trees, grown from such trifles, spread their shade and produce their honey-sweet crop.

The date palm starts to bear from the sixth to eighth year, reaches maturity at about thirty years, and does not decline until the age of about 100. Trees have been known to be fully bearing up to a ripe old age of 150 years.

The striking leadership of Iraq in date production is due to the outstanding natural advantages of the country. Temperature and rainfall provide ideal requirements for a fruit rich in protein, fat and minerals.

There are three kinds of dates. There are soft and juicy ones rich in sugar; ones that are hard and dry, most favoured by the indigenous population; and ones of inferior tough fibrous fruit, low in sugar, which even the poor can afford.

Iraqi dates come to us kneaded together in small cellophane blocks or vivid chip packets. Four varieties go out into the world: the large golden brown Hallawi, the extremely tasty Khadrawi, the small but excellent quality Sayer, and the large amber-coloured Zahdi.

Almost every part of this stately tree is used. Date seeds can be roasted to make a coffee substitute which, before the arrival of the American coffee bean, was a common drink of the desert Bedouin. An oil expressed from the seeds is used to protect the delicate complexions of Bedouin women from the ravages of wind and sand.

There are many ways of eating dates. Many people like them raw. Try making a delectable confection of sliced dates, milled nuts, ground grains, stoned prunes, finely cut figs and dried fruits. If you haven't a food processor, beat into a paste with a large spatula or spoon.

A strengthening beverage can be made by pouring milk over macerated dates and drinking after fermentation. Distilled into date wine, sap from the palm is mighty powerful.

Served with cheese and biscuits, dates make a flavourful alfresco snack. The favourite combination of the desert Arab is a drink of goat's milk and a handful of dates.

They combine well with cottage cheese in a green salad. When did you last taste date and lettuce sandwiches?

The fruit is so versatile that there's no end to its attractions: sliced on vegetable and fruit salads, sliced on cereals or stuffed into cored apples they make a pleasing 'sweet'. Children find them a nice chewy topping for a sundae. An imaginative cook will remember them as a welcome extra ingredient for a milk shake, ice cream, bread pudding, or for giving 'body' to cakes and cookies.

Date Cake

This is the recipe for my wife's favourite date cake.

110g (4oz) Margarine or butter
110g (4oz) Muscovado sugar
1 egg, beaten
175g (6oz) Wholemeal self-raising flour
25g (1oz) Ground almonds
50g (2oz) Walnuts
110g (4oz) Dates, chopped
Milk

Method: Cream the fat and sugar. Gradually mix in the beaten egg. Fold in dry ingredients, adding the milk to make a soft dropping consistency. Place in a loaf tin and bake in 180°C/350°F/gas 4 moderate oven, for about an hour.

In past ages this queen of the Orient was 'poor man's bread' and regarded as part of the natural wealth of the people. Dates help build up your body resistance. Healthy food makes healthy people.

Eggs

You are to be envied if you are fortunate enough to collect your own eggs from the bottom of the garden, or down on the farm. If you do keep hens you will want them to run free range, warmed by the sun and watered by the rain. You are likely to insist that they have freedom to forage the soil for food, exposed to all weathers, yet offered shelter and protection from predators.

Chickens are easy enough to rear on a couple of handfuls of protein food in the morning, and a handful of grain in the evening, together with scraps from the table. A few chickens should keep you well provided with eggs most months of the year. They, too, need their minerals and will respond well to first-class supplements such as bonemeal and soy-bean meal.

Eggs are rich in amino acids, essential to health, iron and vitamins A and B2.[10] When poached or scrambled in one of the golden oils they do not bring about a rise in blood cholesterol. They should never be over-boiled or subjected to excessive heat otherwise their health value will suffer. Rather, they should be cooked over a low heat. When fried or scrambled in an open pan, as much as 48% of the vitamin B2 is lost, whereas no loss occurs where the vessel is covered.

Figs

Though the main property of figs is one of a laxative, they are a rich source of calcium, phosphorus, sulphur, potassium, magnesium and iron. They are welcome in sweet and savoury dishes from starters to desserts. As a snack they are a source of energy, and cut into small dice offer a welcome ingredient to salads.

This fruit reminds us of the slow evolution of all things natural.

'Nothing great is created suddenly, any more than a bunch of grapes or a fig,' wrote Epictetus. 'If you tell me that you desire a fig, I will answer that there must be time. Let it first blossom, then bear fruit, then ripen.'

Fresh fruits and raw vegetables

There's no thrill half so zesty as raising your own lettuces (they require such little space), or picking a punnet of your very own raspberries.

You say you prefer fruit juices? That's fine. But don't forget that before they are canned or bottled they have to be heat-treated. This is bound to destroy some heat-sensitive enzymes. Remember, the more natural you can take your food, the better.

'It was in the Carlsbader Sanatorium in Czechoslovakia that, more than thirty years ago, I discovered the immense healing and invigorating power of freshly made raw juices,' said Gayelord Hauser. 'Since then, I have recommended a daily pint of fresh vegetable juice to every human being I have met. I am convinced, after all these years, that the addition of one pint of vegetable juice to the daily diet is one of the best safeguards against tiredness and premature ageing.'

Fruit juices

Healthy zestful children are a mother's dream. Fruit juices help maintain those rosy cheeks. They are 'mother's milk' to those who are sick and the only fluid refreshment many can take when in extremity.

Toxic accumulations are re-absorbed into the bloodstream. As the blood becomes more alkaline, toxins that have built up in the tissues over many years as a legacy of a faulty diet and lifestyle, are dissolved from body tissues and conveyed to the liver, kidneys, lungs and skin for elimination.

Fruit juices are to be preferred to a milk diet and are a health-giving and welcome alternative to caffeine drinks. They should be regarded as a food, especially for diseases of metabolism due to excessive uric acid.

To shed those extra pounds without fuss or diet sheets, a three-day fruit juice fast is safe and simple. For three days nothing is eaten, but plenty of fruit juices taken. Some people may lose up to six pounds in those few days! By this natural way of taking vitamins, minerals and general supplements you will keep up your energy levels.

Red and white grape juices are a great pick-me-up and energy-booster for workaholics.

Goat's milk

Those who acknowledge the superiority of goat's milk to cow's milk relish its nutty flavour in their cup of tea. Less susceptible to infection than the cow, the goat is very selective in its food, refusing to eat any impure and partially decayed matter.

Many cases of infantile eczema have lost their exasperating irritative skin rash when children have been taken off all dairy products except goat's milk. Cases of asthma have also found relief.

What's so special about goat's milk? It is richer in calcium and phosphorus, thiamine and niacin than cow's milk. True, it is lower in riboflavin and ascorbic acid, but it is easily assimilated and anti-catarrhal. Much catarrh may follow after consuming cow's milk. One used to read of cases of tuberculosis cured by a changeover from cow to goat. When I was a student, it was said that the TB bacillus did not thrive in those who drank goat's milk.

In the old farming days it was customary to run a goat along with cattle to avoid abortion. In parts of the world where orthodox treatments are expensive, country-folk still use a mixture of goat's milk and honey for TB, pyelitis, chronic skin diseases and for normalizing foetid urine. This combination is also believed to be effective for *Bacillus Coli*.

As well as being a useful source of milk and cheese, a nanny will help the family budget in a number of ways – even if only keeping the lawn and hedges cropped!

Golden oils

Corn oil

Today, the USA is the world's leading producer of corn oil. It offers the world a high-quality oil which is very soft – there is nothing harsh about it. The oil is made from wholesome, well-cleaned seeds and yields a good quality golden table oil – an ideal salad dressing taken for culinary or health purposes.

Some cooks like to combine the flavours and virtues of safflower, wheat germ and corn oils.

Foods cooked in corn oil are easier to handle than animal fat. It heats quicker and blends well with other ingredients in baking mixtures. It may come in cans or bottles, thus minimizing deterioration through oxidation. It will keep indefinitely and never carries an undesirable flavour.

The oil makes food easy to digest and is popular among health professionals for the prevention of angina and coronary disease. Milder than most vegetable oils, it initiates an acid reaction where there is excess alkalinity of the blood and tissues. It is well tolerated by the weakest digestion and its kindly influence upon the liver has proved therapeutic in cases of liver induced migraine.

Corn oil is also a major crop in Mexico where tradition supports its reputation as something of a natural-healer. It has been known to 'stand in' for olive oil, although it could never attain olive oil's percentage of oleic acid. It has been substituted for olive oil in the traditional 'olive oil and lemon juice treatment' for expulsion of gallstones.

Olive oil

Olive trees attain a stupendous age. An Italian plantation is supposed to have been yielding in the time of Pliny. The Mount of Olives inherited its name from a noble grove of olive trees which once stood on the western flank, but which has now disappeared. The road which runs down from the Mount ends at St. Stephen's Gate. On the way it passes the Garden of Gethsemane where trees even today are believed to have been living at the time of Christ.

As it is highly nutritious, people living in hot climates have formed the belief that it is more wholesome than animal fats. The oil is found not in the stone but in the pulp itself, from which it is expressed by pressure. As to be expected from so nutritious an article of food, most countries have at some time referred to it as one of heaven's most bounteous gifts to man. In the Middle East it has always been an emblem of peace and plenty. In biblical times, olive branches sometimes formed part of the booths erected at the Jewish Festival of Tabernacles.

Jesuit missionaries, conscious of the olive's ability to sustain life under the most austere conditions, introduced it first into Mexico, then into California where it grows vigorously.

In relation to health, olive oil is considered 'neutral'. It is not saturated like animal fats, but consists mainly of unsaturated fats. It neither boosts our cholesterol intake nor gives us more essential fatty acids.

Attention has again been drawn to this oil as a protection against irradiation and X-rays. Professors Julian Sanz Ibanez and Adolfo Castellanes of the Cajal Institute, Madrid, in the course of a study of X-rays on rats, concluded that olive oil protected them with full efficacy against progressive doses of radiation ranging from 300 to 2,400 roentgens (La Vie Claire).[11]

Not everybody can drink neat oil, even when emulsified by being well shaken-up in fruit juices, but they can eat olives. Most Arabs regard olives, like nuts, as a day-to-day substitute for flesh meats and butter. Those readers who can eat and enjoy olives will be providing their digestive system with a fruit which is a desirable alternative to dairy products. Not only is it easy on the digestion, it is beneficial for over acidity and an irritated stomach. In its own right the olive is a great little healer. Even the stone has a purpose. Cases exist where the swallowing of a black olive stone has eliminated lower back pain within hours and cured gastric ulcers. As the stone dissolves, valuable minerals are released which can rebuild broken-down tissue.

Olive oil is beneficial for a host of ailments, externally and internally, removing toxic conditions of the blood, which are a fertile soil on which rheumatism and arthritis thrive.

Research has shown its cholesterol-lowering properties and ability to reduce the production of artery-damaging low-density lipoprotein (LDL) while leaving unchanged the helpful high-density lipoprotein (HDL).

It is indicated for chronic constipation, malnutrition, stomach and bowel disorders, and even nervous debility! It helps lower the risk of heart disease and hardening of the arteries.

Masamitsu Ichihashi and his colleagues from Kobe University's School of Medicine, Japan, found that virgin olive oil used as an after-sun lotion could protect against skin cancer.

Researchers at University Hospital Germans Trias i Pujol, Barcelona,

Spain, discovered that olive oil in the diet may 'significantly inhibit development of colon cancer.'

The Bible advises us to take care of olive oil. It is in heat-treated (ordinary olive oil) that most of the antioxidants are destroyed.

The first pressing of the fruit produces the finest and sweetest oil. Ask for extra virgin olive oil for its antioxidants, as produced to the Soil Association Standards Organic Certification UK.

Store your oil in a closed bottle, in a cool dry place, away from strong sunlight and odours. It may go cloudy when cold, but will clear when stored at room temperature. Olive oil does not like to be refrigerated – except in very hot weather.

The elusive flavour means it can be used freely on pastas and as a garnish on everything from soups to omelets.

In Roman times the oil was well known for keeping the skin and hair in good condition. Even the poor rubbed it into their hair and skin without the scented and expensive ingredients the wealthy could afford. Roman athletes and gladiators anointed their bodies with it.

I believe every member of the family commencing with the baby should have a little of this pure food supplement daily.

Safflower seed oil

Were you to see safflower in its natural habitat, you couldn't miss those flaming orange-red flower discs. Ancient Egypt, China and India were not alone in their appreciation of its beauty and nutritive properties. Seeds have been found in ancient tombs. What they didn't know was that it contained linoleic acid to promote health of the arteries. That is why safflower oil should form part of our diet. It contains a higher level of this acid than all other edible oils.

Today, safflower has suddenly come in out of the cold. As an alternative to animal fats it lends itself to the manufacture of an excellent quality vegetable margarine, which helps to keep down cholesterol levels.

The West has never had it so good. At no time in history have people been offered such a conglomerate of proteins, starches and fats.

Sesame seed oil

Sesame seeds and honey were part of the iron rations of Roman soldiers, enabling them to perform some of the longest route marches in history. They prized it as a blood purifier of some power and for its reputation to promote physical and mental endurance.

Sesame seeds contain vitamin T, another agent that enriches the blood and initiates a rise in the blood platelet count.[12] They ripen in Turkey, Afghanistan, India and the Far East, being very particular on what soil they grow. They like it well-drained and fertile, and were grown in the south-east USA as early as the seventeenth century by African slaves who brought the seed with them from Africa.

In these countries it is ground into butter called tahini. Almost all vegetable oils turn rancid on contact with the air. Not so, sesame oil. In Latin America, where it is called 'Queen of the Natural Oils' it can still be seen spread on bread as we use butter. It combines well with raisins and makes a splendid health-giving protein addition to starchy courses.

A difficult symptom to eradicate is tinnitus (noises in the ear), but sesame often relieves it. Because of its high-level calcium content, sesame has no acid-forming effect. In fact, it is good for acid stomachs, being a most alkaline and digestive protein food.

Soy-bean oil

Is the world too crowded? It is a sobering thought that the number of people on this planet increases at an astronomical rate.

It is not just the medical and social services that will find it difficult to keep pace with expansion. More people cannot find food to eat and soon the world population will have almost doubled.

Animal protein resources do not grow any larger. Grazing land now used for animals could produce ten times the amount of vegetable protein when grown on the same acreage. Present world agriculture requires more millions to be spent on animal investment than any nation can afford. Its greatest need is to expand production. What some developing countries need is a fast-growing, cheaply grown cereal so rich in protein and fats that it can take the place of meat.

This is where the soy-bean comes to the rescue as a potential lifesaver. What is so special about soya?

This tiny bean, the size of a pea, is unique in its non-cholesterol, high protein, mineral-rich legume. From it comes a flour with a protein content of 40%, a fat content of 20%. (An older generation of Chinese landworkers called it 'meat from the soil'.) Perhaps its greatest offering is lecithin, the artery protector.

Have you ever wondered how those thin workers of the Far East perform feats of endurance in the field? How can flesh and blood survive such hard labour all hours of the day, with such little fatigue? The West pitied them for their lack of meat, for their laughable daily ration of a handful of soya. Little did they know that those straight-from-the-soil pods generated a power-house of energy and body maintenance material.

The question has often been raised: why was the Far Eastern farmer comparatively free from heart and circulatory troubles? It is now known this was due to the precious linoleic acid (over 50% in the soy-bean oil). Such a huge amount could cope with the highest levels of cholesterol.

In 1854 the year that Henry Thoreau wrote *Walden* – an account of his life in the backwoods of Massachusetts – beans were brought from China and planted in the Deep South. They grew well. Not knowing what to do with the crop, farmers fed it to livestock. It bred super-steers. But it didn't occur to anyone that it might do the same thing for them.

Sunflower seed oil

When early migrants from Europe moved westwards across the Atlantic coast they encountered native Indian settlements where they were surprised to find gigantic daisies – *helianthus* – so called because of the gorgeous yellow flowers which radiate from a fiery-brown disc. When they got to know the native Indians better they learnt how oil from the seeds increased their powers of endurance when spending long hours in the saddle.

Ripened seeds were pounded in a primitive pestle and mortar to make native Indian bread, but they had many uses. The seeds provided a sustaining snack eaten in the saddle, and their children's strong white teeth were attributed to them. Newcomers were not slow to learn from the native Indians who, making a flour from the seeds, were able to keep themselves alive when food was scarce.

There were no scientists in those days to tell them the seeds contained a fantastic 30% high-quality muscle-building material. For this reason alone it has much to offer the developing countries of today.

The oil, as a rich nutrient, has made its way into the diet of most primitive communities, and is believed to have made a contribution to the beauty of Cleopatra.

Like wheat grains, sunflower seeds have survived for centuries stored in earthenware jars unearthed by archaeologists 2,000 years later. They are native to tropical America. The stem is thick and rough; the flowers solitary, from one to two feet in diameter. Forty-five per cent unsaturated fatty acids is to be welcomed in any natural edible oil. But that was not the only thing discovered. *Helianthus annuus* is high in calcium for robust muscle tone and firm bones, phosphorus for strong teeth, iron for healthy red blood cells, natural fluorine for hard tooth enamel, thiamine for sound nerves and vitamin D, which needs no introduction. It has so many good points, that the lesser ones get forgotten – such as its assistance in sterility.

The flowers abound in nectar, and are much sought by bees. They have the astonishing ability to follow the face of the sun from sunrise to sunset. All that life-sustaining sunlight goes into the oil.

But there is another important reason why nutritionists get excited about the sunflower. Its root system is very deep, enabling the plant to take up trace minerals not always available on the surface. Sunflowers are 'strong' food and medicine, saturated with sunshine from above, and fortified with minerals from below.

Sunflowers are never seen in the wild. Since early civilizations it has always been a plant to exist under cultivation. It seems to respond well to care from the hand of man.

Many people have discovered its use as an ideal salad and cooking oil. Western Europe, America, South Africa and Australia market a huge tonnage which almost doubles each passing year. Yet still, they have a long way to go to catch up with the stupendous acreage under cultivation in Russia.

Wheat germ oil

In our efforts to partake of natural foods and discard the ones that are emasculated and artificial, stoneground whole-wheat flour should take pride of place on our tables. However, there are occasions when, through travel, holidays or social custom, we have to fall in with the crowd.

When this happens we know it is only sensible to try to make good the deficiency by intelligent supplementation. This is where wheat germ oil can come to the rescue. Perhaps the easiest way to take it is as an ingredient of salad dressing.

Quick Salad Dressing

One of the simplest is made from four tablespoonfuls of wheat germ oil, half a tablespoonful of lemon juice, and a small teaspoonful of honey (optional). Mix together and shake vigorously.

Or, you can make a simple egg mayonnaise, consisting of 300ml (10fl oz) of wheat germ oil, two tablespoonfuls of fresh lemon juice, two egg yolks, and a little salt to taste.

French Dressing

For a French dressing, mix one tablespoonful of cider vinegar with two tablespoonfuls of wheat-germ oil and whisk. Add a slight touch of salt, pepper and a teaspoonful of French mustard. Smaller quantities can be made with proportional reduction of ingredients.

There are few things like wheat germ and other vegetable oils to neutralize acid/toxic wastes which may encumber and clog our tissues. They cause the albumen to coagulate and convert it into fibrin, a tough substance resulting in fibrous rigidity and improper nerve function. To maintain a youthful spine, bones and muscles without impaired mobility, wheat germ oil will make its substantial contribution.

While breastfeeding, new mothers must have enough vitamin E or they will not be able to make sufficient milk. Animals low in this vitamin cannot suckle their young. Wheat germ oil is a 'must' for the nursing mother. Breast milk is Nature's best natural food.

It has so much to offer the expectant mother also. Scientists have found that, more than any other nutrient, wheat germ is the one which carries the vital substance to prevent miscarriage. It plays an important part in maintaining health of the mother and foetus.

Mothers of bottle-fed babies should give their babies ten or more drops daily of wheat germ oil.

Wheat germ oil in the diet can safeguard the body against eczema, indigestion, varicose veins and toxaemia. It is an oil which makes you feel really alive and is vital to the sustained intelligence of old and young.

Green buckwheat

During the Second World War, Francis Picket made the exciting discovery of the latent power in green buckwheat, which grew so richly in the fields of Kent, and to which he said he owed the last fifteen years of his life.

In 1942, wracked by overwork, he suffered a stroke. He came to hear of the beneficial effect of a substance called rutin, which was a flavonoid extracted from plants and trees.

Scientists at the Eastern Regional Research Laboratory of the United States Department of Agriculture had confirmed, after hundreds of experiments, that rutin causes blood vessels to become more flexible and overcomes capillary fragility. This helped to protect the body against strokes and problems of weakened blood vessels caused by X-rays. Rutin was given to American servicemen and other personnel who might have suffered from internal haemorrhage caused by contact with atomic fission products and the effects of atomic radiation.

One of the main commercially viable sources of rutin is buckwheat, so in 1947 Pickett decided to grow buckwheat on his farm and produce tea in a modest way from the dried leaves and flowers. His health improved as he continued to drink a glassful of infusion of green buckwheat tea every day. Every herbalist is familiar with green buckwheat – a source of the anti-coagulant rutin with an ability to thin the blood.

Symptoms of leukaemia include bleeding of the gums, nose, stomach and rectum and bruising of the skin. Rutin has been used to alleviate these symptoms.

Green tea

To which kind of tea do you turn when spirits flag, when looking for an antidote to trouble?

Green tea does not only lower the blood sugar of diabetics, but it also reduces the incidence of cancer. Studies show how green tea can reduce cancer by as much as 50%. By reducing cholesterol in the blood it is kind to our arteries, preventing them from narrowing and causing them to expand.

Regular consumption of green tea is believed to protect against prostate cancer. 'Green tea-fed mice experienced a decrease in the weight of the prostate gland itself, an inhibitor of various harmful cancer growth factors, and a reduction of some of the markers and proliferating prostate cells.' *PNAS*, 2001, 98: 10350–5.

Weight watchers will be glad to learn that the tea without milk and sugar contains no calories at all! It even improves our teeth!

Fish

If you are not a vegetarian, fish has some impressive advantages over meat. For one thing, it's low in fat, except when fried. An important reason why we should all eat more fish is because it contains a complex of those vital minerals absent in many non-seafoods: zinc, selenium and iodine. (Sea-vegetables, kelp and dulse also carry these salts.)

Malnutrition is a world problem. Fish is seldom advanced as a practical solution. Consumption ranges from 100g (4oz) a head in Norway to 30g (1oz) a head in Britain. Although fish is a universally accepted food, its value needs to be more widely known. Its source of vitamins A and D is too often overlooked.

Fish oil has one great advantage: it is much more unsaturated than vege-table oils. Mackerel, herring, salmon and sardines all have a high oil content. You may be surprised to learn that cod liver oil is much more effective in lowering plasma cholesterol levels than vegetable oil from corn.

Sprats caught off the coast of England are delicious, but they are far from being a top-selling item at the fish counter. Yet few fish are as nutritious as sprats. No wonder Russian factory ships call at a certain season to fill their holds with them. I hope you will not despise 'Jack Spratt' for being cheap but prize him for the excellent quality of protein he offers. Besides, he's a tasty little fellow. We ought to eat a whole lot more. Cod fillet on the other hand costs more than three times as much.

Fish oils

Fish oils are advised to protect against coronary heart disease, thrombosis and high cholesterol levels. Premature babies fed on an infant formula enriched with fish oil had healthy eyes and mental alertness. Fish oils are rich in vitamin E, beta–carotene and selenium. Mackerel and sardines contain zinc and the co-enzyme Q10.

It has long been known that such oils may help prevent a second heart attack and even improve the quality of life in old age.

Flaxseed – *see* Linseed

Honey

We have to search the past for records of the extraordinary properties of honey. Hundreds of references exist on papyri and manuscripts around the world. Add to these the findings of today's scientific foundations, and we have a formidable assembly of evidence which the thoughtful investigator finds difficult to ignore.

When asked by Emperor Augustus to what he attributed his ripe old age, Rumilius Pollio said he daily anointed himself with oil and ate liberal amounts of honey. 'Onions and honey' was a favourite among the Chaldeans for protection against infection.

Perhaps the greatest enthusiasts for this food-medicine were the Greeks. They advised it for prolonging youth in rhythm and movement – even into old age. This agreeable sweet was a constant subject of praise by philosophers, one of whom went as far as prescribing it as a panacea for almost anything.

Hippocrates made a special study of honey, which played a major part in his natural treatments. He recommended it to many of his patients. He himself took it every day of his life. Among his many references were: 'Honey heats the body, cleanses sores and ulcers. It relieves difficult breathing, being an expectorant which loosens phlegm. When taken with raw fruits and vegetables it nourishes and freshens the complexion.'

Banana, Date and Honey Loaf

A great teatime and picnic cake which becomes moister with a day or two of keeping.

175g (6oz) margarine
11g (4oz) soft brown sugar
2 tablespoons heather honey
Few drops vanilla essence
1 tablespoon lemon juice
3 bananas, mashed
3 eggs, beaten together
11g (8oz) stoned dates, chopped
225g (8oz) self-raising flour

Pre-heat the oven to 160°C/325°F/gas 3.

Method:

(1) Cream the margarine and sugar until light and fluffy. Beat the honey, vanilla and bananas together, then blend into the margarine and sugar.
(2) Beat in the eggs gently, and fold in the dates 3 bananas and flour. When everything is well blended, spoon into a 900g (2lb) loaf tin or an 20cm (8in) cake tin with a greaseproof base.
(3) Bake for about one hour or until firm to the touch. Cool for 10 minutes in the tin before turning out to cool on a rack.

Serves 6–8 Banana, date and honey cake with buttered slice. (*Food Features* +44 012 52 735240).

According to Samuel Purchas (1575–1626) in his *A Theatre of Political Flying Insects*,[13] bees made their home in the sepulchre of Hippocrates for some time after his death. Mothers of sick children took them there to be anointed with honey and be fed with the comb. It is recorded there were impressive cures. In those days honey had the reputation for inducing clear vision. Even today some cases of cataracts have been known to 'dissolve' and the vision improve.

All civilizations had their beekeepers. Pliny the Elder, (AD 23–79), who was killed in the eruption of Vesuvius that burned Pompeii, was fascinated by news that people living round the basin of the River Po were able to work in the fields at great ages. He couldn't resist going on a pilgrimage to see for himself.

He discovered that 124 of these people were over 100 years old. Two were 125 years, and seven over 135 years. Following his visit, he was able to record: 'Honey invigorates the body, is soothing to the stomach, and reduces fevers.'

The Greek surgeon Dioscorides (born about AD 20) was another who couldn't resist honey. How right he was when he advised this thermal booster for the aged with a weak circulation! He reckoned it made new blood. Even today it has been shown to brighten up a poor blood picture.

Early in Arabian medicine, it was recognized for wasting diseases. Avicenna, the tenth century Persian physician, gave it to his 'heart' cases, advising honey and pomegranate. In the sixteenth chapter of the Koran we read:[14] 'There proceeds from the bee a liqueur of diverse colours, wherein is rare medicine for men.' Muhammad avers: 'Honey is a remedy for all diseases.' The Prophet had a high opinion of it as a beverage. 'Not only because it is sustaining and healing, but because it is believed to sharpen the intelligence.' The Jews also used it for mental exhaustion, for example, when preparing long scrolls of the scriptures. The same belief was common among scholars and monastic scribes engaged for hours inscribing and painting gloriously illuminated *Books of Hours*, which have come down to us from the tenth century. It is not coincidental that present-day researchers claim it good for brain fatigue.

The land of Israel was a land flowing with milk and honey. This reference appears twenty-five times in the Bible. Jonathan, son of Saul, war-weary in his efforts against the Philistines, plunged his spear into a cache of honey, ate it and drew strength to finish the fight.

King Solomon praised it – 'My son, eat honey, for it is good.' At the Jewish New Year, apple dipped in honey is eaten, a combination of fruit and honey symbolizing peace and prosperity. King Nebuchadnezzar had a healthy appetite for it.

At the time of Jesus of Nazareth there lived a tribe of hardy ascetic Hebrews called the Essenes. Their foods were raw, natural and unheated. The community was well served with beekeepers. Records testify to their long life.

Dr D. C. Jarvis, writing in his *Folk Medicine* gives one convincing reason for use of honey. 'Taking honey each day is advised in order to keep the lymph flowing at its normal tempo and thus avoid degenerative disease which shortens life. The real value of honey is to maintain a normal flow of tissue fluid called lymph. When this flow rate slows down, then calcium and iron are precipitated as sediment. When the lymph flow is stagnant, then harmful micro-organisms invade the body and sickness appears.'

Dr W. G. Sackett, well-known bacteriologist, once put honey to the test. Frankly he did not believe honey could destroy disease bacteria. So in his laboratory, he placed various disease germs in a pure honey medium and waited. Results were astounding. Each single one of these disease organisms died within a few hours, or at most in a few days.

Before I took up my work in the natural health field, I spent fifteen years in a number of general hospitals, including the Norfolk and Norwich Hospital, where Dr Michael Bulman, obstetrician and gynaecological surgeon perfected a technique using honey dressings to treat post-operative cases.

Dr Bulman treated carcinoma of the breast with honey dressings, reporting them to be self-sterile, nutritive, non-toxic, non-irritating, bactericidal, easily applied and cheap.

Perhaps the greatest benefit honey has to offer is the strengthening and sustaining power it brings to a tired heart. There are practitioners who believe it is one of the finest cardiac foods the world has known.

Who else uses honey? From hard personal experience it is daily proved of value to arduous mountaineers, deep-sea divers and long distance runners. For the superhuman performance of Battle of Britain pilots, honey proved an infallible source of quick energy and a natural stimulant.

Honey is unquestionably one of the most remarkably safe and natural substances known to man. Any untutored layman can help his family or livestock with this simple food-medicine.

Kelp and other seaweeds

World population statistics soar. Despite the best of man's endeavours, future output is likely to be inadequate and illusory when measured against actual needs. The steep upward trend in population increases shows no sign of falling off. The gap between food production and the developing nations has widened rather than narrowed. The West, jealous of its privileges and consuming the largest share of the cake in its efforts to bolster up a greedy civilization, is so wasteful that it can no longer be regarded as a model to a world on the verge of famine.

We encourage our schoolchildren in the belief that science and technology will one day remove the basic drudgery from human life. A twenty-hour working week will ensure we have all the time in the world for cultural pursuits and getting to know one another. It will be a way of life free from fear and want.

Our knowledge will be infinitely superior to the ancients, establishing a stable society, a universal literacy and an adequate food supply for everyone.

However, how many of us take the trouble to assess the earth's resources? Not one of us really wants to face up to the facts of diminishing supplies of fossil fuels, timber and minerals. How easy it is to be lulled into complacency by accepting what the experts have to say about the world's tremendous food potential. But how are we meeting today's demands?

Feeding the world's hungry is presumably no problem in the minds of those agricultural scientists who visualize conversion of the Arctic wastes into titanic food-producing hothouses heated by atomic power.

Off the coasts of every continent billions of tons of protein-rich seaweeds (kelps) await harvesting and processing. Kelp is another name for seaweeds of the order *Laminarales* which have been used for food for untold centuries by primitive peoples of the world.

There are supposed to be more than 300 varieties of seaweed. Many of these form hollow air vesicles (bladders) which allow plants to rise plants to the sea-surface for contact with the air to take part in Nature's universal cleansing operation known as photosynthesis. There are, however, some kelps which never see the surface.

Off the coast of California grow the largest kelps on earth. Huge redwoods of the oceans throw up vast primitive forests, some with stems over 45 (150ft) long. Divers get lost among the branches wavering in the wake of ocean tides washing this great submarine jungle. Other kelps are so small that, exquisite in design as a wild flower, they reach no higher than 1.8m (6ft) from the seabed.

All kelps are rich in potash, which is a top-line priority nutrient for man and animals. We have seen, elsewhere, the importance of the grit or mineral content of our foods. In kelp we have the richest of all foods in mineral content, and scientists confirm this as no exaggeration. We can understand practitioners who wax eloquent over an analysis of this marine treasury. Twenty-four vital elements present in one single edible plant makes impressive reading, especially when they include high percentages of calcium, potassium, magnesium, sodium, phosphorus and sulphur.

As the world's cheapest food it can be one of its most nourishing. Besides minerals, it offers no less than twenty different amino acids, from alginate to tryptophane.

Many people take iodized salt (a mixture of sodium chloride and iodine) for the health of their thyroid glands. How much better it is when we obtain our iodine intake from its natural source – seaweed! Kelp seaweeds grow in the richest 'soil' in the world and have so much more to offer than straight iodised sodium chloride.

Norway leads the world in the seaweed industry. Her kelp is gathered from such depths below the country's fiords that it doesn't see the light of day until harvesting time when it reaches the surface. Water in such depths is loaded with a wide variety of minerals eroded from different geological stratas fragmented along those subterranean mountain slopes. Having no atomic programme, and consequently no effluent problem, Norway's kelp is in great demand and is regarded as the purest obtainable.

Were it not for this versatile non-land plant, diabetics might be less than adequately nourished. Kelp crops up in so many places in our lives. It is as common in your cosmetic cream as it is in your daughter's hair styling products, and can be a substitute for sugar in a calorie-controlled diet.

Kelp has a popular close cousin – Irish moss (*carragheen*). Your first encounter might have been when you were young, when the cook of the house would be seen using it to put the spine into a jelly. Today, tons are consumed in ice cream – its texture is so smooth, those amino acids giving 'body' and substance.

Another relative is *agar-agar*, a seaweed gelatine from the East. It is used in the confectionery trade for cake icing, in dentistry for plate-making and in pathology as a medium for incubating bacteria. New uses are discovered every day.

Perhaps the most famous of the kelp family is the one especially at home around the coasts of Japan.

The history of nori seaweed goes back into the distant past. Settlers from the Philippines brought stories of its life-sustaining and medicinal properties. Highly nutritious, this traditional sea-vegetable is believed to be partly responsible for the exceptional longevity of some of the Japanese people. Even were the nation cut off from the world's food supply, if they had access to their underwater granaries, it would be possible for them to survive.

In 1948 came a crisis. Sea pollution and artificial fertilizers, whipped up by an unprecedented series of violent storms, transformed coastlands into disaster areas. Fifty per cent of the nation's larder was devastated. Nori disappeared. In those anxious months after the last war when standards of living took a plunge into demoralizing poverty, many starved.

Little were they aware that quietly working in a small holiday cottage in North Wales a Quaker with a first-class honours degree in botany was wrestling with the mystery of the red algae family of seaweeds. Dr Kathleen Mary Drew, a graduate from Manchester University, spent most of her time close to the rocks trying to piece together the life cycle of *Porphynia umbilicalis* which grows off the shores of North Wales and which is a close relative to nori. From it, the Welsh bake a 'laver' loaf of bread which can be very sustaining in the absence of first class protein. As in Japan, it had been a reliable food staple for centuries.

Just when it appeared that the Japanese nori would become extinct, Dr Kathleen made a spectacular 'breakthrough'. She discovered the missing link.

The plant spores (asexual reproduction bodies) seemed to get lost in summer. Scientists lost track of them from the time they were discharged from the mature plant to the time when these 'seeds' took root and germinated.

Nobody had been able to trace them in the sea or in fronds of the plants. That was the season when they were most vulnerable to storm and pollutants. Just where they went during the summer season was an unsolved mystery – solve that, and get the spores into action again, might save the plant.

Dr Drew discovered that these tiny spores burrow into the pores of shells, clams, oysters or even eggs, where they spend those missing months. In the autumn, at the onset of the cold, they emerge to cling to any rock or marine debris where they reproduce at a fantastic rate.

An account of Dr Kathleen's work was passed on to the Japanese authorities who immediately started to grow the spores on eggs and oyster shells among the fronds with great success. A dying industry revived and once again people of limited means had enough to eat.

Not long afterwards the science of human nutrition confirmed the traditional experience of centuries – that seaweeds are among some of the world's cheapest and most nourishing foods. In Japan today, it would be difficult to enter a restaurant in which seaweed food combinations are absent. Some people believe this may account for the tireless energy, lively intellect and challenging impact their businessmen and workforce are making upon the world economic scene.

Kelp is harvested in special trawlers equipped with a huge hook which hauls the seaweed fronds out of the sea. Powerful steel cutters mow off tops of the plants, which are handled by a conveyor belt and stored in the hold. At the onshore processing factory the weed is fine-chopped, dried and shredded. At no point is it boiled or subjected to heat; thus all minerals remain in the original plant.

The international team of sailors under Thor Heyerdahl subsisted entirely on algae, seaweeds and fish during their memorable Kon-Tiki expedition.[15] Feats of energy necessary for survival were quite out of proportion to the elemental diet they followed. It was said that some even gained in strength. All agreed they'd never felt fitter.

When scientists found the intestines of penguins to be practically free from harmful bacteria, they studied the bird's principal food, a tiny shrimp-like creature called a euphausid. In its turn, this creature depended upon one of the tiniest seaweeds known, *phytoplankton*. This plant yielded a new antibiotic.

As a source of pharmaceutical remedies, oceans of the world are practically limitless, incalculably rich, full of surprises – and all virtually untouched!

Chlorella, a one-celled algae is so powerful against certain forms of bacteria that it can convert sewage into a safely disposable waste to be got rid of through such channels as rivers and streams. Another form of algae, a green pond scum, is shown to have a positive therapeutic factor in the diet of lepers.

Bearing in mind that many present-day disorders are regarded as deficiency diseases, and because each of such diseases is due to a lack of vital elements in the diet, the sea has so much to offer. The thyroid requires iodine, the anterior pituitary gland needs manganese, the parathyroid gland must have cobalt and nickel, the posterior lobe of the pituitary demands chlorine, and the gonads insist upon iron if our bodies are to function at optimum health. All are present in seaweed.

The sea is an untapped reservoir of answers to many of our nutritional problems. Rachel Carson writes that the ocean floor is the earth's greatest storehouse of minerals.[16]

Only Nature has all the answers. Science has only some. Until first class protein and other vital food components are available in much greater quantities, sea-plant nutrition may be the answer the developing countries are seeking. The future food supply of tomorrow's unborn millions may already be waiting for the marine developer among those trackless forests of the deep.

The history of mankind is fraught with famine. While ecologists remind us of the limitations of agriculture on land, they are not the first to lead our attention elsewhere. Maybe we are not far off those prophetic words of Herman Melville in that extraordinary epic *Moby Dick*. At the end of the book he recalls a group of people standing on a high hill overlooking the ocean.

In that last decade of the nineteenth century they were witnessing the unforgettable spectacle of a school of exuberant whales tossing and tumbling, threshing the air with their waterspouts for the sheer joy of living. A man pointed to the sea: 'There is the green pasture where our children's grandchildren will go for bread.'

Lecithin

The evidence that lecithin is a useful supplement in low calorie diets for weight loss continues to mount, even when debates wax hotter and hotter. But in the midst of the controversy its important role in body health must now be accepted.

Just what is lecithin?

Lecithin is a complex mixture of fats and minerals called phospholipids containing inositol and choline. Not a cell in our bodies can do without it. Every health enthusiast will want to welcome its place in a cholesterol-free, low-saturated fat diet. When fat is deposited on walls of arteries there is always too much blood cholesterol and too little lecithin. Lecithin is an emulsifying agent prevent that is hardening of our arteries.

Although fats cannot be dissolved in blood any more than in water, the presence of lecithin causes cholesterol to break up into microscopic globules that circulate in suspension in the blood until burnt up as energy. Lecithin keeps them 'on the move' so they are not dumped and again allowed to accumulate on artery walls.

It comes as no surprise to learn that soy-bean is the most prolific source of lecithin. Most natural food lecithin preparations are made from soy beans.

Soya lecithin is a dark viscous liquid bought in capsules as a supplement. This is the natural form. If you buy it in granules make sure they are made from a 'solvent extraction' of this liquid, because some of the granules are minus the enzymes, minerals, vitamins and oils naturally present in soya lecithin.

Lelord Kordel, the well-known nutritionist, writes:[17] 'Lecithin is a food, not a drug! It is a food substance found to be an essential constituent of the human brain and nervous system and also of the endocrine glands and muscles of the heart and kidneys. Nervous, mental and glandular over-activity can use up lecithin faster than it is replaced. Then you become irritable, exhausted – a nervous breakdown can result. Lecithin deficiency is a common condition today, especially among men. The nervous strain associated with competitive business, often combined with the mental insecurity of a distasteful job or an unhappy home life, uses up lecithin in a man's body faster than it can be produced.

Added to the daily diet, lecithin helps overcome headaches, insomnia and nutritionally induced impotence, sterility and senility.'

Kordel continues: 'Many of your nerve fibres are surrounded by a sheath of somewhat fatty substance, the myelin sheath. This protective sheath is rich in lecithin, which nourishes your nerve cells and supplies them with motive force. In lecithin deficiency, this fatty sheath is depleted and we know some of the results: fatigue, nervous exhaustion, even a complete breakdown.'

Overweight and obesity are blamed for shortening life. They are an enemy to a healthy heart. The older generation of Chinese and Japanese who worked on the land and did menial jobs usually managed to avoid heart trouble – not only because they regularly worked-off any excess fat – but because their staple diet included the soy-bean, their 'holy bean', which was rich in lecithin. To them it was an alternative to fish, flesh or fowl. They also used the soy-bean oil for cooking purposes. Very few suffered from heart trouble.

Eggs are high in lecithin, but they are also high in cholesterol. That ought not to discourage us from taking this first-class protein. Those subject to migraine, liver and kidney weakness are wise to avoid them.

Lecithin, cider vinegar, kelp and vitamin B6 are regarded as a magic foursome that not only helps you to shed pounds faster than ever before, but also lifts you out of all those depressing dieters' dumps.

'The special magic of these four friends is that while you eat almost what you like (within reason), they do the hard work for your body, breaking down fatty acids and burning up calories faster than ever before.' Dieter's Notebook.

Lettuce

'Lettuce cools the heat of the stomach, called heartburn; and helps when it is troubled with choler (bile). It quenches thirst and causes sleep. Lettuce makes a pleasant salad, being eaten raw with vinegar, oil and a little salt.' Master Gerard (Herbalist), 1597.

Linseed (*Linum usitatissimum*)

Also known as flaxseed. Rich in fibre and essential fatty acids including Omega-3, flaxseed contains demulcent mucins, coating intestines causing them to swell thus adding bulk to combat constipation. A valuable source of linoleic acid which keeps cholesterol under control.

It is splendid for coughs and bronchitis. Helps to reduce the risk of atherosclerosis and thrombosis.

One tablespoonful may be taken three times daily with breakfast cereal, yoghurt, sprinkled on salads, soups and vegetables or as an ingredient of muesli.

Make sure you choose a brand cultivated without the use of artificial fertilisers, pesticides and growth regulators.

Macrobiotics

In the 1940s George Ohsawa, a Japanese man, was told he had very little time to live and that he would die from tuberculosis. But he was determined to live and studied traditional oriental medicine. This led him to diet as the chief curative factor. From it he evolved a personal philosophy and a healing therapy.

He didn't die but lived to create a centre for his teaching in Hitoyoshi, Japan, which was to become a Mecca for the sick and those responding to the intuitive way of eating as practised by religious and ancient cultures.

It was not long before his philosophy became a way of life for thousands of followers and a fascinating development in the health field of recent years. The essence of his teaching is the unity between correct diet and good health.

It is more than a system of sensible eating, being regarded both as a preventive and cure of disease. Followers go as far as equating it to personal behaviour, claiming that many social ills arise from wrong feeding. The diet is believed to predispose to non-violence and peacekeeping communities, the baser animal instincts being stimulated by meat and flesh-foods. 'Our diet,' it is claimed, 'contains all the nutrients necessary to health.' Some nutritionists however draw attention to its deficiency in certain nutrients.

Choice of food is based on the active yang and the passive yin – the Chinese doctrine of 'antagonistic but complementary opposites', as in acids and alkalies, hot and cold, etc.

This principle of unity split in two has always been a way of life, and their food is no exception. Like electricity, it is said to possess a negative or a positive charge (yin or yang). In the West, we go along with this theory when it comes to electricity, believing that all natural phenomena is accompanied by positive or negative electrical charges. Some do not find it difficult to believe that the life of every organism depends upon the correct balance (the sum total of yin and yang of its various parts).

The great secret in macrobiotics is to balance the yin and the yang foods. When treating disease by food therapy it is important to find the appropriate food to match up with the body condition. Disease is believed to be caused by a disturbance of the balance of the yin and yang in the body.

Lassitude, depression, nerve and skeletal weakness, and feeble digestion are conditions requiring yang foods: meat, certain 'strong' grains and fish.

If your nerves are irritable, your disposition impatient, angry, with actions erratic, and you're probably carrying high blood pressure symptoms, correction is possible by a switch to the yin foods: oats, wheat, green leaf salads, raw vegetables, fruit, honey and rice.

All this is done with a view to establishing a 'balance'. When interpreted it means that man is in complete harmony with himself and with the universe.

For those living in hot climates, yin foods are recommended. Those living in the cold north are likely to require the yang foods. A manual worker is better sustained with yang foods; the sedentary worker, yin foods.

The true believer will exclude animal foods of the West: meat, cheese, milk and butter, which are said to be harmful to health. Because tea and coffee are strong nerve stimulants they are avoided, and are replaced with simple herb teas such as thyme, mint, lime flowers, ginseng and lotus.

Twig tea, from the bancha shrub, is a favourite but excessive drinking is discouraged, especially the old custom of drinking to 'flush' the kidneys.

A number of roots rich in minerals are used as an alternative to coffee: dandelion and burdock and calamus. Making an entry on the American and European scene is the Japanese coffee substitute, yannoh, made from roasted grains and beans. And very refreshing, too.

From soy-beans is made a very palatable creamy mixture known as Tamari for adding to soups. Another fascinating item to brighten the table is tahini (sesame butter) for making fine sauces and sandwich spreads, said to sustain the brain. These are popular in macrobiotic foods.

Vitamin-rich sesame seeds are used for making biscuits while cooks discover more intriguing menus for arrowroot. Devotees claim a non-toxic alternative to ordinary salt. They make it from sesame seeds and sea salt, known as gomasio.

Most are very particular about the source of supply of their vegetables, coming down heavily in favour of organic gardening and natural farming methods without 'artificials'. Seasoning is an area in which they excel, being known for their delicious flavours.

Maybe there is something to be said for living on food grown only on one's own soil, though few of us would wish to give up the exotic spices of the East. As it is almost impossible to follow the ideal diet in a complex society, it is important to see that the foods we eat possess the adequate nutrients we need. Grains seem to meet this requirement wherever one lives. Macrotics eat them at every meal.

Unpreserved foods are 'alive' and 'active' and remain so until cooked. That is one reason why processing and refining is discouraged and most foods eaten raw. Usually those who adopt the diet do so for religious or other conscientious reasons and are often of a high moral tone in a permissive and profane society. They need to be of some strength of character because their diet requires a certain amount of time spent in preparation. However, their results not only look extremely colourful and attractive but carry with them added nutrition.

Not all the medical men go along with the macrobiotic diet. Some say a diet exclusivly of plant foods may lack vitamin B12, leading to a form of anaemia. But supplements of this vitamin are on sale at most health shops and pharmacies.

Some enthusiasts may go too far, when they run into a vitamin C shortage (the anti-infective vitamin). A deficiency of vitamin A is possible. Vitamin A is required not only for the eyes, but for teeth and all body cells.

A deficiency of vitamin D is another possibility. Without it our bones would become de-calcified and thin. In age, this can increase the risk of falling and fracturing the thigh bone.

However, those on the diet appear to maintain a good health record, though there may be the occasional hazard of deficiency disorder. At least statistics tend to show that they miss out on most of the degenerative diseases: diabetes, heart disease and cancer. They are among the world's longest living people.

It is to macrobiotics that we in the West owe the advent of many nutritive substances, some of which have entered the vocabulary of the 'sprouters' whose main kitchen pastime is to germinate seeds and grains for health. These include: mung beans, black-eye beans, adzuki beans, lentils, chick-peas, rye flakes, maize (corn), brown rice, wheat, oat flakes, millet, barley flakes and black beans.

This science of eating is still young. It does not pay to be too rigid in outlook. Experiment, read up and become acquainted with the yin and yang theory and your life may be enriched.

Melon

Although this fruit contains over 90% water, it is good to start a meal by getting the digestive juices flowing. A useful calorie-free fruit, its flavour is enhanced by ginger. Diced into fruit dishes together with segments of orange, cherries or banana, with ice cream it adds to the pleasure of a meal with friends.

Molasses

If you learnt the piano as a child you may remember 'Water Wagtail', a favourite among music teachers. It was composed by Cyril Scott, whose enchanting harmonies were much in vogue in the 1920s. He was the man who introduced molasses into Britain as an item of diet and wrote the first book on it.

Molasses had, of course, been imported into Britain many years before, but only as an ingredient in silage for cattle fodder.

A delicate child, Scott was a martyr to anaemia. Physical fatigue caused by a lack of iron, left him an easy prey to depression and nervous exhaustion. Resigned to a life of limited vitality he chanced to consult a naturopath in the days when it was a courageous thing to do. He was surprised to find himself put on a 'molasses treatment', which left him rather sceptical.

However, he persevered. He never felt better in his life and found results 'astonishingly beneficial'. His blood picture improved to a level which brought new life to body and mind. He felt it was his mission to make it known far and wide.

Subsequent investigation showed how it was the iron and calcium content which wrought the seeming miracle. Unable to keep it to himself, he wrote a book on it with sales climbing to more than a million copies since the late thirties. It is still going strong, although there are more authoritative books on the market today.[18]

Modern research confirms its contents of calcium, iron, copper, magnesium, phosphoric acid and most of the B vitamins. It is high in inositol and B6, and few foods can touch it for potassium.

Nutritionists agree that it has attained a place among the elite of wonder-foods including star performers like brewer's yeast and cider vinegar. It has earned its reputation because it contains more 'good health essentials' than most foods.

Some people have kidneys that cannot eliminate salt as efficiently as others and as a result suffer from high blood pressure. One alternative to reducing salt intake is to include in the diet more potassium-rich foods, and molasses does this admirably.

It is sometimes believed that adequate potash salts can be found in raw green foods. This is not always true. For one thing, there may be insufficient potassium in fresh vegetables to counteract a heavy salt intake. Cyril Scott believed that a deranged salt metabolism could be one of the causes of rheumatism and arthritis. An abundance of potassium in molasses can help make good its loss through heavy salt intake. Thus, in some cases of high blood pressure it would appear that molasses could be a good thing.

Dr Forbes Ross caused quite a stir when he published his report on molasses and cancer. He observed how workers on sugar cane plantations, who ate plenty of crude sugar, seldom went down with the disease. He put this immunity down to the presence of potash salts in the raw cane and which are removed in any refining process into white sugar.

It was Dr Ross's theory that the cause of the disease was a deficiency of potassium salts in the blood and tissue cells. He enjoyed a number of positive results which were published, but which excited acrimony from his colleagues. He was particularly successful in dispelling neoplasm on the tongue by way of direct therapy. Molasses was held in the mouth for long periods until the offending mass came away. Since his efforts, others in the field have tried to prove the veracity of his claims but have met with limited success.

Muesli

Thinking of breakfast, have you discovered muesli? This healthful repast makes a good nourishing breakfast in place of bacon and eggs. Try a mixture of rolled oats, dried fruit, dates, golden linseed and nuts. Five almonds and two Brazils will provide a whole day's allowance of selenium, calcium, zinc and iron. All you have to do is to add some milk or fresh fruit – chopped apples do quite nicely!

Nutmeg (*Myristica Fragrans*)

This is the fruit of an evergreen tree native of the Molucca Islands, Indonesia. The powder or fine grindings can be used as a stimulant to a sluggish circulation and sustain the heart under tension. They are usually bought whole and should be grated as-and-when required because their efficacy is believed to decline on long exposure to air.

Freshly grated nutmeg adds a distinctive warm flavour to food and drink.

Nuts

Nuts are exceptionally rich in nutrients and can sustain in the place of meat. Traditionally, nuts and seeds were supposed to strengthen both mind and memory. This belief acquires some credibility when we reflect that nuts contain ten times more phosphorus than fish.

Iron deficiency anaemia is one of the enigmas of the modern scene. Nuts and seeds are a source of this metal. Nut foods maintain strong nerves from the magnesium they contain. Nuts also contain zinc, necessary for the healthy function of the male reproductive system.

The natural oils in nuts build firm connective tissue to keep us well toned and alert. This is especially true of the almond. Dr J. DeWitt found that twelve almonds a day strengthened his wife's fingernails and prevented cracking. He says almonds make for sound teeth, strong bones and bouncing babies. It is the most completely alkaline of all nuts. For as long as can be remembered, almond oil has been a favourite cosmetic and healing lotion.

Peanut butter, flour or peanut oil are all nourishing and have no lack of vitamins B1 and E. When you cannot obtain wheat flour, peanut flour is a good 'stand-in'.

Tiger nuts, or earth almonds, have a reputation for fertility and milk production, which explains why they were eaten by nursing mothers of ancient Egypt. When ground, they offer a new dimension of sweetness to breakfast muesli.

Stuff of dreams

A new simple remedy against insomnia has been discovered by a French doctor. He says: 'Cut out salt from your meals after midday, then you stand a very good chance of peaceful sleep.' It took him thousands of laboratory tests and five years of study to come to this conclusion.

A man who claimed that he had not slept for forty-five years came forward to make his case known, after reading of the death of a woman who said she had not slept for twenty years.

continued

> While not wishing to raise false hopes we would like to offer from our own casebook a man who said he had not slept for forty-one and a half years, but who went off like a dormouse when he discontinued ordinary tea and coffee and started drinking lime-flower tea. He also took five yeast tablets at mealtimes by way of topping up his vitamin B reserves. So you see, there's hope for you!

During the American Civil War soldiers soon became aware of the food value locked up in the pecan nut. To roast them over campfires was to discover a taste much to their liking. Pecans are rich in vitamin B6. Twelve pecans a day for six weeks may make an impression on cases of nagging neuritis.

You can easily make nut butter at home if you have an electric blender. The resulting meal may be somewhat coarse but it can be mixed with a little corn oil or other vegetable oil. The proportion is roughly one tablespoonful of oil to five tablespoonfuls of nuts (ground). If a little too thick to be spread-able, add more oil, or vice versa. Nut butters are a palatable alternative to butter and margarine. Small quantities can be made, and you will know it is free from doubtful preservatives.

Nuts are free from waste products, uric acid, urea, carnine and other tissue wastes. Nuts are aseptic, free from putrefactive bacteria, and do not readily undergo decay either in the body or outside of it.

The fat of nuts exists in a finely divided state, and in the chewing of nuts a fine emulsion is produced, so that nuts enter the stomach in a form best adapted for prompt digestion.

The protein of nuts is perfect and is superior in quality to that of ordinary vegetables or meat. Nuts present the choicest and most concentrated nutriment of all food substances. They also contain a large proportion of albumin and fats. Most nuts contain 50% or more of an absolutely pure and easily digested fat. Nuts also contain a large proportion of proteins, or albumins, so much that 450g (1lb) of nuts contains nearly as much albumin as 900g (2lb) of beefsteak. Albumin and fats are two of the most essential food substances. They are necessary elements for building fat and blood. It is because meat supplies these elements that it holds so high a place in the popular esteem. Nuts supply these elements in more abundant quantity than do meats, and in a more nourishing form. 'The nut is the choicest aggregation of the materials essential for the building of sound human tissue, done up in a hermetically-sealed package, ready to be delivered by the gracious hand of Nature to those who are fortunate enough to appreciate the value of the finest of earth's bounties,' says Dr J. H. Kellog.

Nuts are high in vitamin E, zinc, selenium and fatty acids. Aim to eat 30g daily.

Oats

Fine, medium or coarse oatmeal all have the same food value. When we eat oats we lower the levels of cholesterol and glucose in the blood and therefore lessen the risk of diabetes and heart disease. Oats are a valuable source of fibre which, when eaten as part of a low-fat diet, promote a healthy heart and circulation.

Our mothers told us to eat up our porridge because it was good for us. Like it or not, we ate it. Now we can see she was right all the time. Modern research proves how this common grain keeps our cholesterol under control.

Oatmeal biscuits offer a substantial snack in place of gooey cakes, and have a high-energy value.

Oatmeal is useful for thickening soups. To speed up cooking, soak oatmeal overnight.

Parsley (*Petroselinum crispum*)

Although a common herb known by everyone, parsley provides more vitamin A than carrots. It is renal-friendly as a diuretic for some kidney problems, retention of urine and for those who pass water only at long intervals.

It is a splendid remedy to activate the adrenal and thyroid glands, and to reduce the discomfort of prostatitis.

All parts of the plant can be used: seeds, roots and leaves, eaten raw or in cooking. Menstrual problems may be resolved by drinking parsley tea.

Parsley Tea

Place one heaped teaspoonful of dried or 3–4 teaspoonful of fresh parsley in a small saucepan (not aluminium) and pour on a tumbler of cold water. Bring to the boil. Simmer for one minute. Strain when cold. Drink ½–1 tumblerful 2–3 times daily.

If you are a rheumatic, it is a must for salads – delicious when chopped up fine – and also for flavouring soups and fish.

Pears

Pears are an interesting fruit with a distinctive flavour. Conference, Comice and Williams pears include iron, magnesium, calcium, potassium, phosphorus, sodium and silicon – an impressive array of minerals!

A good source of fibre and vitamin C, they can be enjoyed as a seasonal fruit. To eat pears daily is said to reduce cholesterol levels.

Over the years I have received letters from readers who say they have been able to assuage the pains of shingles by wiping over the affected area with a cut juicy pear.

A pear can be delicious when eaten with cheese at the end of a meal.

Pineapple (*Ananassa sativa*)

Pineapples contain sourced of *Bromelain* a proteolytic enzyme that can be derived from the stem of the plant. This is a favourite among the women because of its effect upon cellulitis for the removal of fat, and ability to solve menstrual problems.

Pineapple juice contains natural enzymes that can be effective for digestive problems, sore throats and rheumatism. It can also clear clogged-up sinuses.

Pineapple juice contains both anti-inflammatory and anti-bacterial properties. Being rich in minerals it is said to assist the union of fractured bones and to allay the onset of osteoporosis.

Pollen

> 'Pollen is the substance of all life in the world. Each gram contains every important substance necessary to a living body ... there would be no life without pollen.'
> Dr Naum F Joirisch, Russian Academy of Science

The *Oxford English Dictionary* describes pollen as the 'fine granular or powdery substance produced by and discharged from the anther of a flower, constituting the male element destined for the fertilization of the ovules'.

In Britain, attention was drawn to it in The *Observer* in 1974, when it was reported that Judy Vernon, a chance outsider suddenly jumped into the limelight when she became hurdles champion. She admitted she had plenty of energy to spare after the race, and that she hadn't had a cold since taking pollen.

After a crash-research programme it was found pollen was one of the few substances on earth to contain the widest range of vital elements – minerals, vitamins and enzymes – known to man.

Some American and European businessmen take pollen to enable them to be still on their feet after long arduous hours of duty. Why? Because each single grain contains eleven enzymes, six carbohydrates, fourteen minerals, sixteen fatty acids and nineteen amino acids. What more could you want?

Countries where pollen is gathered and eaten as a protein food include India, Russia, China, Peru and the Polynesian islands. Pollen grains are the chief debris swept up by scavenger bees for dumping purposes. Known as 'honey-scrap' this rubble, with the viscosity of sump oil, is eaten by, and said to be responsible for great ages of, centenarians in such isolated communities such as Georgia in Southern Russia, reputed to be the world's oldest people.

A paratrooper escaping from a Japanese prison camp was picked up in Burma in an emaciated condition by local people who fed him on nothing but pollen floating on the surface of the river before guiding him to safety.

On examination by European doctors, he was found in an energetic and well-nourished state, and all of his former weight had been restored!

There are as many different kinds of pollens as there are plants and flowers. The plant itself will last for ten years. Some say its life is longer. Sweden leads the world in pollen production; in that country thousands of doctors prescribe it for various complaints. As a natural healer and food supplement, it is widely sought for its curative abilities by the medical profession and for its bodybuilding powers by athletes.

Potatoes

Don't take the humble potato for granted. To refer to it as a 'spud' shows great disrespect to one of the plus-foods of an essential diet.

We each consume about 300lbs of this rich source of potassium, calcium, iron, carbohydrate and a small amount of protein a year.

But that is not all. High in vitamins, they offer us nicotinic acid, thiamine of the B group as well as vitamin C. Low in fat, low in calories; high in fibre they are a slimmer's aid. Whether you use them for roasting, in salads or as a barbecue treat for the children, they always make healthy eating. They have only sixty-six calories compared with rice which has 138 calories.

In a Canadian study, the nutritional and healing qualities of potatoes was revealed.

Agnes T. Andrews healed herself of ovarian cancer on a potato-based diet. (*Canadian J. Herbalism* 2001, 22[4]: 21–25). *Greenfiles*.

Do you conserve the goodness of your potatoes by baking or steaming them whenever possible? If you haven't a steamer, a colander placed over a saucepan of boiling water covered with the lid will suffice.

Stuffed Baked Potatoes

Take a large baked potato, cut in half lengthwise, scoop out most of the inside and mix in a basin with pepper and salt and about 50 g (2oz) grated cheese. Pile the mixture into the potato cases and sprinkle the tops with a little more grated cheese. Return to the oven to brown.

Alternatively, mix a scooped-out potato with about 110g (4oz) cooked fish, finely chopped. Season with salt and pepper and pile back into the case. Sprinkle with chopped parsley and reheat in the oven.

Even leftovers can be made attractive. Cut into thick slices and place under the grill in a mixture of butter and olive oil until golden brown, turning once. A little fresh mint injects that extra zing.

Prunes – powerhouse of nutrition

Prunes are one of the few fruits allowed to ripen fully on the tree before gathering. This means they reach the consumer full of wholesome nutrients and replete with their vital energies.

Prunes are rich in vitamins A, B1, B3 and C, potassium, phosphorus, calcium, magnesium, iron and manganese. They are higher in vitamin B (now known as riboflavin) for mental health and emotional balance than any other fruit. Prunes will restore normal haemoglobin levels and red cell counts in many cases of iron and copper deficiency.

Because prunes are rich in magnesium, they cause excess calcium to be eliminated by the kidneys. This action is useful for the prevention of hardening of the arteries. In the same way, conditions resulting from the deposit of calcium salts in joints and muscles, as in arthritis, may be indirectly benefited.[19]

The most famous prune is the Californian French, a descendant of the original La Petite d'Argen from France. The romance of the Californian prune industry is a fascinating success story. In the 1850s, a French nurseryman named Louis Pellier, severely smitten with gold fever, spent weary months in lonely prospecting – all of which ended in disappointment. If he was lucky in love, it didn't show up in his pan. Watching neighbours strike it rich could be a galling experience to a man who couldn't afford a plate of beans.

Why he didn't pack-up and go home, we shall never know. For some unaccountable reason he bought a parcel of land and started a nursery. It was not long before he was joined by his brother Pierre and the two pooled their resources.

Now, Pierre was in sore need of a wife, but couldn't find anyone to take him on. So he went back to France to find someone to share his destiny.

The world was to hear nothing about Mrs Pierre, but was to follow with amazement the meteoric rise of a man who arrived back in America with an armful of cuttings of the La Petite d'Argen plum. Grafting them onto rootstocks of the American wild plum, the Pelliers grew a forest of nutritional dynamite and the mighty prune was born.

Experiments proved Pellier's black gold to be the perfect vehicle for the treasures of the Californian sun by day and of the starlit cosmos at night. Mineral-rich, quick-energy black bullets flourished in those rich green valleys – a sight to gladden the eye as well as the bloodstream. To this day, few other fruits can chalk up such a rich mineral content.

Radishes

Radishes contain vitamin C and other useful minerals, especially potassium, which assists the liver in its control of the level of fluids in the body.

As dispersers of catarrh, they clean-up mucous surfaces: congested throats and sinuses. Used for centuries by herbalists for gall and kidney stones, they increase the flow of bile.

At one time leaves of the vegetables were brewed as a tea for indigestion. Place a handful of leaves into a teapot (not used for making traditional tea) and allow to stand for fifteen or more minutes. Drink freely for any of the above ailments. Perhaps their most valuable mineral is sulphur, believed to delay the onset of malignant disease.

Radishes should be avoided for internal ulceration.

Raisins

Raisins are dried black grapes and are good sources of fibre, magnesium, copper, iron, zinc, sulphur and vitamin B6. They are useful for the reduction of cholesterol and their potassium content helps prevent fluid retention.

Raisins are high in sugar and therefore a ready source of energy during rigorous physical exercise. However, like other forms of sugar, they may destroy the enamel of teeth when taken in excess. Hydrocarbon chemicals are sometimes added, so they should be washed before eating.

Raspberries

Raspberries are not only delicious, but they offer us a rich source of calcium, phosphorus, potassium, magnesium, and vitamins B3 and C. They also add fibre, which helps the alimentary canal.

They are rich in bioflavonoides which are protective to heart and circulatory vessels. Their mineral content ensures healthy nails, teeth, bones and hair.

Powerful antioxidant properties in raspberry fruits are of value for rheumatoid arthritis and to sustain the immune system. They are also a help to overcome chronic constipation, and as a detox agent for internal cleansing.

Herbalists of the past prescribed the leaves for menstrual problems and for easy delivery at childbirth. *See also* Raspberry leaves (p. 255).

Rooibos tea

Rooibos tea has increasing sales in the health shops due to its freedom from caffeine. It has a very low content of tannin as found in traditional black tea. It is made from the leaves of a South African shrub, which is an effective antioxidant and anti-allergy and may reduce the mild-degree pain of rheumatism.

'The Hottentots who lived in Cape Province were the first to discover the properties of the Redbush, which grows on the slopes of Cedar Mountains. They attributed certain magical powers to the tea. Today, you simply make the deliciously rosy-gold brew in an ordinary teapot. Serve neat, with milk, or a slice of lemon. Many people prefer to taste the tea itself, enjoying it especially at night – when the last thing you want is caffeine.' The London Herb and Spice Company

Seeds

Alfalfa seeds
With ten times more mineral value than any other grain, the roots of this plant go down as far as 36m (120ft), unplumbed by other vegetation. It is the richest source of the widest possible range of vitamins including: A, C, D, E, K, B1, B2, B3, B6, B12, folic acid, inositol, pantothenic acid and biotin.

The seeds respond well to 'sprouting' by yielding fifty times more vitamins than found in any other seed. They increase enormously in bulk so that a half teacupful per person is plenty. This quantity is said to contain as much vitamin C (an added bonus) as six glasses of orange juice.

It used to be called 'the great healer' on the South American Pampas. When pioneering farmers began to settle there, they watched their cattle grow fit and healthy without the realizing that it would do the same for them.

Alfalfa is one of the earth's most impressive links between the power of the sun and the elements of the soil. No other plant contains so many minerals in such high proportions. Only Nature could produce such a balanced food.

Aniseed

Some cooks sprinkle the seeds into dough when making bread. It is also used for flavouring meats and cakes. It may even be added to vegetables and fruit salads. As a garnish it has much to commend it – if only for its anti-burp factor. If you have occasions when you have to tuck in your chin and thump your chest – then aniseed is for you.

A host of herbs exist for wind trouble; they are as old as mankind. They include peppermint, ginger and dill carminatives bringing a rosy flush to the stomach wall. With these, aniseed tea has one thing in common – it induces a straightforward belch when your stomach is under pressure.

Coriander seeds

Even in Elizabethan times folks made corny jokes of the seed-cake containing coriander. There was a time when buns and cakes were sprinkled with the seeds. Today, its use has widened to flavour rice dishes, grilled fish and gingerbread.

The Neolithic peoples of Britain flavoured their barley porridge with it. Today's macrobiotic followers suggest it renders lentil soup more exciting. With exotic menus introduced by immigrants from the East, coriander sales have soared. They may be used singly or in combination with hot spices: chillies, mustard, turmeric or mixed pickling spice.

Writers of the Arabian Nights regarded it with distinction, possibly because of its power as an aphrodisiac. The well-known Eau de Carmes, heart cordial, was prepared by monks of the Carmelite Order from lemon peel, cinnamon, nutmeg, cloves and coriander seeds steeped in strong wine.

Coriander was known to the Old Testament Hebrews during their desert wanderings. We read that the manna they gathered at sunrise had the appearance of coriander seed. It features in the Talmud, where it is regarded as a special food and medicine to those of the Jewish faith.

Its dry ripe fruits are extremely good for flatulence. Judging by the number of times the subject is mentioned in their literature, the Romans must have been a very windy lot!

One of its most important uses is in curry powder. All oriental spices are health-promoting as well as epicurean. Some are preventive – allaying infection by stimulating the body against mild ailments and giving heart to the digestive organs.

There may be times when you feel a little light-headed, or sense the room going up and down, round and round. There are many different causes of dizziness. Coriander acquired the folk name of 'dizzy corn' because, when crushed, it exuded an aroma believed to allay mild dizziness.

Fenugreek seeds

Shortage of protein is no longer restricted to isolated ethnic groups but to all high-level civilizations, spreading through poorer urban districts. At this end of the social scale, the same foods may be the main staples because of having to forego sound protein foods (eggs, milk, meat) in order to make ends meet.

That is why high-protein fenugreek seeds now receive more attention in the West – and in the East. They will ripen almost anywhere, so one day it could help feed all nations.

The aromatic seed of an Asiatic herb, it is bought in large quantities by racehorse breeders who find it provides their animals with extra stamina. This is also true for the two-legged species.

With a content of 21% protein (as well as iron and lecithin) it augurs well for future food supplies. The seeds contain roughly 35% calcium and 12% phosphorus. Hence their value for the brain.

Being mucilaginous, they have a soothing effect upon the alimentary canal. After having been soaked for a few hours they yield much mucilage, which is drunk for peptic ulcer and inflamed intestines. Parts of the Arab world still use the steeped seeds as a poultice for external ulcers and an unhealthy skin (one ounce of seeds to one pint of water, left to soak overnight).

When you run your car engine too long without a change of oil the sump will fill with sludge, so your mechanic will have to flush it out and replace it with thin, fresh oil. When your body's sump gets bogged down with catarrh it demands a solvent. This is where fenugreek tea can move in to disperse the obstructive mass.

Wherever there is irritation from stagnant mucus, as in mucous colitis or diverticulitis, this smooth silent bowel besom has much to commend it.

Dominican Father Sebastian Kneipp (1821–97), pioneer of hydrotherapy, was successful in curing chronic throat troubles by applying a cold pack around the throat and prescribing frequent gargles of fenugreek tea.

'My son's breath is so bad,' confided an anxious mother, 'that he can't keep a girlfriend. He is so embarrassed that it is developing into a psychological problem.' Fortunately, he was amenable to mother's fenugreek tea, took it for a week and was cured of the distressing condition.

Are you one who finds it harder to put on weight than your fatter friends to lose it? If you are a 'thinny' and seek a curve or two, take a leaf out of the Arabian Nights. Even today, some Turkish women prepare a mixture of honey, milk and ground fenugreek seeds which they eat with relish as a kind of sweetmeat to preserve.

Fenugreek tea is still given to nursing mothers in the Lebanon for the purpose of more milk secretion for their breast-fed babies. It was prized in Old Arabia for 'an alluring roundness of the breasts', while Roman matrons used it as a soap before stepping into steaming spa baths.

Sesame seeds

Tahini, a paste made from sesame seeds, can be an interesting addition to a number of courses. Houmous is now a well-established item of diet, a blend of tahini, and chickpeas. Sesame seeds have a mild nutty flavour and are splendid for decorating and flavouring breads and cakes.

They are perfect for adding to salads, poultry and vegetables. Sesame oil is golden from unroasted seed and used in cooking. All preparations help enhance immunity and lower cholesterol level.

The seeds are anti-bacterial, anti-inflammatory and antioxidant. Rich in calcium, they offer a welcome alternative to dairy products for those who seek protection from brittle-bone disease.

Sesame seeds embrace a wealth of health-benefits in the form of minerals, lecithin and fatty acids, linoleic acid and alpha linoleic acid.

Like sunflower seeds, sesame are full of vitamin E, selenium and zinc. Eat a tablespoonful a day to maintain optimum heath – sprinkled on cereals, salads or vegetables. Also, try coating your fish with seeds before cooking.

Sprouting seeds

Are you aware of revitalizing elements waiting to be liberated in your kitchen? Unless you have discovered them for yourself, you may not know what nutrient treasures await you.

Grains, seeds, beans and peas are packed with minerals and vitamins waiting to be tapped. Sprouting seeds can convert your green meals into super-salads. If not yet acquainted with this fascinating activity, why not move into production and acquire a new exciting pastime?

Seeds can be germinated on beds of damp linen, cheesecloth or plastic trays. A number of aids exist for growing these miniature cornfields in your own kitchen. The least expensive equipment is a wide-mouthed jar (say, an empty honey jar) and a piece of an old nylon pair of stockings.

Place the required amount of seeds, grains, etc., in the jar and fill with water to about one third. Your piece of nylon, sufficient to cover the mouth of the jar, is secured by a rubber band. Soak for a few hours. You may wish to prepare at bedtime, leaving to soak overnight.

The next morning, strain off the excess water. Rinse the seeds and leave them to germinate. Briskly rinse with water two or three times a day but do not allow them to stand in water. Just rinse and drain. All they need is to be kept moist.

Each time you rinse, gently agitate to see that the contents are well spaced. Allow them to germinate until the appearance of slender green spears, then wash off the husk or pod in a colander. They are ready for use at the table or can be stored in the refrigerator for up to four or five days.

Some seeds or grains need to be rinsed more than others. The secret is in the rinsing. Do not forget them, otherwise they will dry up and die. Adzuki, mung and kidney beans, chickpeas and sesame seeds need a good douche under the tap four or five times a day. Soy-beans, even more. But three times daily is sufficient for most.

We know friends who have a row of jars under cultivation, each containing a different seed 'on the go', all the time. You can go into business with a selection from sesame seed, chick peas, garden peas, wheat/oat/barley/rye grains, maize (corn), beans (kidney, mung, lima, etc), cress, mustard, lentils, millet, sunflower seeds – the list is endless.

If you prefer tall shoots, raise them in a dark closed cupboard for three or four days before bringing them out into the light for a further day to 'green-off' with extra chlorophyll.

This low-cost form of nutrition is much cheaper than expensive vitamin preparations, and much better for you, too.

Spices of life

From the spice-laden lands of Malaysia are exported cardamom seeds, the world's second most favoured spice – the first is saffron. Hindus use it for their exotic dishes, Muslims for ritual and Germans for their time-honoured burghers and sausages.

Saffron itself was the zesty colouring matter used in hot cross buns for hundreds of years. It was used also to add colour and flavour to butter, cheese and confectionery. But no one knew it contained vitamin B2 (riboflavin).

Not so very long ago a traveller might enjoy the thrill of trading runs, visiting past oriental spice forests and returning with the most romantic of cargoes. Who would not envy the sailor before the spicy breezes off the coast of Ceylon with its cinnamon plantations? In the harbour of the island of Zanzibar dried flower buds of the clove tree have been loaded for European ports for years. Cloves are used for cakes and other purposes in the kitchen. Oil of cloves, a mild painkiller, was a past remedy for toothache.

Spices owe their aroma and pungency to the essential oils they contain. Caraway seeds are the fragrant carpels of the caraway plant, for sprinkling into dough or seedcake for flavour and digestive aid. From the tubers of the curcuma plant is obtained a dark yellow powder – turmeric – favourite ingredient of curries.

Aniseed is used to flavour soups, stews and boiled potatoes. Nutmeg has a sweet, warm, spicy taste when freshly grated and is a popular seasoning for rice and soya dishes. A few grains of grated nutmeg have been known to revive a failing heart and is still sometimes helpful for dizziness.

Koran and Hindu literature refer to sacred spices: cinnamon, cloves, nutmeg, allspice, turmeric, garlic, mace, paprika, white pepper, black pepper, ginger and cayenne.

Ginger no longer travels westwards by camel caravan but its vitamin C still serves a purpose in protection against some minor complaints. The Egyptians were the first to mix it into wheat to make gingerbread. It is a stimulating diffusive for discomfort in the bowels.

Cayenne pods (chillies) yield a vivid orange-red powder known as cayenne pepper, also rich in vitamin C. In winter it is warming and sustaining; some finding it a helpful aid against cramp and neuralgia.

The National Institute of Medical Herbalists in England insists that cayenne is one of the purest, safest and most powerful heart stimulants known. They say that a pinch or two (or a drop of the tincture) increases arterial force, enlarges calibre of the blood vessels, and enables the blood to travel through the body more freely.

Much of the old spicy wisdom is still very much alive. Living under conditions of over-refinement of foods can bring about the destruction of vital elements. In a very real sense, spices can make an important contribution, often making up for losses. Some, if not all, have marked healing properties.

Sweet potato

The edible root of a tropical plant, this vegetable comes in two varieties – white and yellow. The yellow is rich in carotenoids which have the ability to be converted into retinol (vitamin A). Apricots, pumpkin, melon, cantaloupe and carrots all have a distinctive colour – a bright orange or yellow – and are all sources of carotene. Sweet potato is known for its high levels of vitamin A to help the body deal with infection and maintain a healthy immune response.

This potato is one of the most powerful antioxidants and anti-virals. Its beta-carotene is advised against risk of stroke, cataracts and heart disease.

It is also valued as a source of vitamin E. Why not include it in your diet once a week?

Tomatoes

Tomatoes are one of today's top nutrients. They contain lycopene, an active anti-cancer agent, as well as carotenoid, which gives them the rich red colour.

> 'A study carried out by Harvard University revealed that men who ate tomatoes and tomato products more than ten servings a week, enjoyed a reduction in the risk of prostate cancer by as much as 50%.'
>
> *Journal National Cancer Institute*, 1995, 87 21767 76.

Tomatoes are packed with antioxidants. A high blood level of lycopene means you are less at risk from some forms of cancer including its appearance in the pancreas, colon, rectum, bladder and especially the lungs. It helps prevent heart disease by reducing stickiness of the blood, which can block blood vessels.

Including vitamins A and C, tomatoes boost resistance to infection, promote a healthy skin and protect part of the eye from damage by light.

It is said that people living on the Mediterranean men eat up to ten servings a week, which is believed to be responsible for the fact that they suffer from 50% less cancer than people elsewhere.

> 'Tomatoes cooked in virgin olive oil have been found to be a valuable source of readily absorbable lycopene, a powerful antioxidant, which may help to prevent heart disease and cancer. Tomatoes eaten raw, however, yield up very little of their lycopene.'
>
> *Greenfiles*, 1 September 1996 p.29.

Cooking releases five times more lycopene than raw tomatoes.

Make sure your tomatoes are sun-dried. They develop a sweeter flavour when ripened on the vine. Home-grown have much to commend them.

The life of a tomato is prolonged when stored stem side-down. If you suffer from rheumatoid arthritis or food allergy the tomato should be eaten sparingly as they may worsen symptoms.

Rita Greer, the wholefood cook, says: 'Buy firm fruit. They will go on ripening after you have bought them, so use within two or three days, or buy less ripe ones and keep them a few days before you use them. Always wash tomatoes as they will most likely have been sprayed. Remove the stalks. Slice or chop with either a very sharp knife or a small one with a serrated edge.'

Rita describes her tomato starter: 'Only make this when you have really good tomatoes available. Homegrown ones are ideal. Allow 1 or 2 per person. Wash and slice thinly on to a plate. Sprinkle with a little finely chopped onion, a few pinches of sugar, freshly ground black pepper to taste and a little freshly chopped parsley. Serve with homemade, wholewheat bread and butter, sliced thinly. Sounds too simple but it is really delicious if the tomatoes are extra good.'

Turnips

Turnips are a diaphoretic (produce sweating) as part of a detox programme for body cleansing when eaten raw. They are known to bring ease in respiratory congestion and are useful for use in cardiovascular disorders.

Leaves are rich in chlorophyl and carotenoids, which are anti-carcinogens to fortify the immune system against invasion by cancer.

Vegan diet

For some discerning people, veganism is a way of life. Careful planning is needed to ensure that calorie intake is adequate and the food rich in variety.

One great advantage of a vegan diet is that it contains no cholesterol and is low in fat. Researchers have found that both vegan and vegetarian diets reduce the risk of heart disease, diabetes, osteoporosis and cancer.

However, the absorption of iron (present in meat) may prove a problem. The experienced vegan will consume an adequate amount of vitamin C. This vitamin appears in tomatoes, green leafy vegetables, oranges and other citrus fruits, enhancing the absorption of iron.

The flesh of animals is regarded as an important source of iron, but iron is also present in reduced amounts in pulses and whole grains. A deficiency of iron or vitamin B12 may lead to anaemia, so some vegan and vegetarian foods have them added.

It may be necessary to single out foods rich in calcium or take calcium supplements. Calcium absorption is reduced by oxalic acid found in beet, greens, spinach and rhubarb.

Vitamin D intake may also need to be monitored closely, and might need to be accompanied by exposure to direct sunlight or calcium and vitamin D supplements.

For fats, the chief nutrients are plant oils (olive oil, etc.) avocado and nuts. Popular foods include: chickpeas, lentils, spaghetti, macaroni, apples, oatmeal, wholemeal bread and toast, cereals, dates, lasagne, peanut butter, almond butter, soya, salads, orange juice, baked beans (organic vegetarian), seeds, pulses, legumes and figs. Many of these contain an adequate supply of B vitamins.

Vegetable juice therapy

Vegetables contain vital substances that act as catalysts to minerals and trace elements to regenerate body tissues. Vegetable juices are great inner-cleansers. Some stubborn ailments frequently respond to raw juice therapy. To drink a glass or two of raw, unpreserved juice daily ensures a continuous detoxifying process throughout the whole system.

- **Dermatitis:** beet, carrot, celery and parsley.
- **Gallstones:** tomato.
- **Heart trouble:** carrot, cucumber, spinach, and parsley.
- **Thyroid gland:** spinach, lettuce, radish and watercress.
- **Headache:** parsley, beet, carrot, spinach, lettuce.
- **Rheumatism, Gout:** celery, parsley, cucumber, carrot and spinach.
- **Hay Fever:** celery, carrot and parsley.
- **Piles:** celery, turnip, carrot and watercress.

Watercress (*Nasturtium officinale*)

Second only to broccoli tops in vegetable food ratings. By adding watercress to your meal you are adding much more than a tangy flavour; it is one of our richest sources of vitamin A, together with trace elements iron, protein and iodine (for the thyroid gland).

Watercress is a natural health food with more vitamin C than lettuce and more calcium than milk. It contains much sulphur, which means it will be an excellent blood purifier, being good for the complexion from pimples to freckles. Containing 20% potassium, it is alkaline and therefore kind to sensitive digestions.

The Romans blended this 'poor man's pepper' with vinegar in the belief that it helped those with mental illness. Watercress offers us a high nutritional salad vegetable, which goes well with sliced cucumber and celery. The vitamin C of an added orange ensures absorption of the iron from the watercress.

This versatile plant is obtainable throughout the whole year. Savour its goodness by eating raw and fresh. Stir into mayonnaise or salad cream a tablespoon of chopped fresh watercress.

The Crusaders are said to have valued it as a food to make up blood lost through wounds of battle. Old Culpepper, seventeenth-century herbalist, said: 'It is a powerful blood purifier as well as warming a cold and weak stomach, restoring appetite and assisting digestion.'

This spicy-hot, tasty little plant is a rich source of beta-carotene, an antioxidant which is advised as a preventative of rheumatic disorder.

Yoghurt – the prevention food

Yoghurt is perhaps the most popular of all health foods. Yoghurt is delicious and helps digest food. It is now part of the diet in many hospitals for protein in a pre-digested form. The bacilli form a 'laboratory' of beneficial bacteria in our intestines, producing B vitamins.

Yoghurt is one of our most natural foods for the acidophilus or 'friendly' bacteria in the colon. It was recommended in the Sanskrit and in the Koran, and was made from the milk of goats and asses. It can be made from any kind of milk and is today consumed by more than 500 million people, many of whom make it at home. Its value far surpasses that of plain milk.

Little wonder a 'health cult' has grown up around this lactic acid ferment. Some common ailments have been known to clear up automatically. Treating a case of colitis, a Swedish doctor was surprised to learn his patient lost her incipient migraine. One of the less wholesome effects of regular milk is an allergic reaction, giving rise to flatulence, liver and bowel disorders, which is absent in yoghurt.

When taking a combination of yoghurt and prune whip, no laxatives were required for 95% of the patients of a hospital. People who suffered from wind, belching and stomach rumbling mostly found relief after a month, eating 300m (10fl oz) of yoghurt a day.

Blend soaked prunes to a puree, add 3 tablespoonfuls yoghurt to each serving. For honey yoghurt, stir some honey into some plain yoghurt. Pineapple yoghurt is also delicious, and can be made by stirring in pulped unsweetened pineapple before serving.

Those looking for a substitute for milk (as in coronary disease) will find yoghurt excellent. Making this food, using a culture, is no more trouble than making a cup of tea. To make it yourself is to bypass many dubious products on the market which masquerade as the genuine article. For high-quality protein, it is something of a wonder-food.

Detox

Time to make a clean start. Are there times when you feel below par? Maybe you have put on a few pounds! If so, now's the time to shed them. Why not enhance your sense of well-being by this safe and natural way of achieving fitness.

Here's how to rest your digestion and give your body a well-earned rest. Plan your day to include a fifteen to thirty minute walk when you can breathe deeply which, in itself, is revitalising.

Spend the first three days on a diet of fresh fruit and green vegetables alone. Take no alcohol, coffee, tea, milk, sugar or salt. If you smoke, give it up.

Apples are rich in pectin and move on any accumulations of decayed residue from foods.

Pineapples contain the enzyme bromelain which purifies the stomach and destroys offensive bacteria.

Grapes cleanse mucous surfaces of catarrh.

Drink plenty of water, five or more glasses a day to flush out toxins. In this way you would be properly hydrated and on the ball. Boil tap water or drink bottled water to replenish the balance between trace elements.

On the day after your three-day fast prepare a green salad containing parsley (which contains zinc) and ensures good bladder health. watercress to assist the liver in neutralising noxious pollutants entering the body by food; grated beetroot for boosting production of red blood cells.

Don't overlook the sulphurous onions and garlic, which are powerful blood purifiers. Treat yourself to a cup of dandelion coffee to stimulate the flow of bile.

From the fifth day onwards, enjoy your favourite breakfast with a drizzle of honey or crude black molasses and a cup of dandelion coffee if desired. Have a salad as above, to which you can add unsalted nuts. Introduce whole-grains, bread and butter. If you are not on a gluten-free diet add oats, rye or barley. For your main meal eat cooked vegetables and oily fish – salmon, sardines and mackerel – though any kind of fish is acceptable.

From the next day you should be able to see colour return to your complexion, feeling restored in body and rejuvenated in mind and spirits. Be sure to continue taking fresh fruit and vegetables every day.

The Mediterranean diet

The 'natural nutrition public' becomes increasingly aware of the Mediterranean diet which appears to offer so much towards optimum health.

Scientists prove that the food we eat today becomes the bone and tissue of tomorrow. They insist that a vast volume of disease follows a diet high in fats and sugars, low in vitamins and minerals. Little wonder problem diseases, dental caries, liver and gall bladder disease and coronaries impose a heavy burden on our over-worked hospitals.

Today, added to junk food, we have to face the practice of gamma irradiation for prolonging the life of foods. Much of our diet is threatened at the fountainhead.

How does all this compare with foods consumed in countries bordering the Mediterranean? How is it that some of the poorer countries enjoy a measure of health above that of northern Europe, including the UK? In spite of saturated fats, alcohol and excessive smoking, they do not suffer from the chronic diseases of arthritis and of the heart.

Why?

The answer must be because they consume large amounts of 'superfoods'. What are these must-eat-foods?

In the first place come apples, good for the heart; artichokes for the liver and gall bladder; carrots for good eyesight; olive oil, rich in vitamin E and a protective against arthritis; grapefruit for a smooth and easy digestion; onions for urinary infections; grapes, powerful antioxidants; avocados, a nourishing fruit for relief of stress; yoghurt, protection against thrush; tomatoes, the key carotenoid containing lycopene without which olive oil cannot be absorbed; rice to lower cholesterol; garlic, antibacterial properties covering a wide range of infections; bananas, for their potassium; greens, anti-cancer and maintenance of a healthy bloodstream to allay the onset of anaemia and chronic blood disorders; pulses, (dried beans, lentils, peas) for vitamins and minerals; nuts, for B vitamins.

All these foods, fresh, unpolluted and unprocessed, provide an adequate intake of protein, fat, carbohydrate, vitamins and minerals. Even the poor may consume a measure of these foods, being unable to afford the glamorous processed food of the West.

It is interesting to note that constipation is not as prevalent as in northern Europe and the UK because their nourishment contains an abundance of fibre, which aids elimination of body wastes.

For healthy eating it's not so much what we eat, as what our food contains – or leaves out – that is important.

Once you have become interested in Mediterranean foods you will start on a never-ending source of enjoyment with good nutrition as the end product.

5

Fitness for Life

To succeed in business, domestic and social life you must be fit. This is not such a difficult condition to attain. If you want to be fit, you must look to your innermost self.

Anxious thoughts and fearful emotions can wreak havoc on your health, create wrinkles where none appeared before, and lower the body's defence system. If you are to enjoy whatever life brings, you need to create a lifestyle in which it is fun to be fit. It all depends on how you keep in shape, and shape up. To enjoy the glow of good health, you must exercise.

You don't have to be a 1500m (4900ft) Olympic gold medallist, but you may wish to break your own record at walking, cycling, gardening, swimming, dancing . . . even calisthenics! All you need is a few minutes a day – something to get up for in the morning.

Is exercise really necessary? Yes, says William James, psychologist, 'Muscular exercise will always be needed to furnish the background for sanity, serenity and cheerfulness – to give elasticity to our disposition – to round off the wiry edge of our fretfulness.'

When we are physically fit we are alert. Regular exercise increases our powers of endurance and muscle strength. It maintains our lungs, blood vessels and heart in top condition, keeps our weight under control, promotes flexibility of the spine and joints and releases tensions of body and mind.

If you are active with some form of daily exercise you are less likely to develop trouble with the heart or circulation. You will have more endurance and not tire so easily. Something you do not hear is – that regular daily exercise cuts down your capacity for worry. Active people are seldom depressed, moody or anxious. You are more likely to meet day-to-day problems with common sense, make intelligent decisions if you are not bugged with stress disorders.

Stress is something we all have to contend with in today's world. Management feels the strains of constant responsibility. All over, people are less satisfied with their lot and harassed by thoughts of unemployment. An active person makes his or her own exercise and finds pleasure in firming-up loose muscles, tightening up a sagging skin and making the most of life.

He will learn how to balance rest against effort, calmness against strain, quiet against confusion. He will have discovered how rhythm and style are an inseparable part of exercise. Sir Roger Bannister, the first man to run the four minute mile, wrote: 'I think there are reasons for the basic satisfaction of rhythm and style in our lives. They are an essential ingredient of the skills which underlie sporting performances and we reach a point at which high sporting skill is almost an art form. If we watch Olga Korbut, for example, in her gymnastics, the rhythm, the skill, the style indicate a level of co-ordination which involves her whole capacity both mentally and physically. It is a delight to the performer because she feels that she is releasing the total innate potential of her body. It is a delight to the spectators who are able to see in this almost an art form and who therefore experience a satisfaction that they might also experience when listening to music or watching ballet. I hope this causes the desire to emulate.'

Whatever our form of exercise, it is when we bring into it rhythmic flow and harmonious movement that it becomes an art form of great emotional satisfaction. Just as we make time for work, we should make time for exercise.

To feel our best, and to be at our best, every cell in our body requires oxygen. We cannot survive more than five minutes without it. The last cause of disease is oxygen starvation, and the most effective way of meeting the demand is exercise, to produce a better functioning heart. If we follow a sedentary lifestyle our oxygen level will need constant boosting with gentle exercise.

The heart and lungs are concerned with the distribution of oxygen, but sometimes they are not able to do so. The heart may not have the strength to propel blood through the arteries to meet the demands of muscles. The arteries, themselves, may be so narrowed by fatty deposits on their walls, that the flow of oxygen is impeded. Thus capillaries that convey oxygen to the tissues cannot do their job.

It is seldom we have a surfeit of oxygen. The golden key which unlocks its release is 'exercise'. 'Oxygen debt' is a term known to athletes which causes muscle fatigue through lactic acid pile-up. But it is extremely unlikely your daily dozen would reach anywhere near this state for which trainers of professional sportsmen prescribe the super-vitamin B15.

Breathing

Without breath there is no life. Even plant life depends upon the air for its existence. Life is made up of a series of breaths.

People need no instruction in the act of breathing. They are children of civilization, acquiring ruinous attitudes to standing, sitting and walking. To breathe naturally is his birthright; this we have sold for a mess of posture.

All pay a high price for the civilized comforts we enjoy but there is one small way in which we can redress the balance – by making a personal effort to breathe correctly.

Why is deep-breathing so necessary? Because upon it depends vitality in the veins, the 'tone' of our muscles, the clarity of our thinking, keen eyesight and even our moral sense! Nothing saps morale worse than slowing down the body processes. A feeble respiratory function breeds its own set of vexations.

In Asian cultures it has long been believed that fresh air contains an intangible ingredient: Prana. This is the most primitive form of energy known. They believe that circulating air is made up of much more than oxygen, hydrogen and a bit of inert nitrogen.

By controlled rhythmical breathing we can bring ourselves into harmony with the world and enjoy the bracing curative properties inherent in the air we breathe. Can you sense the importance of giving your lungs a methodical 'work-out' at least once a day? It need only involve five minutes, yet once you start you are likely to want to pursue the exercise at any odd moment.

I need hardly tell you that the more oxygen we take from the air the greater its efficacy for the entire circulation: impure blood is rapidly cleansed, the lymph system stimulated for the expulsion of toxins, liver is given the squeeze it needs and the abdomen firmly massaged. Of what profit is it if we vigorously exercise the external muscles and ignore the internal organs?

Deep breaths

In the simple act of breathing Nature has taken care of everything. She does it through the diaphragm. It is when we further assist her movements by conscious constructive breathing that we open up a whole new field of internal harmony and well-being.

STEP 1:
Stand erect, hands on hips. Raising the shoulders high, inhale slowly. Allow the shoulders to drop and exhale slowly.

STEP 2:
Stand erect, arms at sides. Rise on the toes, at the same time inhale, and raise the arms forward and upward. Clasp hands above the head. Exhale, lowering the heels and sweeping the hands downward in a wide circle until they reach the thighs.

STEP 3:
Seated in a chair with hands on your thighs, try to make your shoulder blades meet; you will not accomplish this, but will take up the right position. Fully relaxed, breathe slowly yet deeply.

STEP 4:
Sit upright during the whole of the exercise, legs at an easy angle. Let the lips be closed and all breathing done through the nose. At the end of each inhalation raise the shoulders to allow some of the air to pass into the upper lobe of the right lung. This is smaller than the other lobes and the haunt for lurking tribes of germs, especially the TB bacillus when conditions are favourable and when a feeble vital capacity follows shallow breathing.

Try to keep the movement rhythmic and continuous, the entire rib-cage expands in a uniform movement. Let your expansion start from the abdomen and rise up to the chest. Draw in all the air possible to the count of seven, hold for seven, and exhale to the count of seven. This is known as the Rule of Sevens and is one of the many methods used by athletes.

Cleansing breath

STEP 1:
Close your mouth. Engage in rapid staccato in-and-out short sharp breaths (panting through the nose).

STEP 2:
Take a complete breath as deeply as possible. Hold the air to the count of seven. Constrict the mouth as in the act of whistling. Through the puckered lips vigorously blow out a little air. Stop. Hold the air. Blow out a little. Stop. Repeat the stop/start process until air is exhausted. Inhale deeply and repeat.

Try out either of the above exercises to revive jaded spirits in a fug-laden atmosphere.

They are particularly beneficial if your workplace is overpoweringly hot or dust-laden. Where possible, you should try to avoid central heating.

Singer's joy

The golden road to perfect breathing is, of course, through singing. Every organ and capillary receives a dynamic oxygen booster when you sing By stimulating the thyroid and pituitary glands (both concerned with the body's defence mechanism) the singer is less susceptible to respiratory disorders – even colds and flu!

This is because when you sing you have to keep your diaphragm up. By keeping up your diaphragm you will have less weight on your stomach, thus facilitating digestion. Try to open your mouth and go through the motions of eating when you are singing. Organised singing exerts an influence on body development. My wife put on two inches in height on taking up singing lessons, after the age of forty.

You say you can't get your top notes! Yawn your way over them. Open your 'yawn' and get over the top. The higher you go in the scale the less breath required. Don't attack a note – get over the top of it. Like the advice of an experienced steeplechaser approaching a difficult jump, 'Before you jump, first lift your heart over the fence.'

It is the same with singing. Lift up your diaphragm. In spirit, lift up your heart. When the voice cracks, you've lost your diaphragmatic support.

What is said about singing can be repeated for the act of humming. If you can't sing – hum. Hum till your lips tingle. If you do ten minutes of humming before starting to sing, you'll be surprised how much better your top notes sound.

Remember, hum to relieve stuffed sinuses and loosen catarrh. You say you're too old to do either! Well, you're only as old as you feel.

Why do I carry on about singing and humming? Because I think you should know how they act as a charm on tired nerves. After gentle elation, they are Nature's own sweet restorer. Learn to make the most of your voice through controlled breathing.

I'm lucky enough to live in a part of the world where facilities for keeping fit are all around. Almost every village and town has its share of sports, games and pastimes.

Bowls

For instance, take bowls, an energetic game for you! Most people think of it as a game for adults only – and some, pretty old ones at that! Not so. There is an increasing interest in bowling in young families – an ideal game where children can play with their parents and grandparents. Some young people make rings round their elders!

Here is a splendid exercise for your low back provided you follow the recognized stance – both knees bent and flexible, neither rigid nor inflexible.

All you need are flat soft-soled shoes, like plimsolls. In hot weather bowlers like to wear a hat. Don't get sunstroke.

Jogging

There were over ten million people watching the London Marathon, in which there were over 60,000 competitors.

Jogging is still all the rage in most countries of the West. In some cities as many as 20,000 people may take part in a single event. Even the disabled have their chair-propelling marathons where shoulder brawn decides the issue. Jogging in such a procession, you are not likely to suffer from the loneliness of the long-distance runner.

A few doctors regard the craze as a medical disaster area, but most of them are all for it.

'I can still remember quite vividly,' said Sir Roger Bannister, 'a time when as a child I ran barefoot along the damp, firm sand by the seashore. The sound of the breakers on the shore shut out all others, and I was startled and almost frightened by the tremendous excitement a few steps could create. It was an intense moment of discovery of a source of power and beauty that one previously hardly dreamed existed . . . The sense of exercise is an extra sense, or perhaps a subtle combination of all the others.'

Everybody has a right to breathe. Even young asthma sufferers say they have found relief, even victory, over their affliction when taking up jogging.

By no means is it everybody's cure, yet excellent results have been obtained under medical supervision. Olympic silver medallist Alan Pascoe, a sufferer from the age of eighteen months, is one of their successes.

Does jogging shake up the womb? Women of today enjoy running, if the 10,000 entries in a woman's marathon is anything to go by. Some find it quickly burns up the old flab and helps reduce weight. Record studies show that athletic women have fewer menstrual and pregnancy problems than their sedentary sisters.

Cycling

In 1979, Tom, a bearded overweight man, pedalled his 120kg (19 stone) the length of France.

Fat, unfit and forty, he felt he was not long for this world. Then he picked up a prehistoric bicycle at an Oxfam shop for a fiver. First using it for shopping, it wasn't long before he was cycling to work. After years of driving a car he found it a rattling good way to travel.

Like other motorists he had spent hours racing from A to B, seeing nothing more than concrete roads and frustrated drivers. Now he's thoroughly hooked. He pedals along enjoying the fresh air, nodding to acquaintances and listening to the birds.

So addicted to riding his bike, he embarked on a 1530km (950 miles) tour of France. He says: 'France is the land of the bicycle. An Englishman riding through the French countryside on a bike somehow expresses the relationship of the two nations.' He struck lucky for weather, not minding the rain – all ten minutes of it – and now he has a 'supremely pleasurable' memory to look back on.

Cycling awakens you to a life you have all but forgotten. Cyclists are rich in stories about folk they encounter along the way – fellow cyclists, naturalists and friendly villagers. If you are not interested in knocking-up an impressive mileage you have more time to stop for a chat. More than most travellers, you will see a rare selection of old-world villages, cathedrals and secluded spots.

The cyclist really gets about and meets people. It need take only a little time to leave the big towns where fast trains wait to carry you to attractive cycling country. Transport costs for your bike are nominal and fold-away cycles can easily be tucked away in the boot of the car. I heard of a Canadian girl who has taken her fold-away bike by air on fascinating cycling holidays in China, New Zealand and Japan, and she is typical of a growing army of cyclists who travel the world for recreation and refreshment.

Popularity of the cycle has led to the formation of clubs. Holiday groups of enthusiastic cyclists spring up everywhere, especially among ecologists who take their belief seriously. Travel agents have a bigger and more varied selection of cycling holidays than ever before.

Rhythmical pedal-power is the fastest growing leisure industry in China, Germany, France and Italy. Every summer Britain is invaded by two-wheeler travellers from the Continent who find the country irresistible.

John Farquhar, professor of medicine at Stanford University, California, and Director of the Stanford Heart Disease Association admits: 'I gave up smoking and I weigh what I did twenty years ago. I ride my bicycle to and from work unless it's raining. When it rains I get a fifteen-minute workout on my exercise bicycle while I read the newspaper. I swim twenty minutes three times a week, and have eliminated high fat from my diet, eat fewer animal products and refined sugar, and more fibre-rich foods.'

The cyclist will know the thrill of achievement and joys that come out of rough going. You cannot be a cyclist without the spirit of adventure. The philosophy of the cyclist shines through a letter by an unknown author who made this discovery: 'Those who ride bicycles say it is easier to ride up a hill at night than it is during daylight. Hills that are impossible of ascent may be negotiated at night. At night the cyclist can see but a few feet in front of him, and the faint glow of his lamp gives him the illusion that the hill is either level or not steep. He feels he can go the few feet more than his light shows, and in this manner keeps on and on, while in the daytime he sees the whole hill, the whole problem, and it seems so steep to climb that his courage fails him.'

Next time you queue at the bus-stop in the rain or wait in a traffic jam, remember that in Holland four out of every ten people go to work on a bike. In Britain only two out of ten use them.

Can you think of anything better to firm-up your major muscle groups and keep you fit at so small a cost? Your bike doesn't consume fuel so it's non-polluting. Manufacturers now turn out more bicycles than cars. In fact, we are witnessing the biggest cycling boom since the 1920s.

Cycling is good for you. It compels you to breathe deeply. You will be exercising your heart, muscles and blood vessels, strengthening them and improving their performance. Who knows, it may stretch your life span!

Dancing

We live in an age of increasing leisure, so it is good to know how to balance work and play. It is physically and mentally good for us to be active and productive, such as in earning a living and the means to enjoy play. We have so much to learn from dancing, such as balance, harmony and rhythm of movement.

Shyness and anxiety in the presence of others are actually very common. It is good to have a modicum of inhibition to guard us from excesses, but when we make our lives miserable with social stresses, real or imaginary, there is nothing like the tension-free zone of the dance floor to help us regain poise.

In the Middle Ages, dancing would break out in the streets and go on for hours. Today, there are those who believe it arrests progressive deterioration of the mental faculties. Others find a great sense of physical release in dancing, recommending it for neurosis.

Some claim its therapeutic effect, forming a national association to organize schools of dancing. They think dancing can help restore hormonal balance in a woman suffering from pre-menstrual tension.

Emotional instability is seldom improved by sitting down and doing nothing. How much better are walking or dancing! Suppressed grief is better brought to the surface and let out of the spirit. Everybody, especially adolescents, have a black mood from time to time. There are few things like dancing to restore mental buoyancy.

A widow, weighed down with intense despair, was invited out for an evening dance. She got so carried away that her acute anxiety disappeared. 'At one time, she was so apathetic,' said her friend, 'that I couldn't reach her. Now, since accompanying me at dancing classes she is more talkative, and a pleasure to know.'

When we tend to be too preoccupied with ourselves, blowing-up minor incidents into major disasters, when we lie awake mulling over our past or dreading our future, it may be a good thing for us to find an agreeable partner and dance these things out of our system.

It may even be the answer to fuel problems!

Money was so scarce and his poverty so austere that Mozart and his wife had only one room into which was crammed a piano, a table, a bed and a chest of drawers. Visiting friends would find them dancing to keep warm.

Inhibitions, especially in the social sphere, can cramp our lifestyle. They place an uneven strain on husband and wife. They cause depression and loneliness. Some people can be the object of hours of well-intentioned 'counselling' but overlook the advantages of learning to dance, thus sweating out their inhibitions on the dance floor. Apart from ballroom dancing there are vigorous Scottish country dance and countless other dance societies in many counties.

What can dancing do? It can stretch and strengthen our muscles. If we are victims of stress, it may be the antidote we need. When more strenuous forms of exercise are denied us, it could be one of Nature's gentle alternatives. Who knows – it might be the special form of recreation we need to relax, revive and restore.

Laughter

There is a story of a family which suffered from persistent bad fortune. For long years they had been so overshadowed by sickness, financial losses, disappointments and set-backs of one sort and another that they lived in constant sadness and depression.

One day, after a fresh piece of bad news, somehow the mother suddenly saw the comical aspect of the situation, and began to laugh. The rest of the family had no idea what she was laughing at, but her laughter was infectious, and they started to laugh too.

When they stopped laughing to recover their breath, they felt happier than they had for years. And that was the turning point in their history. From that time on, whenever anything went wrong, as it often did, they laughed at it. Before long, things started to improve, and they entered upon a new chapter of prosperity.

This story from real life illustrates a truth which is not sufficiently recognized. Of course, it is well known that any mood tends to produce the corresponding facial expression. If you feel miserable you will look miserable; if you feel happy, you look happy. It is not so well known, however, that if you state this truth in the reverse way it is equally true. The facial expression will produce the mood. If you make yourself look miserable, you will feel miserable, and if you make yourself look cheerful, you will feel cheerful.

Put it to a practical test. Stand before a mirror some day when you are in the dumps and, after noting your melancholy countenance, elevate the corners of your mouth into a smile. Make your lips form ten minutes to two instead of twenty past eight! Wear that ten minutes to two look for a moment or so, and then see if you don't already feel better!

It may sound very trivial, but it really isn't. It is an experiment well worth trying. The laughter cure is really effective. Laughter is one of God's best gifts, and it is one of the surest solvents for the hardships of life. A sense of humour, which has been defined as 'the capacity of seeing the amusing side of the tiresome and trying events of life,' is a great asset on our mortal journey. The Bible is right when it says that 'a merry heart doeth good like a medicine.'

Britain's Bible Magazine

Daily exercises

Do you get your fair share of exercise? It is when we are inactive that the heart will not develop resistance to shield us from a number of cardiovascular and lung conditions lessening our chances of health.

So much depends upon stamina. Make no mistake, the next thing to correct diet is stamina and good general all-round fitness. The heart and lungs need to be sufficiently 'stretched' to increase the pulse rate and bring about some degree of breathlessness at least once a day. If we feel unfit after switching the heartbeat into a higher gear, then exercises (except those for breathing) should be avoided.

Soaring energy costs can be a cause of depression when considering heating of our home. The question is, in winter, how to keep warm? But it's an ill wind that doesn't blow some good. The energy you generate yourself by simple exercise is the cheapest and most plentiful source of fuel imaginable.

Always start with deep breathing and relaxation, then test your agility. To receive benefits, a fifteen to twenty minutes exercise period will produce valuable results. If you can afford the time, make it once a day; if not, once every two days.

Always be conscious of posture during your exercises: sit and walk tall. Try to keep the chin back and down, not forward and up.

Clench your fingers into a tight fist; relax, and stretch them as far as possible in a spread-eagled span. Do the same for any other joint that moves: knees, shoulders (shrugging), arms (rotating), hips (one hand on a chair for balance), lift the foot from the ground and rotate the hip socket and spine. The advice of an old arthritis consultant was this: 'anything that moves, keep it moving.'

If you are not used to exercises, give your pulse a spot-check until you get into the swing: the normal pulse rate in maturity is seventy-two beats per minute. This number will be increased in exercise, but if a raised rate persists until long after your exercises are finished, it may be an indication that you are overdoing it.

Arm swinging

STEP 1:
Stand with your feet wide apart and your arms by your sides.

STEP 2:
Raise your arms forward, upwards, backwards and sideways in a circle. Make it a breathing exercise at the same time by inhaling as you go forwards and upwards, and exhaling on the way down.

STEP 3:
Try to keep your upper arms as near to your head as possible on the upward sweep.

Side bending

STEP 1:
Stand with your feet wide apart and your hands on your hips.

STEP 2:
Bend to the left, then to the right, keeping your head at right angles to your hips. Exhale on bending; inhale deeply on rising.

Taking the chair

STEP 1:
Take a chair and stand facing the back of it. Rest your hands on the back for balance.

STEP 2:
Slowly raise your left knee and simultaneously lower your forehead until both meet. Hold this position for a few seconds.

STEP 3:
Repeat the exercise with the right knee, concentrating on the growing strength of your pelvis.

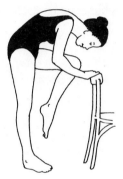

More chair drill

STEP 1:
Hold the back of a chair to perform knee, hip and trunk bending. If you feel energetic enough for 'push-ups' by lowering your chin or chest to touch the back of a chair (a table is more stable), you will be exercising your body to its maximum.

Spine rotation

STEP 1:
Stand with your feet wide apart and your arms extended sideways.

STEP 2:
Rotate the whole of your trunk towards the left, while turning your head in the same direction.

STEP 3:
Repeat the exercise towards the right. This exerts a beneficial longitudinal torsion-strain on your spine which may resolve any temporary rigidity or impacted lesion acquired through heavy lifting, falls or blows etc. The secret is for the head to rotate as far back as possible, as if you're see behind your back.

Dorsal bracer

STEP 1:
Stand with your feet wide apart and your hands clasped behind your head.

STEP 2:
Relax your shoulder muscles but draw up your diaphragm.

STEP 3:
Swing the upper part of your body into a circle, returning to the starting position. Inhale on the way up, exhaling on the way down.

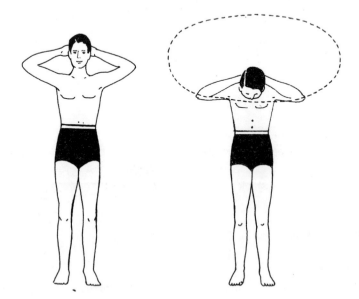

STEP 4:
To the left circle ten times, to the right ten times, or as many as can be comfortably performed. In all exercises keep your chest out and your stomach in. Your diaphragm is the 'bellows' mechanism which keeps you breathing. It sucks that vital life-giving oxygen into your lungs.

Skyscraper – to exercise the joints

STEP 1:
Stand with your feet very wide apart and your hands at your sides.

STEP 2:
Inhale deeply, at the same time stretching your arms sideways and upwards as if 'reaching the sky'. Rise onto your toes to give that little extra skyward stretch.

STEP 3:
Keeping your arms stiff and straight, and exhaling as you go down, bend your knees and touch the floor with the back of your hands as far behind your heels as you can get. In this position, give your hips and back a slight stretch.

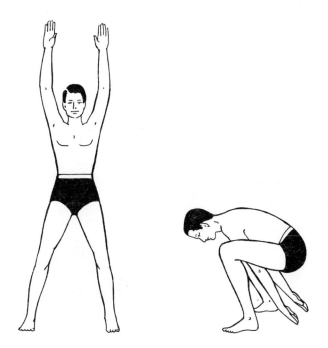

STEP 4:
Repeat as many times as you can. This exercise is a powerful strengthener to the back, thighs and leg muscles.

Ankle reach – to flatten tummy muscles

STEP 1:
Stand with your feet wide apart, and both hands resting on the left upper thigh.

STEP 2:
Exhale as you allow your trunk to slump forward, sliding both hands down your leg to your ankle or mid-leg height. Inhale, returning to the upright position. Repeat on the right.

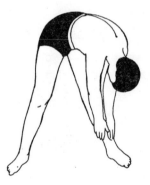

Anti-stress

STEP 1:
Lie face-down on the floor. Clasp your hands in small of your back. Stretch your arms out behind your back.

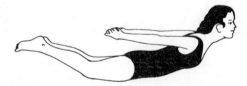

STEP 2:

With your elbows straight, pull back your shoulder blades until they touch. Simultaneously, endeavour to raise your upper body and legs from the floor, strongly pulling back with your arms. Hold the position for the count of three. Relax. Repeat, trying to raise your legs and upper half of your body as high as possible each time.

STEP 3:

Do this six or seven times on the bedroom floor before going down for your evening meal. Relax well after the last effort. Soon, you'll be sitting on top of the world. Do you sometimes feel like that?

Upside-down bike

STEP 1:

Lie on floor with your arms at your side. Raise both of your legs simultaneously until they are at right angles to the body, then pedal away to your heart's delight. Keep your trunk still. This exercise strengthens the back and buttocks.

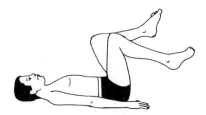

Neat seat

STEP 1:

Lie on your back with your legs up the wall. With your buttocks touching the wall and knees straight, rest your legs at right angles to the body. The perfect relaxing position – It even permits reading!

Foot drop

STEP 1:

Lie on your back with your legs up against the wall. Flex one foot causing it to drop forward. Give the tendon a stretch by pressing the ankle forwards and downwards.

STEP 2:

While you are doing this, give the foot nearest to the wall a strong forward stretch (extension). Reverse the position of the feet, and repeat a number of times. Restful for the arches and good for varicose veins. Your feet will thank you for it.

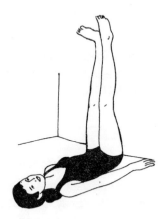

Cat stretch

STEP 1:

Get down onto your hands and knees.
Let your head slump and arch your back like a cat.

STEP 2:

Raise your head and flatten your back.

STEP 3:

Lastly, lean forward, touching the floor with your chin and chest, while keeping your elbows uppermost. Repeat the series.

This three-part performance exercise will strengthen chest muscles and correct bad posture. It is excellent for piles, bowel troubles and to alleviate breathing difficulties.

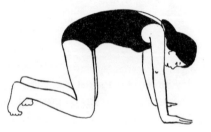

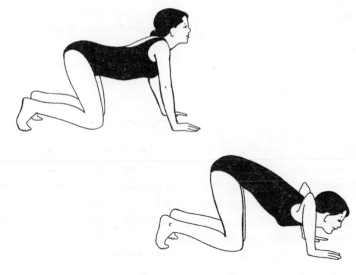

Secretary spasm

When sitting for a long time it is possible to lose sensation in the buttocks or suffer from stiff legs. 'Secretary spasm' might be due to an uncomfortable seat or to poor general circulation.

STEP 1:
Raise one leg in front of you, keeping your knee rigid and flex your foot forward. Rotate your ankle in a circle a number of times. Do alternate legs, then give both legs a long stretch together.

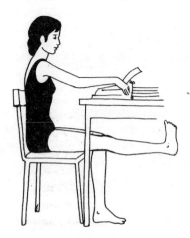

129

STEP 2:
Take a series of deep breaths, forcibly raising and lowering your diaphragm, and at the same time pulling in your stomach.

Secretary back

We all spend too much of our time sitting on chairs. The greater part of our lives seems to be spent in the sitting position on chairs of shocking design. Prolonged inactivity destroys good posture (which ensures a healthy functioning of our internal organs) and causes a collapse of the abdominal walls. Neither is it good for the back to be arched, which puts extra strain on the hips. Adjustable back rests giving support to the small of the back are commonplace in offices and factories today; if not, insist on one. It should be possible to operate your computer without bending over. There is only one answer to stiffness or 'pins and needles' in your backside and that is to get up and walk about.

STEP 1:
Sticking your neck out. Sit comfortably with your hands resting on your hips, in the erect position.

STEP 2:
Commence a slow nodding by allowing your chin to slump into your chest. Raise your head up and over until it rests on the nape of your neck, eyes looking back over your head as far as possible. Repeat this slow nodding fifteen or more times.

STEP 3:
Next, turn your head to the left as far as it will travel. Give it a series of gentle jerks to increase its range. Turn your head to the right and repeat.

STEP 4:
With your shoulders at rest, sit comfortably and draw a circle with the tip of your nose. Commence in a clockwise direction and follow with one in an anti-clockwise direction. Repeat smoothly each pair of circles fifteen or more times. (Do not do a series of clockwise circles all together because of possible giddiness. Follow each clockwise circle by an anti-clockwise one.)

STEP 5:
Looking towards the front, draw a circle with your nose but with your head pushed forward a few centimetres. Do both – clockwise and anti-clockwise circles. Repeat fifteen or more times.

STEP 6:
Looking towards the ceiling, draw fifteen or more clockwise and anti-clockwise circles.

STEP 7:
Eyes front, press your chin back and down, and draw fifteen or less circles (by that time you will just about have had enough of this exercise!). Restore your head to the normal position and finish off with circles each way.

You may be surprised to hear crepitations (crunching in the tiny joints). Regard this as a good sign. You will be breaking-down deposits, your joint movements becoming smooth and mobile. These back exercises have been successful in dispersing certain kinds of headaches as well as stiffness of rheumatism and arthritis. When you stick your neck out in this way you might well be helping visual problems, too!

Take every opportunity to have a good stretch, using the whole of your body. Breathe deeply, stretching upwards, breathing out as you come down. Breathe in as you rise from a chair, keeping the top of your head tilted slightly forward. When you stoop, bend at the 'hinges' of your hips and knees. Use the back of a chair for the support of your spine.

You may not wish to perform all the exercises at any one time; you yourself are the best person to make the best selection. At the end of your exercises you should be feeling great. With perseverance you can increase your lung capacity within six weeks.

When did you last warm up with a little skipping?

How to get strong

'Nobody can live successfully in this world without being strong', said Dr Norman Vincent Peale (1898–1993), one of the most widely-read inspirational writers of his time. 'You may be pampered and protected when you are a child, but you have to learn to be strong as you mature because sooner or later life will throw the book at you. Sometimes it will throw the whole book at once. I sometimes think that the greatest virtue of all is to be strong.'

Do you know of any way of reaching fitness without engaging in some

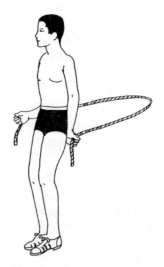

kind of sport? It does not really matter whether you choose to ski, sail an ocean-going yacht or polish up your skills at ten-pin bowling as long as you live an active life.

What is your choice? Horse-riding, basketball, golf, rowing, tennis, squash, badminton, bowls or even skipping? Perhaps you are a skater enjoying amenities at a winter resort.

Some people have a passion for sawing wood. You may be different – how about all-in-wrestling? If you're a bike courier or fitness instructor your job will trim your figure down to size. But if you're a shop assistant, clerk, machinist or teacher you'll need all the exercise you can get.

Thousands have the ability to succeed in sport but few have the inclination to devote time and practice to achieve their goal. As in other spheres of life success is made up of inspiration and perspiration.

Exercise develops. Lack of it causes us to be breathless from the slightest exertion. Whether gentle or vigorous it is always an insurance against nervous tension. Under-exercise means flabby muscles which Nature never intended.

What is your sport? cricket? baseball? Can you honestly walk past a game without stopping to watch? There is nothing more exhilarating or more fun than playing games in the park or back garden with a group of children.

Always warm up before trying to swing a golf club to avoid sprains and pulled muscles. Games help reduce the risk of heart attack, especially if you give up smoking and avoid fatty foods.

Whatever your sport, when you're down, it will lift you up; and when you are up, it will enable you to 'take off'. You simply can't help feeling good when vigorous exercises lower your cholesterol level. A quickened circulation at regular intervals, can be a powerful body incinerator – burning up waste materials and cleansing the bloodstream.

Do you want a stronger heart? Whatever our age exercise will improve its mechanical efficiency. It will do more. It opens the vessels to ensure a better flow through the coronary arteries.

Even in cases of angina, carefully controlled exercise can relieve that nasty chest pain caused by decreased blood flow to the heart muscle. This is why a regular brisk walk with deep breathing can add years to your life.

Out of eight years of her keep fit shows on TV, Eileen Fowler, broadcaster, singled out one exercise above all the rest: 'Raise the arms above your head and stretch up hard with one, then the other, as if climbing a ladder. Go up on your toes, too.'

Asked what was her beauty secret, she replied: 'Olive oil. I always used it for cleansing my face and for massaging my neck every night.'

What are the basic essentials of exercise – in a nutshell?

Suck in your stomach by raising the contents of the abdomen as far as you can into the chest and holding it. Bend your legs, as in squatting. Give your skin a dry friction rub with the palms of the hands, all over. Use your arms: flail, reach and circle in all directions. Roll your neck in a circle, clockwise and anticlockwise. Straighten your spine by pressing the small of your back against a wall. Endeavour to walk tall. Breathe deeply by expanding the chest at all times when opportunity permits.

Invisible exercises will help you keep fit. You can do them any place. You can shrug your shoulders, contract your stomach, stretch your Achilles' tendons, walk on your toes, and press together your knees to give tone to flabby inner thigh muscles.

Play a piano concerto with your toes, giving each a good wiggle in turn. Go up and down the scale. When you listen to the radio, wiggle your toes in time with the music. In all these things stretch as much as you can – at all times. It will relax tension and is the most natural exercise in the world.

For some there are not enough hours in the day. For others, there are too many. Don't go to seed. Find something to get up for in the morning.

Whatever your age, your joints can be relined and made more flexible. You'll be surprised how much more bounce you'll get to the ounce!

Swimming

One form of exercise which may bring you handsome rewards in the health sphere is swimming. If you already enjoy this activity you will know how good it is for your heart and lungs. There's nothing like swimming to give your spinal muscles just that little extra 'stretch' they need.

Few sports are more invigorating, leaving you feeling so fresh and relaxed, and swimming is good for the figure.

So it is twenty years since you donned a swimsuit? A woman hadn't swum for twenty years and decided to do it again. To her horror she became terribly breathless after a few strokes. Retreating, she felt she was too old for that game. However, on her daughter's persuasion she visited the pool a second and a third time after which she could swim without effort.

After five-minutes breast-stroke, she discovered, all traces of her backache and stiffness had disappeared.

Being able to swim is like riding a bicycle; once you have learnt, you never forget it.

Only when swimming – as any osteopath or chiropractor will tell you – is the spine and all its components completely relaxed.

A boy of twelve developed rheumatoid arthritis after excelling in cricket. Can you imagine the mental trauma to a once-active child? Closed to him were the gymnasium and that exciting expanse of green turf that sets a boy's heart racing. Even walking was painful.

One day the whole family decided to take a trip to the baths. Mother swam with the two girls while Dad and the boy sat as interested spectators. Antics of the swimmers were screamingly funny. They laughed their heads off. Mother scrambled up the steps out of the water to hold a brief conference with Dad. They would try an experiment.

Dad went off to hire a swimsuit from the attendant and they persuaded Mark to take to the water. At first, he hesitated. Then, with the aid of his parents he joined the thrashing throng.

The fun was terrific. He splashed the girls with his powerful arms while mother held him up. The frolic would have gone on for ever but they lifted him out when he became breathless. He was so elated he'd forgotten his pain before they wheeled him home in his chair.

The session was repeated the following Saturday with no adverse effects. Mark still has his rigid limbs but has discovered a new activity in which he can excel. He still has to be supported in the water, but it is difficult to keep him out of it.

Maybe, you haven't been inside a swimming pool for years. How about renewing this simple, inexpensive pleasure?

Summer is the best time to learn. Beginners' classes are organized at most local pools. Look out for adverts in your local newspaper or at the pool. Whenever you go swimming, remember pool attendants are there to help you if you get into difficulties.

If the chemicals they put into the water to keep it clean irritate your eyes, use protective goggles. Vitamin E cream should effectively deal with any infection picked up. Wear gossamer-light rubber swim-shoes where you can.

To avoid cramps, don't swim for at least an hour after a meal.

This is a pastime for which you will require no partner. It's up to you to change your way of life, if needs be; and change it you can.

Walking

If you have little time for regular exercise then walking is the thing for you. It costs nothing, requires no special gear or tools. All you need is a comfortable pair of shoes, flat-soled and soft welted.

Walking for health is something each one of us can enjoy at any odd moment. Fewer folk seem to take a walk before bedtime to encourage sleep. There is something to be said for a saunter after an evening meal to assist digestion. Some people find they can walk themselves out of depression and anxiety.

Is it better to walk than to drive? Cervantes thought so. 'The road,' he said, 'is always better than the point of arrival. Once you get into the country there is no substitute for legs.' That is true when drinking in 3km (2 miles) of oxygen: the medicine that vitalizes all ages.

All over the world, single or in groups, you can see purposeful people setting off for the cheapest relaxation. Ramblers' associations include fans from every walk of life: clerks, miners, secretaries, shopkeepers, solicitors and academics are among their members. One special feature is the number of octogenarians window-shopping on Nature: walking the novice off his feet in the pursuit of some rare native bird or wild flower.

If you've two healthy legs there's nothing to stop you joining them. Have you ever considered it to warm cold feet, cool hot heads, flush feeble lungs and to cure a bad temper? It is a medicine that never fails.

When not stepping out briskly along country lanes, you'll find there are fascinating scenes everywhere in the towns, better explored on foot. London is the walker's paradise. Most of its sights are well worth a visit, and admirers of Sir Christopher Wren have about thirty of the master's churches to visit plus, of course, his masterpiece – St. Paul's. The same applies to other great cities.

Whenever Bob Hope had spare time between shows, one of his greatest pleasures was walking the streets of small towns and New York, savouring new sights and enjoying the gardens. Sending his baggage on ahead, he told of how he walked through 'clean little towns with white picket fences and neat lawns, the smell of the good earth in the air.' He said: 'I'd meet lots of folks just walking along, and it always made me feel glad I was a comedian and could bring them a little laughter. But I found out what they brought me was more than I brought them.'

Getting into step with your new lifestyle. When did you last indulge barefoot walking on dewy grass? Old Father Kneipp, whose cures comprised nothing but cold water and herbs, had his patients walk barefoot on the wet grass for weakness and feeble health. Later in the day the lawns would be watered with a hose.

He prescribed this when patients were nervous and tense and before the days of tranquillizers. He reckoned moderate exercise improved body tone, enhancing the general feeling of well-being.

If you go for long walks with a rucksack or backpack make sure it is not too heavy. Carrying too much weight, for too long, can cause vertebrae to become 'impacted' with abnormal pressure on the nerve roots and blood vessels. Every osteopath and chiropractor is aware of this and offers special spinal adjustments.

None of us is likely to undervalue the convenience of our car for comfort and business purposes. But life can be bearable without it. Discontinuing a habit you once thought essential can bring a new set of values.

A word about walking-sticks. You don't have to be an old codger to use a stick. It can be a treasured companion on any walk. It is no evidence of weakness in a man or a woman to be seen walking with a stick. All those with a sense of rhythm, for instance dancers, will not wish to deny themselves the zest of getting into the swing of it.

It is a pity walking sticks are less common today, but really it could be as important as a pair of tough shoes. Leigh Hunt observed: 'Deprive a man of his stick, who is accustomed to carry one, and with what diminished sense of vigour and gracefulness he issues out of the house. Wanting a stick, he wants himself.'

No, you are not decrepit when you add an extra spring to your step in this way. Some use it as a precaution against falling on an uneven sidewalk. Whenever I am sightseeing in the open country my trusty ash stick adds pleasure to the occasion. Much younger walkers may envy my stick when negotiating a slippery bank after the rain and the puny defence it offers against inquisitive farm animals. And, of course, it may come to the rescue clearing a way through the brambles.

There is nothing like organizing your own programme. Do you take public transport to work? Why not walk further than you have to, and catch a bus at a later stop along the route? You may be lucky enough to be able to walk the whole of the way to and from work. That means your ration of oxygen will be greater.

If you have an opportunity to take a brief leg-stretcher during the lunch hour, do so. A healthy circulation at work means much. Consciously stretch your legs, inhale deeply, and walk tall.

If you are on a calorie-controlled diet, you may wish to consider that 5km (3 miles) at the average speed, burn up just under 1255kj (300 calories).

There's nothing like walking in a group for unloosing tongues and stimulating brains. The fitter you are the more you will enjoy it. And walking alone gives you time to think. Dogs love walking and make the perfect outdoor companion, especially before bedtime. Let him send you to bed healthily tired. After seeing him settled for the night, help yourself to a hot milk-and-honey drink to take care of any sleep problems.

Yoga

When a televised programme on yoga was beamed in Britain, over six million viewers sat glued to their sets. The astounding series went on to become one of the most successful programmes.

What is the essence of this ancient/modern culture which has hit the West? If its purpose could be summed up in one word, it might be harmony. Followers seem to acquire a peaceful outlook on life. Some say it goes deeper than that. They claim self-realization and an expansion of body awareness. Health and happiness, they say, depend upon the harmony existing between body and mind.

The yoga generally taught in the West is hatha yoga (body fitness). Its teachers regard it as a philosophy and way of life. A profusion of books of instruction on the market tell of tens of thousands of people who find yoga helps them to cope with their problems.

I suppose its main usefulness is that it helps us to help ourselves. Yogis are mostly a peace-loving community and can be found almost anywhere in the world. While instructors and study groups abound in our cities, there is no reason why you should not practise this most tranquil of arts in the privacy of your own home.

There are those who take it up from the clinical angle to overcome functional disorders, but to most people it is a non-violent way of keeping fit. Some claim that it stimulates the body's immune system, strengthening our bodies' defences against infection.

It is the hope of every committed yogi that the art will enable his mind to pass upwards to higher levels of consciousness. However, you do not have to be a disciple of a wise man from the East to adopt this attitude of mental quiet. Not all seek an awakening of the intuition or wish to explore the mysterious Overself, yet all can acquire a greater capacity for health and happiness. It is, however, better to have a teacher at least to start with.

Some approach it to increase their 'personal magnetism' by bringing their bodies into close contact with the earth. Its disciples regard Nature as a friend. They will run barefoot as a child over a grassy lawn or lie down flat on their back on Mother earth.

They are likely to believe that the energy of man comes not only from the food people eat but from the earth, and that the earth is one huge global battery from which they recharge spent energy. In this age of stress-induced illness this can be a restful and relaxing activity. It requires no specialized equipment and very little floor space.

Young and healthy of both sexes combine in the pursuit of stillness and serenity. Some say it makes for a balanced function of the body's many parts and is good preventive practice.

Many great athletes and sportsmen have found themselves unconsciously adopting Yoga principles when developing their bodies to a peak of perfection. Swimming and yoga have much in common. If you are a swimmer, used to the breath control it demands, you should excel at yoga.

My 'let go' pose

STEP 1:
Firstly, have a good stretch all over.

STEP 2:
Lie flat on your back, legs apart, arms a few centimetres away from your body and palms upturned. Insert a cushion in the nape of your neck and a rolled-up towel under both your hips and the small of your back.

STEP 3:
Relax. When you're comfortable, allow your mind to wander from head to toe. You may feel some muscles still tense. Tell them to fully relax. Feel your nerves at rest.

STEP 4:
Close your eyes: Breathe rhythmically and lie quietly. Start with your toes; tell them to relax completely. Work upwards, letting go bit by bit. It is not as easy as it appears. Is your jaw still too tense? Is your neck too rigid?

STEP 5:
Imagine you are lying on a warm, soft, sandy shore in the sun and that your limbs are as heavy as lead. Repeat these words a number of times: 'As heavy as lead . . . heavy as lead.' Feel your tongue withdrawing to the back of your

mouth. Breathe in slowly through the nose. Allow the stomach to expand and find its own level, at the same time breathing deeper and deeper. Fill the whole of your lungs with air. Sink deeper into the sand. Think of a sleeping child.

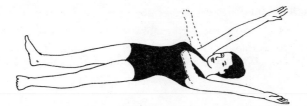

Lotus pose

For meditation and conscious breathing. Once your legs and pelvis have been educated into this position you may obtain a satisfying body awareness and firm-up leg muscles at the same time.

STEP 1:
Sit on the floor. Fit your right foot into the left groin. Take your left foot into your hands and fit it into the fold of your right leg.

STEP 2:
When you are comfortable, relax as long as you wish, hands resting on your knees.

Reverse the procedure. Where your joints do not permit the manoeuvre in comfort, do the next best thing: sit with a straight back, knees outstretched sideways, soles of the feet together. Close your feet into the groin and bear downwards with the knees towards the floor.

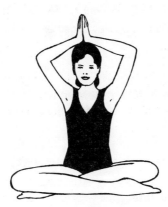

Spinal twist

STEP 1:
Sit on the floor, knees straight. Carry your right leg over your opposite thigh, with the foot flat on the floor.

STEP 2:
Bend the left knee completely so that the foot rests beneath the buttocks.

STEP 3:
Turn your trunk towards the right, exerting a strong torsion twist on the spine. Carry the left arm over the outside of the right knee, the left hand clasping the right foot.

STEP 4:
With your right hand on the floor to give added support, turn your head sideways over your right shoulder. Hold the pose for as long as comfortable. Unlock yourself and repeat on the opposite side.

The plough

STEP 1:
Lie on your back with your arms at your sides and your palms facing downwards.

STEP 2:
Keeping your legs straight, tense the abdominal muscles sufficiently to sustain an effort of slowly raising the legs to form a right angle to the body.

STEP 3:
Push down with the hands. Endeavour to raise your hips and pelvis from the floor. Make sure you keep your legs together. Hold the pose. Slowly return your legs to the ground. Rest.

STEP 4:
To carry this one stage further, raise your legs to the right-angle position. Hold, then carry the legs as far over your head as possible. Hold the pose.

STEP 5:
After having practised this a number of times with success, try to touch the floor behind you with your toes. Hold for a few seconds before gradually unwinding to the resting position.

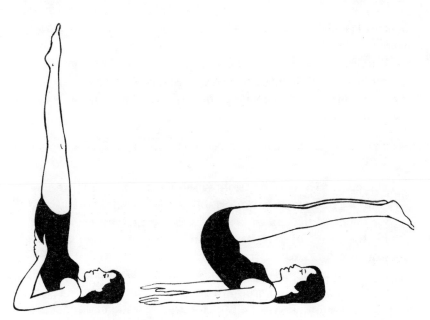

This exercise will improve your sense of balance, strengthen your spine and increase flexibility of each separate vertebrae. It is not indicated for high blood pressure but is ideal for increasing body warmth by stimulating the circulation.

At an age when most men want to put their feet up, Sir Francis Chichester, hatha yoga follower, sailed alone around the world. Once he was found reading the draft of his book *How to be Fit* – while standing on his head.

All this may demand as little as ten minutes a day. If you can add to this two hours in a weekly class, that may be all a busy person needs. All movements should be carried out very slowly. If you are a tense person you may find yoga difficult until you get into the hang of it.

If it is not possible for you to take more vigorous exercise, Yoga may be the kind of activity you are looking for – to help you look and feel good. It can bring a richer blood supply to parts where circulation is feeble. If this happens to be face and neck, Yoga helps ease out furrows and wrinkles. You should feel the benefit almost immediately.

They say it stops your joints stiffening. Perhaps that's why its adherents suggest it holds back old age.

These are days when birth centres can be found in most Western capitals, promoting natural childbirth. Expectant mothers who have practised yoga throughout their pregnancy often have much easier deliveries.

After the baby is born, post-natal exercises help mothers to get back into shape.

If you feel a little irritable or neurotic at times, don't reach for the tranquillizer bottle, just slip into a simple relaxation pose.

There's something in yoga for everyone – it's safe and satisfying for all ages. You are never too old for yoga.

Palming

If you'd like to have better sight without glasses, try this exercise. First of all, sit down in a comfortable chair. Second relax and clear your mind. Loosen up completely. Close your eyes. Cover them with the palms of your hands, leaving the nose free. Without undue pressure exclude the light and concentrate on inky blackness. Think blackness. Any posture may be taken provided it is comfortable, and that arms are supported. Do this from ten to twenty minutes. This is helpful for squint, astigmatism, short-sightedness, eye fatigue and eye strain.

6

A Guide to Complementary Medicine – Getting Well Naturally

There are two ways of overcoming disease. One is combative; the other, preventative.

Modern medical practice is almost wholly combative. But in many cases, disease is actually a friend. It amounts to this: there are two ways of being healed – one, suppression of the body's efforts with agents which drive away symptoms; the other, to assist Nature's healing efforts by natural methods.

Do you recognize the true nature of disease as a cleansing process? If so, you are in the vanguard of modern scientific thought. Nature's efforts to bring about a 'change for the better' are seen as being corrective in purpose. Much disease has been found to be assistive, not destructive.

Many forms of acute disease are now regarded as 'healing crises' through which the forces of Nature rise to cleanse and heal. Herbal medicine regards this as part of the constructive principle of Nature which repairs, builds up, and strives for perfection. This is the opposite of the destructive principle which destroys and breaks down human life on the physical, mental and spiritual planes, which inhibit function.

How is it possible to assist the constructive principle of healing?

- Encourage elimination of wastes and toxins without injuring the body.
- Restore a natural environment, and restate normal habits in accord with Nature's laws.
- Support the Life Force in its efforts.
- Ensure that blood is reinforced with natural constituents to assist sound body maintenance.
- Arouse the sick person to make a positive personal effort.

It stands to reason that anything harmful to body tissue cannot be harmonious with the constructive principle of Nature.

What are the basic causes of disease? These include infection, the accumulation of toxic wastes, lowered vitality, and abnormal composition of the blood and lymph.[20] Lymph is a diluted form of plasma (i.e. fluid part) that seeps from blood vessels into tissues and delivers nutrients to local cells; it eventually drains back, carrying with it waste products.

What causes a build-up of waste materials? This may range from overeating, a blameworthy diet, too much tea, coffee, alcohol, drugs, steroids, poison by petrol fumes, chemicals including defective lead plumbing pipes and other environmental hazards. A common cause is the suppression of healing crises manifesting as colds, flu and minor ailments by widely prescribed drugs of the day.

In chronic disease the accumulation of wastes and other factors change the body's chemistry to the point of tissue destruction, when Nature's constructive forces are powerless to react with further efforts of elimination and cleansing.

Why do you suffer from lowered vitality? This is understandable if you are over-stimulated, indulge in too much work, take suppressive measures to dampen down the symptoms of headache, pollute your lungs with smoking, and generally burn the candle at both ends.

How can we get back to normal? By a return to Nature. What will this entail? First, you have to trace your way back to natural habits of breathing, dressing, eating, drinking, working with ample rest, social activity and so on. To these, I would add such elementals as sunshine, air and baths. I would not forget to build up the blood with natural foods, raw fruits and vegetable juices, and plenty of exercise.

Next, I might consult a doctor or other qualified practitioner to search for any mechanical defects in my body, and for them to be resolved by massage, osteopathy, chiropractic and other therapies including surgery – where necessary.

There are other means of raising the body's recuperative powers as have been discovered in the sciences of acupuncture, aromatherapy, biochemics, biofeedback, chiropractice, colour therapy, herbal medicine, homoeopathy, hydrotherapy, hypnosis, macrobiotics, naturopathy, reflexology and spiritual healing.

All these have one thing in common: they recognize that Life Force – referred to as the 'vital force' – pervades our whole being, and upon which our bodies rely for their wholeness.

Since the beginning of the nineteenth century there has been fought a battle between supporters of vitalism and the advocates of mechanism. The mechanist regards the body as a machine, the vitalist sees it as a machine operated by a machinist. Mechanists believe – as I do – that there is a vital force that regulates the body's internal environment, holding in balance the various salts, sugars and constituents, and safeguarding the correct balance between acid and alkaline elements of the blood.

It is all a question of belief. The vitalist cannot measure the power of the vital force because it lies outside the sphere of (exact) science. The orthodox mind cannot accept the existence of an intelligent force within a biological unit. The vitalist (usually the unorthodox) believes the vital force to be the source of all life and the spiritual energy implanted in the body by a wise Creator.

General science looks at life as a manifestation of magnetic, electric and chemical activity. The vitalist believes in a kind of 'healer' within.

You may be surprised to see that a new kind of practitioner has emerged, whose efforts accord with these principles. Instead of aiming at a single organ, his efforts will be directed towards the whole of the person. The patient will be treated as a person – not a case.

The practitioner of the future will not look at a damaged spleen, but explore the whole person, and his or her reactions to family and history. The approach will be 'macro' instead of 'micro', integrating mind and body.

Our bodies possess their own innate healing system, responding to Nature. Let us look at some of these alternative therapies.

The changing face of medicine

'The body has an avid taste for life', says Dr Kenneth Walker in his book of essays. 'It displays great wisdom and experience in its struggle to survive.' 'Who has put wisdom in the inward parts?' asked the writer of Job. The fact that he asked this question shows that he was aware of the skill with which these inward parts surmounted their difficulties.

'This concept of the healing power of Nature is indeed the one fixed point in our ever-changing stream of medical theories. It remains as true in these days of medical science as it was true in the bygone days of medical magic.'

'It is to Nature alone that a sick man can look for cure. If he enlists the help of a doctor, all that his doctor can do is to serve as Nature's assistant. Our work as medical men lies in discovering her ways and in lending her a hand whenever we can. The greatest sin that a doctor can possibly commit is to work at cross-purposes with his great teacher [Mother Nature].'

There is a powerful uplifting force in Nature that is always on the side of health, provided we do not attract Nature's penalties by breaking her laws. Chief among her requirements are proper feeding and efficient elimination of toxic wastes.

Few scientists of the twentieth century came to understand the secrets of natural health more than Dr Alexis Carrel (1873–1944), Nobel-prize-winner (1912) and author of *Man, The Unknown* (1935). He was one of the first bio-ecologists of this century to point to Nature's way.

Are people seeking alternative methods to get well? Medical journals show that they are. In the UK alone it is estimated that twenty million treatments a year are carried out by practitioners of the natural therapies.

The era has arrived when the migraine sufferer is referred by his doctor to an acupuncturist, a crippled back to an osteopath, an asthmatic to a trained herbalist and a stress-racked mother to a school of meditation.

With similar national natural therapy associations in Europe, the stage is set for a harmonious working between orthodox doctors and alternative (also known as complementary) practitioners. This closer co-operation between previously opposing factors is welcomed by the World Health Organization. In it, they see a means of relieving the work-load of hard-pressed doctors.

Some doctors have already undergone a course of training with alternative societies, thus offering their patients an additional dimension of health care.

The great bacteriologists of the nineteenth century equated disease with germs of micro-organisms. They and their followers have led us away from the Hippocratic concept (for better or worse), seeking to prove that each specific disease was caused by a single germ.

Modern medical science is founded on the germ theory of disease. Since Louis Pasteur (1822–95) and Paul Ehrlich (1854–1915) and their microscopes brought to light the apparent evil activity of germs, it has been assumed that they are the direct, primary cause of most diseases. And so the theory became: we must kill the germs in order to cure the disease.

The bio-ecologists think differently. They say these germs cannot be the cause of disease, because they can be found in any healthy bloodstream. There must be another cause. They bring forward some convincing arguments to claim uneliminated wastes provide the soil on which micro-organisms flourish.

They will tell you bacteria are a secondary aspect of disease, and that parasites breed and thrive on any rubbish dump where there are accumulations of waste materials. 'There is but one cause of disease,' said Major General Sir Arbuthnot Lane, MD, famous British abdominal surgeon, 'poison, toxaemia, most of which is created in the body by faulty living habits and faulty elimination.'

E. Hooker Dewey, MD, a well-known American consulting physician, tried to put back the horse before the cart when he said, 'Disease has its origin and development before a germ disturbance in the body can become possible.'

What then is the purpose of germs? They must have some constructive action in the body's biochemistry. Their most likely role is one of the scavenger, ever ready to break down into its elements unhealthy tissue (in the cells or the blood) that the body intelligence wants to get rid of.

'If I could live my life over again,' wrote Dr Rudolph Virchow (1821–1902) bacteriologist of international fame, 'I would devote it to proving that germs seek their natural habitat – disease tissue or a poisonous blood-stream – rather than being the cause of disease tissue or impure blood e.g. mosquitoes seek the stagnant water, but do not cause the pool to become stagnant. Germs are scavengers.'

What then poisons our blood? Lack of exercise, too little oxygen, debilitating personal habits, sophisticated foodstuffs and infection. Destructive emotions, such as anger, envy and jealousy may also change the character of the blood by interfering with the full and harmonious flow of life's vital energies.

Even today, it can be said that the many diseases are really crises of purification, which means toxic elimination. Symptoms are the natural acts of defence of a body under attack. Was Hippocrates right when he said that all diseases are but one? Many MDs are returning to this old concept, believing that most forms of disease may have one root cause, although they manifest themselves by many different symptoms according to the place where they appear. The so-called diseases are really only groups of symptoms.

The endeavours of this new generation of doctors will therefore be to restore health through the cleansing, strengthening and renewing influences of Nature. By removing the cause of sickness, the effect will disappear. Poisons or toxins in the blood are really the waste products of metabolism and cause the body to initiate a healing crisis, or forced elimination.

This is what happens when you have a cold. Your body has accumulated poisons beyond its ability to expel. The immune system then engages in a violent reaction to get rid of the morbid material. Germs will disappear when the need for them disappears. The future doctor will assist the body in its vital effort to dispel obstructions and keep clear the channels of circulation.

The Bible tells us the life is in the blood: not in the heart, brain or nervous system. That is why destructive emotions also strike at the very life principle, creating disturbance in the blood. If it were possible for us to keep our blood in perfect purity, disease should be almost impossible.

The blood is the life of the body. Our mental and physical health and well-being are a reflection of our blood condition, for better or worse.

Tomorrow's doctor is likely to tell us that our healing power is resident deep-down in our own body, and that it is natural to be healthy. He will endeavour to awaken that power through the gentle influences of sunlight, air, water, fasting (which is physiological rest), natural foods, manipulation and positive living.

This art is part of a new lifestyle which encourages self-awareness and self-understanding. A physician says: 'Holistic medicine addresses itself to the quality of a person's life by bringing values, goals and aspirations into a harmony in his life.' It gives consideration to his social and physical environment. This is just the scientist's admission of the part played by the metaphysical – the employment of spiritual resources in the healing process.

All remedies can do is to provide a favourable environment in which the healing power can operate. Chronic disease may start years before symptoms call attention to it. Most likely, it will be the result of inadequate nutrition and poor elimination.

Your new doctor will be a bio-ecologist who will want to:

- Detoxify;
- Adjust deficiencies or excesses in the diet.
- Discover whether the trouble is due to allergy.
- Revitalize the body's defence system.
- Carry out such treatments as may be necessary.
- Sustain body and soul.

He or she will lead his patients to the highest possible level of personal health on each plane of being. Max Gerson was such a practitioner. He proved these points when he cured Dr Albert Schweitzer's wife of a systemic erythematosus (a disease that damages connective tissue) – in the usual way incurable. Mrs Schweitzer attained freedom from the disease as she responded to a balanced diet that provided certain mineral elements that she was lacking.

Many of these points can be followed by the interested layman in his daily routine.

Acupuncture

'You get to the stage when you can't take any more . . . and that was where I stood . . . now, thanks to acupuncture I feel better than I have for years.'

Reading this letter from a grateful patient to an acupuncturist, you may think sticking needles in your feet is an odd way to go about treating migraine. But there are those who say it is painless and works.

Its skills are taught in many medical schools and have become an essential part of orthodox health care systems.

A Northampton doctor's introduction to the art was a patient with a sore throat. In this case he happened to use acupuncture in the hand. Later on that day the sore throat had gone. After that, he read all he could find on the subject and now believes it offers an effective treatment for complaints such as migraine.

A well-known author had a history of multiple injuries during the Burma Campaign in the Second World War, which left him with persistent pain. He tried everything: surgical operation, steel corset, and a barrel of pills. Nothing would dispel it until a doctor stuck two little gold needles into his thigh.

British doctors visiting Shanghai witnessed an operation for the removal of a tumour in the neck of a railway porter and gasped in astonishment as to how it was done. The patient was fully conscious throughout ninety minutes exacting surgery.

A practitioner of this Chinese art, who is also a homoeopath, was appointed to the Queen, who thus confirmed her belief in such forms of treatment.

A doctor who took the official course at the Academy of Traditional Chinese Medicine writes: 'I often practise acupuncture on my patients when I think I can obtain a quick and satisfactory result.'

This therapy, which the Chinese claim has been in use for at least 5,000 years, throws up such impressive results on pains almost anywhere in the body. For facial nerve paralysis, it is found to be singularly successful. But the longer you talk to one of its practitioners, the more heady becomes its achievements including asthma, high blood pressure, painful menstruation and morning sickness. Some say there are few things to equal it for the severe pain after shingles, though it may have to be repeated.

The yin-yang theory that all things have two opposite but complementary parts is applied to medicine. The acupuncturist first diagnoses the case by finding out the yin-yang imbalance and with the use of needles piercing relevant acupuncture points, corrects the internal disease. To arrive at a correct diagnosis the Chinese place importance on an examination of the tongue, pulse and auscultation – listening to the sounds of the body, as with a stethoscope.

Perhaps its most exciting possibilities in the West lie in the field of pain relief in surgery. In China, acupuncture is now used in about 10% of surgical procedures – major as well as minor operations, as with the railway porter. One might be tempted to ask if a Westerner is as stoical about pain as his oriental opposite. It would take an awful lot of endurance in a major operation.

While, on the one hand, Chinese farmers say it boosts fertility on the farm (needles restoring the fertility cycle), its medical practitioners insist it is almost specific in relieving immediately the chronic backache of unknown origin that has defied efforts of scientific medicine for decades.

One thing seems clear: acupuncture has the ability to relax muscle spasms immediately, the cause of pain in rheumatism and arthritis. One practitioner records that he is successful in about 50% of those who try it.

Even the Chinese themselves confess they do not know how it works. They agree it is not dependent on physical factors. They think it has to do with the emotional state of the patient and how he or she can be 'conditioned'. But this can scarcely be acceptable when we consider its use as an anaesthetic in hysterectomy and brain surgery. All this is difficult to relate to orthodox medicine.

Walter H. Thompson, British acupuncturist, writes: 'Gypsies always claimed that the fitting of earrings improved the eyesight. This is interesting that the point of the lobe of the ear pierced for earrings is recognized as an acupuncture point for the eyes. It seems that although the needling and treatment of the ears has been carried out through the ages, the relatively recent discovery by the Chinese of new ear-points and their value as "anaesthesia" points may lead us to a new dimension in surgery and acupuncture.'[21]

Acupressure
There is a kind of half-sister therapy known as acupressure. This is acupuncture without a needle. Instead of needles, finger tip pressures are exerted on acupuncture points. You may have a headache and suffer pain in the neck. When a specific spot of the neck is pressed vigorously with the finger, pain is temporarily relieved.

Every doctor knows of the network of nerves present under the skin. These convey impulses from organs in the body. If an organ is weak or in poor condition, nerve-endings retail that information to the skin. In theory, to press the identical spot causes pain in the distant organ to disappear.

In acupuncture, the organ part is relieved by puncturing the nervous system at a sensitive point on the skin related to the organ. In acupressure it is a matter of pressure alone, and this may sometimes be of a temporary character.

Could rheumatism be a disease which commences in the nervous system? Practitioners believe it might be so. They still create ripples in the medical profession. Why should a needle stuck in the foot relieve the excruciating pain of shingles in the face? This is a question which may one day be answered. But in the meantime, it is a source of fresh hope to those who may have given up.

Chiropractic

Adjustments of the human body by use of the human hand are an ancient form of natural treatment. Since the dawn of history it has been known that spinal and bony distortions can be responsible for pain and disability.

Records show that a form of chiropractic existed in China as early as 2700 BC. The Greeks, also, had a knowledge of the art. It is now known that what they were doing was to relieve pressure on nerves. Spinal segments were 'adjusted' to their normal alignment by a number of methods, one being for a young son to 'walk up and down' father's spine in his bare feet after a laborious day in the fields.

But it wasn't until 1895, the year Roentgen discovered his famous X-rays, that it was founded on a scientific basis. An American doctor called Dr Daniel Palmer worked on magnetic healing until requested to treat a case of total deafness. He happened to notice that one of the vertebral bones on the back of the patient was slightly off centre.

With his hands he was able to restore the bone to its proper alignment. Both patient and practitioner were amazed at the instantaneous return of the man's hearing. Other similar successes followed. Encouraged by results, Palmer dedicated his life to finding the anatomical basis of such cures. From his experiences he evolved a therapy he called 'chiropractic', founding its first college in Iowa, USA.

Palmer had stumbled on the elemental truth that perfect body function depends upon nerve messages in the form of electrical impulses reaching the brain without hindrance from congestion or displaced vertebrae, etc. In simple terms, he explained that chiropractic opens up and repairs channels of communication in the body which have been cut off.

Like the osteopaths, chiropractors claim that when manually corrected, subluxations (minor displacements of the spine) cause related symptoms to disappear – even when such symptoms may appear far from the original lesion.

What are the differences between osteopathy and chiropractic? There may be similarities, but the chiropractors mostly confine their efforts to specific spinal vertebrae by means of a direct 'thrust' made by the hands in a given direction. They will give you an adjustment using a high-velocity, low-amplitude thrust, which is applied directly to a particular point of the body.

Although chiropractors now give detailed treatment to the whole of the bones and spine, there are still many of the old school who single out the cervical region (part of the neck supporting the head) as the most important area.

The major difference is the belief by the osteopaths that their treatment evokes a response from the blood circulation, while that of the chiropractor triggers off a response from the nervous system. Differences between the two manipulative techniques become less apparent with the passage of years.

Chiropractors insist on X-ray examinations for a large number of their patients. This, they believe, obviates any subsequent charges which might be made for negligence or wrong diagnosis which could easily happen as, for instance, giving manipulation to cases of bone infection or tumour.

What conditions can be relieved by chiropractic? It is sought mainly for lower back pain, hip and knee problems, pains in the shoulders, arms and neck, slipped discs, sciatica, and back troubles in general. Like other therapies, it is powerless where there's advanced tissue degeneration.

Colour healing or chromotherapy

Roland Hunt made the extraordinary suggestion that 'the seven major centres in the body each have their own particular rate of vibration. They absorb from the food we eat, the thoughts we think, the emotions we harbour, certain qualities or vibrations whose rate of frequency is identical respectively with each of the seven colours of the spectrum.'[22]

Some therapists believe colour is intimately related to the mind. Just as the constituents of the body are protein, water and mineral, so the nutrients of the mind are colours. By increasing our awareness of colour we are better able to neutralize the deadening effects of our grey, mechanized civilization. There is much to be said for decorating our rooms with a colour, or colours, compatible with our temperament.

As with music, there are times when we prefer calm and quiet colours, and others when we need up-and-doing stimulants. It is not difficult to understand how colour can be related to emotional problems. But physical ones? This is not so easy to accept. However, when we learn of its use for certain bodily ills in the ancient civilizations of Greece and India, maybe we have a case for investigation.

I used to be puzzled by the use of precious stones for the purpose of healing. Surely this was too far-fetched? Now it occurs to me that maybe it is the colour vibrations of the gem that affect the body in some unknown way.

Colour concentration can do some extraordinary things. It has been proved that so long as the pineal gland is functional, blind and colour-blind people do, in fact, react to colour. Without colour, body metabolism slows down.

Theo Gimbel, British colour therapist and expert in the field, stated that colour promotes subtle chemical changes in the body cells. Scientists do not know what causes the nerve endings to release certain chemicals. Chemical imbalance is a known cause of physical discord resolved by exposure of parts of the body to specific colours. 'Disturbances are corrected in the vibrational rate.'[23] Apparently, movement of fine chemical traces can be accelerated or retarded by sound and colour. Sounds sung or words spoken have a strong impact on subtle chemical changes in the blood. Gimbel believes colour has an even deeper impact, being a higher vibration than sound.

Another explanation of its *modus operandi* comes from the esoteric practitioners who suggest that colour has an effect upon the 'etheric' body. They believe colour works on the 'etheric' which clairvoyants can see as an aura surrounding the body. If the body can attract the electromagnetic energies it needs by absorbing colour, how important it is for us to decorate our homes with compatible combinations, and to select our household draperies and even our clothing with care.

Theo Gimbel reminds us that the whole of life is made up of rhythmic vibrations emanating from an electromagnetic field and manifesting as radio waves, infra-red and ultraviolet rays which are found at both ends of the spectrum. He also reminds us that colour healing and meditation blend well. Whereas a therapist may work on your body with colour-lamps, there is something you can do for yourself. He claims that by 'visualizing' colours in the act of meditation, results are possible.

Red

Gimbel believes that red promotes the flow of adrenalin and disposes the blood to the surface of the body. It activates red blood cells and at the same time rouses the sympathetic nervous system. Overpowering reds are best avoided on carpets and furnishings unless you wish to raise your pulse rate. Colour may play tricks on the unwary: yellow fabric seen against a red wall gives the appearance of orange. Red clothing tends to keep you awake and enliven vitality. It is said to be helpful for anaemia. To live in a red room may cause anxiety and emotional restlessness. Colour therapists often associate this colour with blood.

Orange

Orange is an antidote for heaviness of spirit, evoking cheerfulness. It is said to speed up metabolism and influence the digestive system. Children seem at home in this colour, but it is best avoided by the highly sensitive, blue being more restful and of a lower wavelength. Orange is associated with the spleen. This colour might brighten gloomy corners or basement corridors but seldom bedrooms.

Yellow

Theo Gimbel advises against the use of yellow for mentally restless people – it has an unstabilizing effect. He recommends that white be worn by patients undergoing chromotherapy, another name for the art. White reflects the light. Coloured light is beamed onto the body, either by coloured glass filters or from a cinemoid 'gel' as used in stage lighting. The whole body is bathed in colour for a specified time. This therapy is for the relief of mental as well as physical conditions. Yellow is also equated to the lymphatic system.

When engaged on exacting work demanding prolonged use of the 'old grey matter', you may wish to put yellow to the test. Incidentally, it is best avoided in bedrooms and workplaces.

Green

Paracelsus, sixteenth-century alchemist, together with the ancients, equated green with the heart – for emotional stability. Modern esoteric literature associates it with the pituitary gland, which it stimulates. Also, through the glandular system it preserves physical and mental equilibrium.

Green is restful for the eyes, and disposes to inertia and inaction. A mental institution reported its residents were more at peace with themselves and with the world when surrounded by green lawns and green carpets.

Green is the superb sustaining colour of Nature. But rooms bearing dingy greens may take the zip out of a lively disposition. Some people may wonder why they are listless when, all the time, it may be due to the wrong colour of their environment. Changing to a different colour can change a mood.

Green may lift a dull headache and sometimes bring about a welcome release intensive conditions.

Blue

Blue is the colour believed to reflect higher consciousness. It encourages relaxation more than any other, and is used for its anti-stress and calming influences.

Other colours

Other colours used in this fascinating art are: turquoise, to assist the act of breathing; indigo, to free us from fears and inhibitions; violet, to create inner balance and feelings of reverence; and magenta, to give us a sense of dignity and composure.

How does colour affect our lives? Theo Gimbel looks upon it as a subtle restorative process, comparing it with homoeopathy which offers infinitesimal medicines as a means of restoring the body's chemical balance.

Fasting

If you go to a health farm, you are likely to start off with a short fast. Today, this is a much neglected therapy, but going back in history we see how the ancient Egyptians and the Greeks advised abstention from food for the ailing body. Had you observed how a sick animal such as your pet dog or cat promptly goes off his food, but will drink?

Records left by the schools of ancient philosophy and medicine all advise fasting for cleansing of body, mind and spirit. Elijah, Moses and Christ each fasted forty days as part of their preparatory role for exacting work to follow. The Sanskrit and Koran both emphasize its importance for the maintenance of health. Hippocrates said: 'The more you feed a sick body the worse you make it.' Or, as a modern writer puts it: 'Well timed abstinence kills the sickness in embryo and destroys the seeds of disease.'

Here is a wonderful opportunity for the house-cleaning of every internal organ. Its devotees say there is nothing like it for heightening the sense of well-being and sharpening the intelligence.

Fasting has nothing to do with starving, which is denial of food to the body with harmful effects. It means a positive, intelligent abstention from food for a certain purpose – to cure a disease or to cleanse a soul. If you have not tried it, you would be surprised at the extraordinary sense of release from mental and physical encumbrance.

An abundant literature testifies to cures of desperate diseases after two, three or more weeks. Well-conducted fasts can never do harm and among their reward could be more healthy active lives.

But your fast may be for a much shorter period. I used to fast every Friday, and felt like a million dollars on the Saturday. Others prefer a short cleansing fast of three days at intervals of one or two months. If you go to a natural health centre, you may fast from seven to ten days as supportive treatment for obesity, rheumatism and arthritis. Of course, you can go on for two or more months, as did the well-known naturopath, Bob Reddell, to achieve his remarkable cure for osteo-myelitis. Fasting, as part of natural treatment, so changed the whole chemistry of his blood that he became a new man in the place of a candidate for operation after operation. 'It saved my life,' said Bob, 'and after that I felt I had to open my own Health Home and devote the rest of my life to nature-cure.'

An American naturopath called Dr Volhard claimed that fasting is one of the most effective means of treating acute kidney troubles (glomerulo-nephritis). This has often been confirmed. After fasting, all the acute symptoms – high blood pressure and oedema (a collection of fluid in the tissues) rapidly subside.

Hospital controlled fasting is not always successful because of the tendency to prescribe glucose or other sugars to make-good supposed energy losses. This spoils the fast. Sugar-laden soft drinks and other sugary products are a common cause of allergies. The ideal is for no food or drink to be taken, nothing except water and unsweetened lemon juice.

What happens when we fast?

No matter how slim, we all have imperceptible stores of fat tucked away somewhere. Our bodies store glycogen for energy. This bio-sugar is stored in the liver and muscle cells and is released gradually to supply us with energy. When stocks of glycogen run low, the innate body intelligence pillages fat from the fat cells to convert it into energy. This is the way our fat reserves get used up. By running down our body's fat reserves it is almost impossible not to lose weight.

I speak from personal experience when I say that a fast gives your body a well-deserved rest from all the feeding pressures we exert upon it. Few of us have not, at one time or another, added to digestive tension and stress by eating the wrong foods, not to mention added colourings, flavourings and permitted additives.

How shall I fast?

People react differently to fasting. First of all, start with a small fast – maybe for twenty-four to forty-eight hours. Weeks or months later you may wish to extend the time. There should be no real need for you to give up your usual work or play – unless you are an exceptionally strenuous character.

Some people prefer to do it with others and go to a health farm, for instance. Besides having the support of a group, you are likely to meet so many interesting people.

If you have been advised to live on air for two or more weeks for the treatment of some chronic disease, there is always somebody on the same routine to pass the encouraging remark. You will not feel hungry or need any pep-talks when you see with your own eyes the high level vitality and clear-complexions of your new friends leaving for home.

It is not always convenient to forego food at home; the family and other distractions may weaken your will. If you can afford to stay at a health farm offering a well-organized regime, you may live to look back on it as one of the soundest investments you ever made.

Don't be surprised if, for the first few days, your tongue furs-up in a disgusting manner. Your new friends will not mind in the slightest – their breath is likely to be as offensive as yours! Those who know the ropes may tell you that the well diluted natural lemon drinks tend to dissipate this.

They are not far wrong. It all depends upon how much rubbish is being burnt out of your system. Remember, the worse the tongue, the greater the good.

Some may have a transient stage of weakness, but this is not always so. I, myself, have held down a busy practice while fasting for fourteen days at a time. It is perfectly true to record that at the end of it I was just as energetic as when I started.

On a fast you may have a little palpitation due to increased action of the heart. Sometimes there is a slight rise in temperature, which may darken the colour of the urine.

There are many ways of breaking a fast but I would recommend a day on unsweetened fruit juices until the evening, then enjoy three or four ounces of yoghurt, laced with a little wheat germ and honey. Do not pitch into a heavy meal or hanker after getting back to your usual diet too soon.

Follow with 'transition' meals made up of salads, fruits and fruit juices, yoghurt and cottage cheese, for three days. Bring back your alimentary system slowly.

Fasting and meditation is a well-proven combination if you have time for them in this jet age! They will not only increase your body's resilience but strengthen your faith.

In all my sixty years' experience in natural methods of healing I have seen many miracles through fasting. If there is ever a 'cure all', fasting comes near to it.

Home care

All sorts of exciting things are going on around us. Are more people being born with special gifts? Do some people come into the world with some developed special sense? Maybe they do. But healing may be close at hand in a simpler way.

Your home is full of healing. We all remember how mother would dispel sundry aches and pains by the simple act of laying-on her hands. There are some people who can induce restful relaxation, even sleep, by holding your head in their hands. We have known perfectly ordinary people unaware of some hidden gift.

It is possible you have an ability to smooth away pain. Not all possess some heaven-born charisma to take the pain out of a joint. You never know until you try. All you need is a caring attitude and a pair of loving hands.

A young wife expressed surprise when it was suggested she placed one hand on the forehead and the other on the nape of the neck of her six-year-old daughter for an exhausting headache. She has never forgotten the day when, after ten minutes of simple home-care, that terrible pain disappeared.

It has always been known that healing energies can be transmitted from one person to another, as in the classic experiment carried out by Dr Dolores Krieger of New York University.[24] Patients were divided into two groups, one of which was given the routine treatment. In addition, the second group was given a 'laying-on of hands' by nurses. The results of this 'personal therapy' were impressive. All those who received vital energies from the nurses recorded marked increases in haemoglobin, which carries oxygen to the cells in the bloodstream.

Dr Krieger declares that every person, who so wills, has this ability to transmit healing energies to another person by palm-therapy – the laying-on of hands gently over the affected area, and by concentrating their thoughts on making that person well.

Homoeopathy

Homoeopathy was discovered by Dr Samuel Hahnemann (1755–1843), born in Meissen, Germany. Disappointed with the results of conventional drugs and concerned about side-effects and dependency, he gave up his practice and turned to research.

Adolf Lippe, celebrated homoeopath of the eighteenth century, describes Hahnemann as sitting at Leipzig, with his midnight lamp before him, translating Cullen's *Materia Medica*, which was the standard work.

He came to quinine (cinchona bark) but had little faith in Cullen's account. Determined to find out for himself, he prepared and drank an alcoholic tincture of the drug. To Lippe's surprise, the toxic dose he gave himself in health, manifested in his body with symptoms which showed a close similarity to those of fever and ague, cured by him by the same drug.

In a flash Hahnemann realized that a drug will cure an ailment similar to its power to create illness. From that day, he treated a disease with a medicine capable of producing a like condition. He discovered a law, *similia similibus curentur* (like cures like), which he set down in detail in his major work, *Organon of a Rational System of Medicine*, first published in Leipzig in 1810, now regarded as the homeopath's bible.

Two hundred years before this, Paracelsus, a Swiss physician who revolutionized the theoretic basis of medicine, suggested that diseases be classified by the remedy which cured them – the human remedy and natural remedy to correspond.

Today's practitioners believe that the selected remedy has the effect of alerting or 'touching-off' the body's defence system. In the face of this, the immunization theory might fit – a little bit of what's bad for you being good for you.

Medicines used in this science are derived from plants, minerals, metals – and sometimes animals. They have been 'potentiated', meaning the active ingredients have been diluted many times – sometimes over a hundred times – each dilution being well-shaken (succussed) before proceeding to the next. Today, this may be done by machines. Little wonder patients emphasized the safety of the system where over-dosing is impossible. The more these remedies are diluted, the more they increase in strength.

It is necessary for the qualified practitioner to have some knowledge of toxicology of therapeutic substances used in pharmacy. In spite of it being one of the most difficult skills to acquire, younger members of the medical profession continue to come forward in large numbers to undergo additional training in their search for a form of effective treatment without drugs.

Both doctors and laymen attend courses to acquire competency in treating patients or the family with harmless pilules, tablets or tinctures. Books and pocket prescribers abound for the amateur and, because homoeopathic remedies are not subject to prescribing controls, some proficiency is possible. In Britain, treatment is available on the National Health Service.

The mode of administration is particularly convenient for infants and children. For instance, German chamomile (*chamomilla*) is known as the children's remedy – a dose being taken for sleeping and teething troubles.

In Britain, the Royal London Homoeopathic Hospital and many competent laymen kept the science alive during the many years it has been consigned to the 'wilderness' by the orthodox profession. They were assisted in their efforts by members of the Royal Family, commencing with Princess Mary of Teck (later Queen Mary) who opened the above hospital in 1893. Sportsman Prince Charles uses arnica ointment for bruises and stiffness sustained during strenuous physical exercise.

Is there a place for homoeopathy in modern medicine? Those who have received successful treatment are sure there is. You may ask why it is not in wider use. The answer is simple. Homoeopathy cannot be proved by scientific analysis. It is one of those areas lying beyond technical medicine. The medical establishment finds this hard to swallow, while people like Yehudi Menuhin insisted it is a clean, harmless medicine which should be judged by its results.

It is unfortunate that a patient's word or testimonial is not admissible as data in support of efficacy of treatment, but referred to by the term 'anecdotal evidence'.

In most European towns can be found a homoeopathic dispensary from which remedies are available. There are special lightweight packs for teams of explorers and mountaineers, taking up little room and of easy administration.

It has been shown that animals as well as humans can benefit: potentized arsenic comes to the aid of horses, *nux vomica* for dogs, *psorinum* for cats, etc.

Hydrotherapy – the water secret

It is to Hippocrates that we owe the discovery of the healing power of water. But it was Father Sebastian Kneipp, a Bavarian priest, who resuscitated this vital art when he started his clinic in Wörishofen, which attracted attention from all over Europe.

Today, few physicians treat their patients with cold water packs. Herbert Mayo, one-time senior surgeon at the Middlesex Hospital in London, claimed to have been saved from being a complete cripple by his friend, Sir Charles Scudamore, who prescribed the application of rainwater cold packs. Like Hippocrates and Kneipp before him, Sir Charles advised cold packs from fresh sun-soaked rainwater for rheumatism, arthritis, and various aches and pains.

Philosophers of the ancient world placed their faith in Nature. Modern science believes man can improve on her. Though it must have existed, we read little in the history books of terrifying epidemic disease in Rome. During the peak of that virile empire they practised the healing methods of the Greeks. So healthy was Rome, writes Pliny, that with her massive aqueducts of sunlit water, the city was many years without a physician.

One great secret of successful healing with water is its combination with sunlight. Today our supplies reach us from the depths of the earth, not irradiated by the sun – giver of life. It has been claimed that new bone cells can be formed when sunlight reaches the marrow with the aid of cold water packs.

The hydrotherapists remind us that cold packs immediately cool. They have the effect of drawing away blood from the seat of inflammation. But, they do more. They open pores, dissipate heat and cause the body to sweat out impurities.

This therapy is used to stimulate the circulation and nervous system in those robust enough to secure a reaction. The health-inducing properties of common *aqua pura* can be felt in many ways, including outdoor bathing, swimming, hot or cold footbaths, etc.

One favourite of therapists is a foot bath, where you place your feet in cold water up to your ankles. Then there's a limb bath where arms and legs are rubbed vigorously with cold water cupped in the hands. A hip bath is an old routine for shrinking piles, tightening up loose bowels and regulating excessive menstrual bleeding.

A sitz bath is a hip bath built in such a way that the person can sit in it, but with his legs outside. Modern practice at the health farms is to prepare two baths, one with cold and the other with hot water. On the floor in front of the cold bath is a small footbath filled with hot water. On the floor in front of the hot bath is a footbath of cold water. When you take the cold bath, your feet will be in hot water, and when taking the hot bath your feet will be in cold water. The idea is for each bath to be taken alternately (three minutes in the hot and one in the cold), finishing up with the cold.

Such a bath is used for varicose veins, piles and pelvic troubles.

One simple use of water is as a cold compress for bruises, sprains and contusions. For some serious conditions in the sick room, a cold trunk pack may be ordered for reducing inflammation and quietening of a restless patient.

This pack may sometimes reverse a disease process in a surprising way by reducing fever, removing obstruction and raising vital energies. A cold trunk pack is made by wrapping a wet sheet round the body, followed by a large towel, the final covering being a blanket. A length of waterproof sheeting protects the bedclothes.

According to Dr E. E. Osgood, senior consulting physician, cold bathing and massage can increase your white cell count up to 25,000 (normal 7,400) because of contraction of the spleen, which is the reservoir of those little white commandos which are our first line of defence against infection.

The powers of water have, of recent years, enjoyed a renaissance in the spas of Europe. Governments, including Russia, invest huge sums on spa therapy. All natural thermal springs are developed to their maximum potential, proving how much confidence they have in this ancient treatment.

European rheumatologists (with the exception of Britain) have discovered the positive effects of balneology (water therapy) on the progress of rheumatism and arthritis. They are finding it can bring about a reduction in the red cell sedimentation rate, which relies on absorption of certain minerals through the skin.

In his book *Spas that Heal*,[25] Dr William A. R. Thomson quotes a report recording changes in the endocrine system by immersion in the sulphate hot springs at Sukawa Spa in Japan. It was concluded the whole range of body hormonic activity was stimulated.

Attention was also drawn to reports that in Japan 'high temperature' hot springs accelerate gastric activity. They claim bathing in such water is good for digestion, promoting secretion of the gastric juices. This is of special interest because some European spas have, in the past, gained reputations for the successful treatment of these complaints.

Does the water of spas differ greatly from tap water? Evidence shows that it does. Almost each single spa can show a different analysis of its mineral contents. Some waters contain lithium (for depression). Others, such as the Roman baths at Droitwich, good for rheumatism, contain ten times more salt than sea water. Because of the greatly increased buoyancy, underwater manipulation can achieve a wider range of assisted pain-free movement in a joint or spine.

Treatment at a spa or health farm where water treatments are given usually has the advantage of an environment away from domestic and social stresses. The atmosphere is relaxing, where a person can unwind and enjoy congenial company in restful surroundings. All these assist recovery.

Today, health farms have largely taken over the function of the old hydros and provide more comprehensive healing regimes including massage, manipulation, herbal aids, etc.

Turkish baths have all but disappeared before the growing popularity of sauna. When a profuse sweat is induced, the person will take a shower, plunge into water or roll in the snow. Saunas originated in Finland where analgesic properties for assuaging painful and aching limbs are attributed to them.

We should not overlook the benefits of bathing in seawater. This is loaded with minerals – the perfect salt water treatment. Perhaps the most exciting example of hydrotherapy in the world is the Dead Sea which, besides being a major tourist attraction, offers an eagerly sought health service. Israel has always been conscious of the water's unique healing properties. It stimulates positive electro-magnetic energies and is wonderfully toning to the body.

Wherever you live, cold, early-morning sponge-downs can be a rousing day-starter, and a splendid anti-tension device. An occasional hot bath at night might be a perfect relaxant before going to bed.

Osteopathy

In every generation there have been doctors like Sir Herbert Barker – the great surgeon who never used a knife. Before there were professional osteopaths there were bonesetters – men with a gift for manipulation but usually without medical training.

They were men who realized the limitations of the medical establishment. This was brought home forcibly to Dr A.T. Still (1828–1912) who experienced much pain and suffering on the death of his three children from meningitis. All his professional skill failed to save them. The event left a scar slow to heal.

Still was a religious man with the comfort of the Scriptures to support him in his grief. The experience steeled his resolve to find the answer to this and other medical problems of his day. He might not have found the effective treatment for meningitis, but his efforts were rewarded in another direction.

His single-minded approach led him to discover how a number of complaints were related to faulty bone structure. He found how a 'bone out of place' could be responsible for remote pains elsewhere in the body, such as a headache or abdominal discomfort.

Dr Still observed that a healthy spine has a correct alignment in which each vertebra fits accurately into its neighbour. Successful spinal manipulation in some cases of asthma also convinced him that visible illness is not always an isolated happening confined to a single organ.

'Remove the cause,' said Still, 'and the sickness will disappear – sometimes dramatically.' He developed a system of diagnosis by touch (palpation) by which areas of surface body heat (indicating local inflammation) could be traced to misplaced or diseased vertebrae causing the trouble.

Osteopathy means treatment of bones, muscles and joints which may indirectly affect the health of organs. There are some cases where manipulation may be the only way to dispel pain and inflammation. In so many cases, spinal problems have unpleasant consequences elsewhere, and vice versa.

Abnormalities in the spine influence muscles, blood vessels and related organs. It was Still's theory that wherever blood is circulating normally disease cannot take hold. This, he believed, was because our blood is capable of manufacturing all the necessary substances for natural immunity against disease. Where blood flow is arrested by congestion, body discomfort and even disease may follow.

What we believe to be disorders of the skin, stomach and so on, may in reality be due to displaced spinal vertebrae which, when corrected, cause such symptoms to disappear. It was his belief that where spinal misplacements were corrected by manipulation, the blood circulation responded and was able to re-activate afflicted tissues. In this way static blood and other congested fluids (such as lymph) would again enjoy unimpeded circulation.

Osteopaths and chiropractors stretch muscles, ligaments and connective tissue and frequently employ the 'high velocity, low amplitude' thrust to release a joint. Although the patient may hear an audible 'snap' or 'crack' it is usually painless and the spinal tension resolved.

If you cannot afford to be off work from back-pain or sports injuries, a manipulator may be the man or woman you need. National medical associations hold courses designed for doctors. The family doctor gets an enormous number of people in his surgery complaining of back pain. He doesn't always have the time to go through everything in the book, followed by intricate tests; a simple back manipulation may supply the answer to many problems, or a referral to another specialist.

Among the special tests used by manipulators is one where they compare the length of your legs. One shorter than the other would draw his attention to trouble in the pelvis. They may test your reflexes with a patella hammer. Before manipulation, 'soft-tissue' work and massage are used to relax contracted muscles and improve blood supply to affected parts.

People go to the practitioner for back troubles. They may have no deep seated trouble but have just 'ricked' their back through lifting heavy objects, stooping, or been violently thrown off balance. Some people go as they want to avoid drugs.

Cranial osteopathy is a new technique for diagnosis and treatment, in which practitioners endeavour to assess body health by feeling a rhythmical expansion and contraction which they relate to the 'pulse of the cerebrospinal fluid'. With patients lying on their back, practitioners palpate the skull and pelvis and claim to sense the movement of the CS fluid in much the same way as a doctor feels the pulse to find out the condition of the circulatory system.

Some people need only one session and go away relieved. But manipulation does not work miracles all the time. Many cases beyond repair – old broken-down constitutions and chronic cases may fail to respond. Of those cases which have met with success, few are more exciting than one of Dr Still's first attempts, as recorded in his autobiography.

'One of the many interesting cases of my early experience was that of a little boy who had no use in his legs and hips. He was about four years old. His mother, Mrs Truit, brought him to me for six months, in her arms, to be treated for his helpless limbs.

'On examination I found a spine imperfect in form, as I thought from my knowledge of the spine at that time. I proceeded to articulate every vertebrae as best I could, during each two weeks for six months. The mother showed that grit which no one but a mother can show.

All summer she brought him to me, walking a distance of four miles through the hot timber. His father was sceptical about the way of treating, and never helped his wife try to restore the boy, because some old narrow-minded person had told him that Still was crazy and could do the boy no good.

'At the end of six months the family moved West. I heard no more of the boy for ten years. Then came the news of the father's death, also that the poor little fellow had grown to a man weighing 73kg (11 stone). He was running a farm, and supporting his angel-hearted mother as a reward for her life-and-death struggle through heat and cold to save him from remaining a hopeless cripple.

'The story is so marvellous that I could hardly have believed it had I not seen marked signs of improvement in his spine before he left.'

Another dimension

Natural healing may occur in a dimension beyond even the alternative therapies which I have briefly outlined. The complete healing art may need the best of traditional doctors, the best of the newer healing arts, and yet another dimension. This has been well highlighted by Prince Charles, who as President-Elect of the British Medical Association, sent the following message for the Association's 150th anniversary:'I think the members of the medical profession should be reminded occasionally that the words "healing" and "holy" come from the same original idea of "making whole". . .There is a sense, I think, in which medicine today tends to be more and more chemistry and less and less healing in the classical sense. I do not for one moment wish to decry the chemistry because we owe it too much, but I do not want to do it the disservice of pretending that it is the whole answer to the voice of the physician's calling. It can never deal with the sickness of the spirit proliferating with horrific swiftness all around us.'

What is the modern physician's response to the stricken spirit who comes to him with his sick soul disguised as an ailment of the body? Does he allow the faith in him to reawaken the faith in the patient; to join his chemistry for the total recovery of body and spirit?

Paracelsus wrote, "The whole world is an apothecary's shop and God the apothecary in chief." It seems to me that the lack of psychological insight – into the unconscious being of man – is possibly one of the saddest neglects of modern medicine. Has it perhaps been forgotten, too, that the oath which binds a physician pledges him both scientifically and religiously?'

The amazing case of Dorothy Kerin

I shall always remember Dorothy Kerin sitting in our lounge with the sun streaming on her. She had come to Bournemouth to conduct one of her healing sessions in the town. The hall was packed. A surprising number were healed or improved.

Dorothy was full of the happiest laughter. She was endowed with exuberant vitality. I wonder if you have heard the story of Dorothy?[26]

The doctor said she could not live until morning. After five years of hopeless invalidism, she lay dying of tuberculosis. Recovery was seemingly impossible – the end had come at last. For the last fortnight of her illness she had been unconscious and blind. For eight minutes her lungs ceased to breathe, her heart to beat. Many people were praying for her; sixteen of them were assembled at her bedside to await the end.

Just as she was slipping out of this world an incredible thing happened. She had received the last sacrament when suddenly she saw a golden light radiating from the chalice. Becoming no longer conscious of her body, her soul overflowed with a transcendental feeling of supreme happiness.

Her soul passed on and on in space, getting brighter and brighter as she travelled. Then, she saw in front of her a startling formation of angelic beings. Words could not express the ineffable beauty of the scene. Someone called her by name, three times distinctly. She replied, 'Yes, I am listening, who is it?'

The voice said, 'Listen. No, Dorothy, you are not coming yet. But your sufferings are over. Get up and walk.'

Hands were passed over her eyes, ears were touched and she found herself sitting up in bed. Mother and friends were all there looking very frightened, some clutching each other. She said to them: 'I am well now! I want my dressing gown, I want to walk.'

Her mother cried: 'No, Dorothy, you will fall, you must not get up!' While held thus, the angel said a second time, 'Get up and walk.' Just then, a part of the beautiful light, seen only by Dorothy, came and stood at the right side of her bed. With eyes and ears opened, strength returned to her limbs. She threw off the bedclothes and stepped onto the floor.

The light moved forward. She followed, saying to her friends, 'I am following the light.' It led her out of the room and into the presence of her stepfather; she threw her arms around his neck and kissed him. Then it led her back to her room where the whole company were shaking with fear.

In the midst of all this, Dorothy sat down, saying: 'I can't understand why you are all so frightened! I am quite well. Indeed, I feel I would like some supper.' They brought her invalid's food but she refused. 'I've had enough of that. I am well now, and will eat well people's food.'

Food was brought and she sat down to a meal of cold beef and pickled walnuts – after not having tasted solid food for over six months, having been kept alive on injections of opium and starch. That night she slept like a child.

The next day, on hearing the news, Dr Norman, her doctor, hastened to the house where he found Dorothy better and up. 'Can it be possible this is the girl I left dying?' he cried, his hands lifted in astonishment. On recovering from the shock he examined her and found her to be restored to perfect health.

Just to test her muscles, he asked her to walk up a steep stairway. When he saw her run up the stairs, he was astonished and gasped, 'What does all this mean?'

Three days after the healing she had another visitation in the form of a circle of light at the foot of her bed and a voice saying: 'Dorothy, you are quite well now. God has brought you back to use you for a great work – to heal the sick and comfort the sorrowing. My Grace is sufficient.'

From that time Dorothy had a marvellous healing touch which relieved the ills of thousands. Many were present to swear to the truth of this extraordinary phenomenon, confirming the belief of the then Bishop of Coventry that the Creator does intervene in the affairs of those who believe in His ability to heal certain diseases where other means fail. He said: 'Dorothy Kerin was used to heal diseases apparently unresponsive to any other treatments. This is undoubtedly and amply proven.'

After her experience, Dorothy Kerin always had about her a shining, radiant calm, and a strange healing poise. She always insisted that the source of her healing was the Lord Jesus Christ, and always took care never to omit this name in all her healing work.

Today, the Christian hospital Burrswood in Groombridge, located near Tunbridge Wells in Kent, combines the skills of medical science with spiritual ministry. Under the supervision of a physician in charge, a dedicated staff of nurses carry on the work of Dorothy Kerin. Services of healing by the laying on of hands are held by a resident minister and accommodation is available for those seeking temporary rest and retreat.

While many treasure the memory of one whose 'healing touch' assuaged their pain, for me the visit to our home on that bright June day of this truly gentle soul will always be a blessed memory.

Air travel

Do you spend time abroad for your work or holidays? More than twenty million people have problems with airplane travel, ranging from sickness to palm-sweating anxiety.

Here are a few points well-worth bearing in mind.

(1) During the week before your flight, eat a little more oily fish than usual, or take omega-3 fish oil supplements. Take vitamin C in freshly-pressed orange juice, vitamin E (400 iu), and two dolomite tablets together with a good vitamin B complex.

(2) Seize the opportunity to catch-up on your sleep – as much as possible. If sleep is not easy, don't read. Instead, listen to a CD of your favourite music.

(3) Avoid alcohol yet take plenty of fluids. Eat light meals and only during the daytime.

continued

(4) For nausea or sickness chew a piece of crystallized ginger, a ginger biscuit or glass of ginger beer half an hour before the flight and sips at half-hour intervals thereafter. Herb teas are sometimes available: chamomile or lemon balm. Avoid oranges. Some travellers find a teaspoon of honey sufficient. If you really must stay awake, inhale the essential oil of rosemary.

Traveller's tummy

When abroad do not overlook the possibility of travel sickness. How can it be avoided?

The condition may develop suddenly, sometimes violently, causing alarm. Drink only bottled water or beverages that have been boiled. It is good to fast as long as the diarrhoea persists, but if you feel you must eat, avoid shellfish, and raw foods only partially cooked, especially meat, fish, raw salads and vegetables. Only eat fruit that you have peeled yourself.

During an attack, ginger or peppermint tea should prove helpful. To build up resistance after an attack, garlic and zinc may be taken with profit.

If your bowels fail to perform, a tablespoon of linseeds (flaxseeds) usually works the oracle. You may also think of eating an extra two or three prunes at breakfast.

Present-day air travel carries the risk of DVT (deep vein thrombosis) by sitting in a cramped position for long periods. Occasionally, leave your seat and saunter around the plane. Remember, ginkgo avoids blood clots, reducing stickiness of the platelets.

On arrival go to bed, to ensure that your biological time accords with your chronological time.

Do not overlook garlic for its anti-viral action. Echinacea and zinc lozenges during the flight are also of value.

7

Healing Common Conditions and Health Problems

I
t is beyond the scope of this book to provide a thorough survey of all the ailments that can follow in the wake of a faulty diet or unwise lifestyle. There are so many different conditions. However, I feel a word is in place on some of the main health problems that arise in the family.

Cold prevention must be our topline priority in winter and at all times. Vitamin C is one of Nature's guardians. It is on sale almost everywhere. In kitchen medicine it is present in parsley, pimentos, watercress, green peppers, orange juice, blackcurrant juice, tomatoes, Brussels sprouts, raw fruits and vegetables.

Vitamin D is another profitable item of diet for those subject to 'hard coughs'. Why? Because it cuts down infection. For those able to take cod liver oil, it is a splendid source of this sunshine vitamin. In summer-time we are less likely to suffer a deficiency if we spend a reasonable amount of time out of doors, in the sunshine. Vitamin D is synthesized when skin is exposed to the ultra-violet rays of the sun. Sunflower seeds, herrings and fish oils are other sources.

If treated intelligently colds and flu may provide a way of cleansing the body and leaving you much healthier. They may actually do you good! Try to regard them in the light of remarks by that great English physician, Dr Thomas Sydenham: 'An acute disease, in my opinion, however injurious it may be to the body, is no more than a vigorous effort of Nature to throw off toxic or decaying matter, and thus cause the patient to recover.'

Allergies

It can no longer be contradicted that many present-day diseases are caused by foods, especially those of the synthetic supermarket variety fortified with twenty-first century chemicals.

I am amazed at the number of allergies that clear up spontaneously when taking patients off pork, ham, bacon, chocolate, blue cheese, milk, cream, eggs and other 'nasties' to the allergic sufferer. Three-day fasts, elimination diets, and the gradual transition to a basic non-allergenic diet offer attractive rewards to those whose lives are bedevilled by the allergy phenomenon.

Dr Richard Mackarness, British psychiatrist and pioneer in the field of ecological-allergies suspects there are as many as one in three psychiatric patients with allergies that are really symptoms of emotional problems. Now we know that irrational behaviour and mental instability can follow in the path of unwholesome food. Maybe, it's not all in the mind, but in the food![27]

Unbeknown to themselves, patients can get 'hooked' on a chemical or additive in a particular food or aerosol. This might appear necessary to their sense of well-being. However, when they are not taken or used for a day or two, the subject may become conscious of a number of widely different withdrawal symptoms. These are 'masked' allergies.

In reality, almost any symptom may be found to be the result of an allergy. Some manifest as skin irritation, neuralgia of the chest, rheumatism in the joints, vague muscle pains, menstrual disorders, frigidity, hay fever and other conditions.

Two-year-old Paul loved his grandmother, but every time he gave her a cuddle he burst into tears and came out in blotches. For months doctors took tests but failed to come up with a satisfactory answer until it was found the boy was allergic to peanuts. Gran happened to work in a peanut factory; it was not until she had a bath and change of clothes that the blotches failed to appear and he was no longer tearful.

Enigmatical allergies arise from the strangest causes. A woman married to an amateur gardener with a passion for growing hybrid tea roses suffered from severe hay fever every summer, which she never had before. It disappeared when the roses were removed.

A woman sipped a glass of wine at a friend's and began gasping for breath. By insisting in tracking down the cause, she found the makers of the wine had added meta-bisulphate to stop oxidation. Thus, a new allergy was discovered.

Not so long ago it was discovered that house-dust could cause a great deal of nose-blowing and eye-streaming. Particles of this dust are made up of microscopic mites which, when not floating in the air, are found on curtains, clothes and even living in mattresses. Anti-dust measures are called for, such as exposing mattresses to the sun which drastically reduces the mite population.

Although an allergy is not an illness, it can be extremely exasperating. Families with a history of allergies would be advised not to have birds or furry pets in the house. Sufferers find a 'cure' for their allergies in a number of ways.

A nursing sister, working in a cottage hospital adored the countryside but suffered from acute hay fever every summer. Could it be due to the ragwort and grass pollens breathed in at that time? She was successful in landing a new job in a hospital in one of the big cities and was delighted to find her suffering over within days.

Cases abound of hay fever allergies disappearing in children after a switch from cow's to goat's milk. Garlic corms or capsules are not always well-received, but have a reputation for this troublesome condition. With its rich complex of vitamins and minerals, honeycomb is not without its support- . ers. Dan Gunder, journalist, uses castor oil to control his allergy. By putting a few drops in his drink on waking, his hay fever is not so irritating.

Castor oil drops for a stuffed nose and sniffles enable many to breathe easier in bed. Some calm an irritable stomach or bowel by cutting out the gluten foods and substituting rice or corn (maize).

Allergies produce all sorts of social embarrassments. Simple things like visiting friends are made difficult. Even after cutting out the refined sugars and monosodium glutamate there may still be cases that defy relief. It is strange how some food will make us ill, yet the body cries out for it.

There was once a time when an allergy was an itch, and all you had to do was to scratch it. But now we know we are what we eat, especially if it doesn't agree with us.

In his book *Not All in the Mind*, Dr Mackarness shows how it is possible for people to be allergic to ordinary foods like boiled eggs which they can eat every day without trouble. One patient reference illustrates this.

'Many years ago, before I cut eggs out of my diet, I had, like Dr Rinkel, a masked allergy to them. I used to eat them often and I noticed, when I was a student and doing my own cooking, that I could work particularly well after I had eaten an omelet.

'Next morning, after an evening at the textbooks, I would wake depressed, with a headache which lasted until I had eaten two boiled eggs for breakfast. Then I felt fine until the afternoon, when, unless I had eaten eggs for lunch, I would fall asleep during lectures.

'None of this meant anything significant to me while it was happening. Allergy to eggs was the last thing I suspected. I tried to prevent sleeping during lectures by drinking strong coffee after lunch, which I found only partially successful. I now find myself allergic to coffee, so I avoid it also.

'These are the effects of food allergy as it most commonly exists, and they are the reverse of the popular conception of allergic reactions.

'Instead of feeling bad at once, the patient feels better and naturally thinks the food agrees with him. Unpleasant symptoms connected with a masked allergy only appear later, if more of the food is not eaten, and the hang-over stage is entered.'

Alzheimer's disease

Alzheimer's disease is a progressive degenerative disease of the brain involving the destruction of cells. It is a common form of dementia where lesions appear as 'senile plaques', mostly in the nerve cells of the cerebral cortex, the brain's outer layer. The larger the number of plaques and tangles, the greater the disturbance.

Onset of the disease is usually very slow and gradual. Loss of memory and personality changes are common. Evidence is increasing that excessive use of aluminium can contribute to the disease. It has been known for years that patients have levels of aluminium in their brains higher than normal. Replacement of cooking vessels to stainless steel may be helpful.

Improvement of memory has followed the dose of 120mg Ginkgo biloba daily. Recent research confirms the use of Sage (*Salvia officinalis*) for a clear head in old age. Lemon Balm (*Melissa officinalis*) enjoys the same reputation. It would appear that the essential oil of *Melissa*, as used by aromatherapists might have a beneficial effect.

Rosemary is recommended as a powerful antioxidant to counter destruction by oxidants.

A double blind placebo-controlled trial investigating the effects of standardised Ginkgo extract in 309 patients with mild-to-severe dementia associated with Alzheimer's Disease, produced encouraging results.

Le Bars et al, 1997. *The Journal of the American Medical Association* 278: 1327–1332. *Greenfiles*: vol 12: 4, p. 21.

Ginkgo should not be combined with blood-thinning medicines, such as warfarin and aspirin.

In London, at the Maudsley Hospital, some improvement was achieved using large doses of B vitamins. Researchers point out that as we age, absorption of aluminium increases and that vitamin A, E and carotenoids are significantly reduced in Alzheimer's Disease patients.

Propolis, a sticky secretion used by bees to protect the hive from infection is also being investigated for alleviating the distressing symptoms of progressive dementia. The outlook is promising, giving hope to those with the disease and their families.

Backache

Funny how a violent sneeze may trigger a sleeping demon that's been quiescent for weeks. Hairdressers, dentists and all who work in the standing position are particularly at risk of back trouble.

What happens? Affected muscles go into spasm. This may have nothing to do with rheumatism. If movement in one direction is limited it is described as a 'lock'.

As soon as we are aware of unexpected stress – it's a signal for caution. When we become conscious of effort, common sense warns us to take care. Our spine is as strong as its weakest disc.

The man who takes a chance at lifting everything within reach – not knowing his own strength – is a prime target for backache.

The strain some women put on their spine may be just too much for it. Knowledge of how to lift a heavy weight can keep you in the clear. So before you take a deep breath and brace your muscles, place your feet as close to the object as possible. Bend your knees. Keep your shoulders back. Lift with your legs and not with your back.

Watch an experienced furniture-remover. See how he lifts with his legs and thighs. Bending over the load and trying to lift with the back may land you with many bone-wearying months before getting back to normal.

It is an amazing thing how so many people get through life with strictly limited spinal mobility. One person in ten gets by with a third of his possible range of movement. Brought to their notice, patients may tell you they have no ill-effects. This may be so. But they have no reserve for emergencies. Sooner or later, they may find themselves in a situation demanding swift evasive action to protect their body from danger. Then, backache can strike with devastating suddenness.

You may have a car with superb road manners, stylish good looks and impressively low running costs, but if there is insufficient room for your legs, your back may run you into a hefty personal repair bill. Do you have to strain forward?

Back and shoulder muscles will be subject to abnormal strain if your car seat is too far from the steering wheel. The practice of fitting a head-restraint to a car seat is proof against a perilous whiplash injury. Had you noticed how the use of a seatbelt can assist your posture?

Pay a visit to one of those Aladdin's caves, all crimson and chrome, where they sell accessory carparts. There you will find something to take the strain out of motoring. Webbed back rests are invaluable for preserving the natural curve of your spine. As an alternative, you may wish to place an inflatable cushion behind your lumbar region.

Before stepping on and off curbs be observant and carefully judge height.

A day in the office

A golden rule is never to sit in the same position for a long time. For work, always select a firm-backed straight chair. Don't be afraid to invest in a small footstool on which to rest your feet when your back is suspect. It is a good thing to sit with knees higher than hips.

When bending down to the bottom drawer of your filing cabinet, remember, never stoop – squat or kneel instead.

Point of balance

It pays to learn to walk with grace and poise. Incorrect posture is bound to lead to some kind of backache in later life. Good posture is one of the best forms of preventive medicine. Were you ever advised to keep your shoulders high and square? Try separating them as far as possible from the hips.

Do you walk with your head high? Imagine you've a flowerpot on your head. Pursue the idea in the privacy of your own home. Hold your chin up and back, and look straight ahead. By pulling your abdomen backwards and upward you'll flatten the hollow of your back.

Patricia Norris is an expert on posture. Listen to Katie Boyle's description of her.

'Patricia was telling me about her body aligning technique which improves posture . . . no laborious exercise programme. She came "swinging" down the drive to meet me. Yes, she moved beautifully, as though her body worked on well-oiled and perfectly balanced ball-bearing joints. Her shoulders sat back and down effortlessly, her back was straight, her hips and pelvis seemed to form a cradle for the lower tummy, and this, combined with lifting the rib cage, placed stomach and abdominal organs in their right places so there were no bulges where they shouldn't be. When you learn to walk tall, you really do feel the air is purer up there!'

What a perfect example of poise! You have within you the power to look your best, to improve your way of standing and walking. Let your body speak its own language. No need for pretension or artificiality. See in your mind's eye exactly the kind of deportment you wish to adopt. Think of it constantly. Some people are born with engaging presence and appearance. Others have to acquire it. Your whole bearing depends upon your spine.

Talking of pain. On occasion, we have all slept on a soft and yielding mattress. Unfortunately they have a trampoline effect against which long-suffering bones cry out for something hard. Though not necessary to lie flat on the back, you do need to be in the horizontal position. When your back is painful, you are likely to want to turn over more frequently in bed. Leave room to manoeuvre. First roll over. Wriggle to the outer edge. Then, bend your knees, keep your shoulders in line with your hips, and roll from side to side.

Pain may be relieved by lying on your side . . . Draw up one or both knees to shoulder height. A firm, hard bed, preferably with a board under the mattress, offers most relief from pain.

Talking of pain, avoid salty foods before bedtime. Salt stimulates the adrenals. Try chamomile tea with runny honey for a restful night. A slice of lemon adds that little extra flavour.

Of course, if you want to take a leaf out of an old doctor's book, lettuce leaves soothe pain by virtue of the traces of opium they contain. Their effect is more concentrated in soup made from simmering a pound or two of lettuce thinnings with a sliced onion and sufficient water to make a thick soup.

That board under the mattress – how does it work? For one thing, it promotes what is known as lordosis. Remember how pulling your abdomen backwards and upward flattens the hollow of your back? In this lordosis position the spinal discs are less likely to slip, or herniate.

A 'back' patient is likely to wake in the night to seek a more comfortable position. All this means expenditure of effort to relieve stress. Try inserting a pillow in the bed to give side-support. Lying on your back with a pillow under your knees may also bring relief.

If you have been ordered to stay in bed by your practitioner, stay in bed.

Now, supposing muscle-knotted backs want to get out of bed? That can pose a problem. Just grit your teeth and wriggle over to the side. Lying on your side, bend your knees, drop them adroitly over the edge. Push yourself up straight under your own steam and have someone assist you into the upright position.

When we take weight off the lumbar (low spinal) region, as when lying down, we automatically ease low back pain. 'Back' patients are most likely to benefit from sleeping in a hammock. This old naval relic holds the spine in a semi-flexed position, offering maximum relief. The tendency of a hammock to sway from side to side completely relaxes the pelvis.

The whole question of the 'swinging cure' has been rediscovered by an American doctor who believes it will be of first importance to people with chronic back trouble.

Staying with friends in Columbia who put up their guests in hammocks, he tried one for the first time. He had his best night's sleep for months. He woke up free of pain. That did it. Now, nothing could persuade him to sleep on anything else. His backache is cured.

In my rocking chair

Pioneer farmers of the Middle West performed massive workloads. They knew what back strain really meant. Could immunity have been due to the rockingchair? This piece of domestic furniture came over with the early European settlers who found its gentle backward and forward movement ideal relief for a taut exhausted back. Experiments on the nervous system show how the transmission of pain is blocked as long as rocking continues.

There has been a tremendous increase in the number of women who climb mountains, hunt game and fish. In America it is estimated that 21 million women fish. A recent survey at the Yosemite National Park revealed that one-third of the season's backpackers were women. It is an extraordinary thing that women's back troubles from trauma and excessive physical strain have not increased proportionately. Is it because women have stronger backs than generally assumed? Whatever the answer, it appears more women in the southern states are adopting this method of relaxation. One says: 'In my rockingchair a lovely harmony enters my heart, and the cares of my world are forgotten.'

Have you ever had a seized-up back on getting out of bed in the morning? Again, that board under the mattress can do you a power of good by keeping your spine at the correct angle during sleep.

There are times when a back needs a hard surface.

Slipped discs – how do they come about?

'Big oaks from little acorns grow,' is especially true of 'disc' problems. Separating each vertebra along the length of the spine is a pulp-filled washer acting as a cushion. Due to excessive strain the outer coating of one of these cushions may collapse causing part of the pulpy matter to extrude. This may cause excruciating pain and is wrongly referred to as a 'slipped disc'.

If a spine is in poor shape, a disc may be squeezed out of existence and become a case-hardened rim of gristle.

A degenerated disc may obstruct mobility of the two vertebrae it is intended to separate. This exerts pressure on a nerve root at a point where it leaves the spine to serve a distant part of the body. This squeezing pain may radiate down the leg in a condition known as sciatica.

There is convincing evidence to show that a disc prolapse does not come on suddenly. The cause?

An impoverished diet usually heads the list. Those prone to disc problems are recommended to take a diet high in protein.

A healthy disc needs to be sustained by a daily average of at least 500 milligrams of calcium, as well as adequate vitamins D, C and E.

Two glassfuls of milk will supply the body's daily requirements of calcium which the pulp and your bones need.

To facilitate healing of disc tissue you will require plenty of vitamin E (1,000 international units daily). This versatile vitamin is best taken in an oil-based capsule; not only is its life lengthened in a good preserving medium, but it is more easily absorbed. Take for one to three months.

Unless yours is a top-nutrition diet, no bad back can afford to neglect vitamin C, essential for replenishing connective tissue.

Effective relief of backache is now part of the manipulative scene. One reason for its success is the evolution of osteopathy and chiropractic. Experienced practitioners in these fields can 'lock' a disc in place with relief of symptoms.

Are your feet trying to tell you something?
Our feet are made up of a collection of small bones, some of which may get out of line and cause our arches to fall. Anything that causes pain in the feet can be reflected to the back.

Women with backache should avoid high-heeled shoes. A snug pair of well-fitted shoes has relieved many a backache.

The following simple measure may save you pounds in practitioner's fees. Remove your clothes until bare to the waist. Stand in your socks. Ask a friend to stand behind you and take a look at your back.

Is one shoulder lower than the other? Maybe the top of your spine is inclined in that direction. Take a pack of playing cards. Place all the cards under the heel of the foot on the lower side. Reduce the number of cards from the pile until both shoulders are the same height. Slip the cards into an envelope and ask your shoe repairer to raise the level of the heel accordingly. Difference in length of leg is common in those with lower back trouble.

Happy feet sometimes cost money. Your feet may be crying out for a raise.

So you weigh too much!
'I hardly eat a thing, Doctor, but I simply cannot lose weight.' Have you ever said those words? Everyone's dearest wish is to be weighed in the balance and found wanting.

There is nothing funny at all in jokes aimed at fat people. Few realize the torments suffered by weight-bearing joints on those who do not measure up to the fashionable idea of a sylph-like silhouette.

You can add a great deal of strain to your spine if you are overweight. Sometimes a back just cannot stand it. A good slimming diet has cured many backaches in its time.

A woman can profit by going out of her way to safeguard her back. Relaxation, flat on the floor after a midday meal, certainly pays off. Those with a will to give up alcohol, coffee and stimulants are less susceptible to cystitis (inflammation of the bladder) – a common cause of back trouble in women. Prolapsus of the womb may be missed as a cause of lower back pain.

Back in shape

Chronic back trouble may, like arthritis, have been building up over many years. But with care and exercise there is no need for you to get to that stage.

Pain is a warning sign that something is wrong. Always seek professional advice for back, chest, head or abdominal pains immediately. Backache does not always come alone. It is likely to be accompanied by a tribe of hangers-on like aching knees, painful feet, stiff shoulders and headache.

To maintain your normal spinal curve is to remove strain and lessen pain. When your back is playing up, don't take chances with such obvious hazards as lifting heavy objects, bed-making, or standing when you can sit. The Turks have a saying: 'Never stand when you can sit, and never sit when you can lie down.'

Always remember to put on warm protective clothing after exercise, games and gardening. A sensible sportsman or sportswoman takes along extra clothing to combat changes of temperature.

Few bad backs fail to respond – at least temporarily – to the seductive pleasure of a hot bath. If you can add two heaped tablespoonfuls of Epsom's salts to your bath – then you have a perfect relaxant.

Epsom salt baths are fine, but you should go to bed immediately afterwards. These salts make you vulnerable to chills should you go out into the cold. Castor oil packs are known to bring relief from pain, in the long term. In many cases they have brought about extraordinary cures. For acute conditions, cold packs are indicated.

It is surprising how an aching back may be a legacy from an attack of influenza. On such occasions the body makes heavy demands upon the minerals calcium and iron. These are taken from bones and blood, and have to be made-up during convalescence. This is one reason why folk with the flu should stop being heroic in battling their way through their duties at the office or workbench. Not only do they help to spread germs around, but they prejudice their chances of springing back to normal health refreshed, and possibly better for the experience.

An attack of the flu or a bad cold may often be swiftly terminated by going to bed with a stiff dose of vitamin C – If you can drink the juice from freshly squeezed oranges or lemons, then do this rather than taking a Vitamin C tablet or powder Unbroken warmth and total relaxation are healers in their own right.

Backs no longer look after themselves. We expose them to unnecessary hazards unknown to previous generations. In their days, at least, you knew your enemies and could face them in the open.

With progressive deterioration in the national diet through highly refined packaged foods, artificial colourings and additives, more matchstick backs come up for treatment. Vegetarians often claim, 'We become what we eat.' This may or may not be true. But if food we consume daily is lacking in vitality, live minerals and enzymes, how can we keep a strong spine in good repair?

Blood cells begin their lives in the bones. The osseous skeleton is not a mere scaffolding for the flesh. Embedded deep within the matrix of bone are factories for the production of vital components of the blood.

Calcium phosphate, vitamin D and essential minerals are utilized for building strong healthy bones. Mineral deficiencies are first felt within the marrow which, were the truth known, might well prove to be the starting point of chronic disease.

Make the most of the fresh fruit vitamins

Vitamin C is required to make collagen, connective tissue containing fibrils, and these tissues are strengthened by an increased intake. Collagen is an essential constituent of the fibrous cartilage discs.

Moreover, this vitamin is known to strengthen the body's protective system. Dr James Greenwood, Jnr, of Bayler University College of Medicine found that 500–1,000 milligrams of vitamin C taken by mouth daily successfully relieved pain and averted the need for operations in over 500 disc injury patients, including himself.

The acute back

What can I do before the doctor comes? This is where the homely art of homoeopathy is invaluable. Rhus Tox 6 is obtainable from any reputable homoeopathic chemist. Two or more tablets may be taken as indicated. Even if your lesion is not a matter of simple spinal mechanics, this safe remedy may give relief by relaxing tissue under tension. It is prescribed for 'pains better by movement' – the patient is restless and always on the go.

Another effective remedy is Bryonia 6, indicated for pains which are worse by movement. The patient does not want to stir: he stays put.

In acute conditions a cold water pack usually relieves pain and avoids undue swelling. After the first four hours, heat may produce the best results, especially if the condition allows a little gentle massage. The first thing your practitioner will want to do is to satisfy him or herself that no fracture is present.

Stretch your legs

Then there is walking. Some folk have to learn to grow out of a stoop. Whatever our pace, fast or slow, we need to cultivate an even stride. Check yourself in the mirror. Do you shuffle? Don't be afraid to admit to a waddle. Correct your posture every time you pass a shop window. Use of a walking-stick is no sign of invalidism.

Weight of baggage is more evenly distributed when wearing a shoulder-bag, or rucksack. Carrying heavy suitcases is a common cause of bad backs. If you are getting over a bout of pain, don't start it off again by reaching for objects that are too high or suddenly straightening up from the stooping position.

There is no easy way to overcoming back trouble. You have to work at it. Your spine is made up of a host of related components, so that when one part breaks down it cannot be replaced like a blown gasket on your car.

In the new concept of physiology, all parts of the body work together for good. When you come to think of it, these separate parts are served by the same nerve supply, the same blood supply, and the same lymphatic or drainage system. They are all part of this body of flesh and bone.

Treat your back as you would a friend. Give him all the help he needs and he will not let you down when you have to call upon him for that little extra effort in the unexpected emergency.

If you are feeling an odd twinge, it is absolutely necessary for you to inform your subconscious mind what you intend to do.

Breathe with ease and walk with a sense of fulfilment. Bring a swing into every body movement. Picture yourself with the smooth-working chassis you enjoyed before bad posture or injury came on the scene. Sense precious oxygen permeating every cell and tissue of your body.

Every back is a little different. And there is a tendency for back patients to be treated as if they were all the same. Mr A. G. who was over seventy-six years old, suffered unmercifully from attacks of lumbago until he took up rocking and rolling. After only two weeks of shakes and shenanigans his lumbago disappeared.

However painful your back may be, it is comforting to know that it is seldom of crisis proportions. Like many others, we can find out for ourselves how good posture, sound nutrition and exercise pays off handsomely in the long run.

Bioterrorist activity

What can we do to fortify ourselves against biochemical warfare?

I think every one should bear in mind certain nutrients to protect the body against biological weapons. This is an area in which we can do our maximum for personal survival.

The main danger is infection. This calls for a sound immune system ready to spring into action against viruses and bacteria.

It is unlikely that your immune systems would be strengthened within hours through the usual food channels. For rapid absorption, concentrated preparations would be necessary. Consider self-protection by way of the following:

- Perhaps our first essential would be vitamin E, responsible for conserving the body's oxygen supplies. We would need an immediate build-up of enzymes, amino acids, vitamins and minerals.
- One remedy which gave impressive service after Hiroshima was ginseng, known in Chinese medicine over the centuries as 'all heal'. It speedily activates the macrophages with little known toxic effect.
- Garlic is one of our most powerful antibacterials. The bulb may be taken in its natural form. If you *must* have capsules or tablets consider garlic extract 400mg three times a day.
- Turmeric is one of the best remedies for infection. It has a long and impressive history in the Ayurveda pharmacopoeia, the traditional medicine of India. Shake the powder on food as you would using a salt shaker.
- A good multivitamin and mineral supplement is indicated – minus iron which increases bacterial activity – and with plenty of B vitamins.
- Tomatoes are quoted by certain authorities as supportive to the body when in extremity.
- Avoid red meat because of its iron content. Discontinue most of the oils except extra virgin olive oil, and substitute honey for sugar.
- The above are believed to protect against radiation.
- In the meantime, take a fresh look at organic foods. Few things undermine an immune system more than chemical pesticides. The important thing is to build up a sturdy resistance by eating a variety of foods including plenty of fresh fruit and vegetables, fresh oily fish, whole grains and avoiding convenience foods.

High blood pressure

High blood pressure can be controlled but if you want to lower the risk it may be necessary to make some lifestyle changes.

With the stresses of life today, it is wise to keep an eye on your blood pressure. If you have not had your blood pressure checked in the last five years mention it to your doctor or health consultant.

Blood pressure measurements require two readings: the systolic pressure when the heart contracts, and the diastolic pressure when it relaxes between beats. These are recorded in millimetres of mercury (mmHg). The average blood pressure without risk is 120/80mm. High blood pressure is anything over 140/90mm.

How can we lower our pressure? We may have to ask ourselves, 'How much do I smoke?' Smoking narrows the arteries and makes it more difficult for blood for circulate.

Maybe we need to substantially reduce our intake of salt which causes fluid retention, adding stress to the heart and circulation. By increasing the intake of potassium we cause the body to excrete more sodium. *See* under Potassium for potassium-rich foods (celery, tomato, cucumber, potatoes, fish, bananas, watercress etc) pp. 45–46.

Don't add salt to cooking or at the table and reduce your intake to 5mg a day.

If you have a weight problem, you will need to lose a few pounds. A brisk walk daily can prove helpful.

Patients with high blood pressure often feel better when cutting out milk, cream and cheese from their diet. Yeast can 'string-up' blood pressure cases.

It may be necessary for you to consume less animal fat, more fish, and much more raw fresh fruit and vegetables. All these are high in potassium.

Avoid white sugar, fast food and processed foods high in fat. Follow a high-fibre diet where possible. Soya products lower cholesterol levels and high blood pressure. Only moderate amounts of alcohol should be consumed.

High blood pressure is an area where fish oils such as tuna, halibut, mackerel and sardines can prove most helpful. They inhibit the deposition of cholesterol, therefore reducing the risk of stroke and heart disease.

Low blood pressure

Low blood pressure (hypotension) is a condition in which the blood pressure is reduced. Some people have a slightly low pressure which is that person's particular normal pressure. Disorders such as tabes dorsalis and Parkinson's disease may have a low pressure, as do those with thrombosis or in a state of shock.

Symptoms include anxiety, depression, headaches and tiredness, which means the brain suffers from a reduction of glucose and oxygen.

Patients with peripheral neuritis are at risk and successful treatment of low blood pressure may depend upon a treatment of that condition. It is a condition for which more salt may be indicated.

Low blood pressure demands plenty of water to avoid dehydration. Beneficial agents include ginger, garlic, liquorice, panax ginseng and ginkgo – taken only for a short term. Alcohol and smoking should be avoided. In the past, onions were advised by herbalists.

As some hypotensive drugs have side-effects, check with your doctor or health consultant before taking anything. Echinacea and prickly ash bark are recommended by herbalists and naturopaths.

Bronchitis

Arthur was a forty-a-day smoker. He promised himself he would one day give it up, but never seemed to be able to get round to it. At first the doctor's spray-mist would shift the phlegm, but in cold weather he could barely get his breath for days at a time.

Soon, hawking and coughing became a full-time occupation, making it impossible to hold down his job. No longer able to smoke, he was glad of the extra money in his pocket the saving brought. But it was not much use as it all went on medicated sweets. Mother and wife became anxious about his heart, which the doctor said would last him another two or three years at the most if he didn't exert himself. He could no longer go out of the house.

Arthur is typical of many sufferers of chronic bronchitis – an estimated six million in the European countries. It is no longer an Englishman's malady. Can anything be done about it?

Bronchitis is anything but simple. In a nutshell, nose, windpipe and lungs are lined with a delicate protective membrane. Its job is to secrete a fluid to keep the linings moist and to wash out impurities. When the weather is cold, damp or foggy, or when the air we breathe is loaded with dust-borne foreign particles, a part of the brain stimulates these membranes to produce more fluid to kill bacterial invaders and to wash out the tubes.

Thousands of tiny hairs called cilia rise from the membranes, sweeping backwards and forwards in a wave-like motion, thrusting before them any debris and mucus. These may be frustrated in their efforts when wastes build up and the elimination process breaks down.

Worn out by superhuman efforts against the obstructions, they pack-up. Recovery is the rule as soon as the irritant is removed. In many cases the irritant is provided by smoking.

Preventing trouble
Many men and women today are making the effort to give up smoking, and are experiencing success. But Arthur was always one to lean on his luck – this time with disastrous results.

His continued smoking meant endless coughing. Soon, the delicate air-sacs in his nicotine-scarred lungs lost their elasticity. Some ballooned-out like holes in a sponge. When you have seen a man like Arthur in the throes of oxygen starvation you will know what it is like to dice with death.

His mother bought him vitamins. Little did she realize how quickly their benefits were counteracted by the nicotine of tobacco. Without vitamin A the cilia dry up and fail to function. Suffocation becomes a problem. Arthur's response to drugs became weaker. Only oxygen from a cylinder gave relief.

Then somebody casually mentioned lobelia, a common wayside plant used by an older generation of country doctors for chest troubles. His mother at once recalled it from her childhood days. She obtained a supply and persuaded her son to try it.

There's nothing so disturbing as listening to a person's cough at night. One of the properties of this plant is to relax the nerves that make you cough. After only ten days they realized there was less coughing. Nobody was more surprised than the specialist.

Soon, the difference in Arthur's condition was attracting attention. One day he was able to go out – and all because his mother insisted on his taking a teaspoonful of olive oil together with lobelia (in tablet form) washed down with a cup of hot peppermint tea.

Now, the first time for years, he no longer wheezes when he exerts himself. They have a steep hill near their home where actually the fittest neighbours may get out of puff. Lobelia, red-man's medicine, appears to be one of those few anti-tussives which really touches the 'cough centre', relaxing nerves of the cough reflex. Appropriately, its Indian name is tobacco plant.

Arthur is by no means out of the woods. Though he will never be the man he once was, he has found a non-toxic means of relief. He's looking forward to the day when he can climb that hill like a prize greyhound.

Avoiding the cold

For those who suffer from 'chestiness' the safest haven is a warm house. Some houses are naturally damp and draughty; others cold or warm for no known reason. A warm room facing south helps.

If you prefer to sleep in an unheated bedroom it is important to be warm in bed, with particular focus on keeping your feet warm. On cold nights, stuffy noses and blocked sinuses may be alleviated by keeping the head warm. Some may go as far as wearing a nightcap. Desert Bedouin always cover their heads at night to induce sleep and protect them against the cold.

Check the heating in your home for winter. If too dry, you may need a humidifier. Switch on the fire in your bedroom for an hour or two before jumping into bed.

Be concerned about the dryness of your bedlinen. Often, unsuspected in winter months, mattresses may become damp underneath. They may need warming out on radiators, in an airing cupboard, or even in front of a fire until fully dry. Few healthy folk need an electric blanket yet those liable to be chesty may find it a boon.

Is it due to something I eat?
Irvin G. Spiesman, MD, and Lloyd Arnold, MD, described how an experiment investigating cold susceptibility in sixty-three patients at their clinic, for an observation period of three years, proved conclusively that by consuming large quantities of bread, macaroni and other wheat products, cases with breathing difficulties generally worsened.

Some physicians have obtained results after milk has been eliminated from the diet. The child who seems to have one cold after another is nearly always taking too much milk, or has an allergy to it. A number of cases have lost their chronic cough, asthma and colds by cutting out cow's milk and dairy products.

A boy never had a winter free from coughing spasms and spent most of his time in hospital with assistance from an oxygen cylinder and antibiotics. The solution to his problem was found. His doctors regarded it as too ridiculous to contemplate – yet it worked! As a last resort they put the boy on a milk-free diet. He made a rapid recovery and the symptoms returned only when he went back on to dairy products (cheese, eggs, milk and cream).

Cancer

There may come a time in the life of each one of us when we are desperate. We are on our own – out on a limb. The medical profession may honestly admit it has come to the end of its special skills.

In such a situation we have to make up our own minds. There is no time for theories. The whole world is waiting for a cure for cancer. Millions are spent each day on research and treatment. Even if it cannot be cured, have alternative therapies any relief to offer?

A growing number of people believe they can play an important part in body nutrition, sustaining the body's efforts towards recovery, and the relief of pain. Whatever our particular persuasion, orthodox or unorthodox, there are many ways in which we can help ourselves. This is one area where a change in lifestyle may prove beneficial.

Why does a cell turn malignant? This could be due to a number of things, chiefly through a disturbed sodium/potassium metabolism. It is

185

now known that the disease can come when a cell loses its potassium. Sodium and potassium are the two minerals concerned with the body's immune system.

Our bodies require a lot of potassium within the cell but little in the blood. Where the cells and the blood are in a state of correct balance there is a perfect exchange of the two metals, which means that our inner 'electricity' will be flowing without obstruction.

Our first endeavour should therefore be to eat more potassium foods than sodium foods. There is plenty of potassium in fruits, green leafy vegetables, tomatoes, nuts, seeds, peaches, apricots, bananas, oats, corn, broad beans, spinach, carrots, potatoes and wheat. Rice is poor.

One important aspect of the disease is inactivity of the enzyme system caused by too little oxygen or by poisons left over after digestion of meats. Enzymes are substances produced by living cells which initiate chemical change. When our immune system is supported by an efficient enzyme system, our natural vital-force is capable of making short work of any cells which may turn malignant. However, we have to give it a fair chance.

Suppressed grief emotions are said to predispose to cancer. Just how prolonged grief can depress our enzyme system is not known.

Literature on the known causes of the disease run into thousands of volumes. These pages will therefore offer suggestions for helpful home care once the disease has been confirmed.

You will not need any reminder of how smoking makes short work of our body's precious vitamin C, which we shall need in abundance. Neither are you likely to gloss over the fact that it is the most common cause of the disease where it appears in the lungs. Also, nearly every case of cancer is accompanied by liver damage, with subsequent faulty production of bile and vital enzymes. With this in mind, we are unlikely to hanker after alcohol. Herbal teas, vegetable and fruit juices are among the alternatives.

There are some foods that would make your fight back to normal health more difficult. These are the 'dead' foods: canned, bottled or preserved, (*especially shell fish*). A person may find it difficult to give up dairy products.

The patient will need all the B vitamins he or she can get. Sugar leeches them out of the system. Honey and black molasses are good.

Few people can stay well without a proper sodium/potassium balance, and nothing destroys that balance more effectively than an excess of common table salt. To avoid this, a salt-shaker can be filled with powdered kelp or table herbs. Those who have been converted to garlic seldom develop a palate for excessive salt.

Dr George Starr White, Los Angeles physician, believed salt was the cause of some 'lumps in the breast' as well as inflamed conditions under the armpits and between the thighs. 'This has been proved,' he said, 'from the fact that a lot of these disturbances cleared up when all refined salt was removed from the diet.'

A non-meat diet should carry less pollutants in the form of antibiotics which are given to most animals, and which may have an adverse biological effect upon the body. We should sustain the body with life-vitalizing vitamins and minerals, which are mostly missing in tinned foods. We need the best nutrition we can get for the maintenance of the body's internal defences.

Like plants, our bodies need lime, phosphates, potash and other minerals. Just as a healthy plant depends on having a good supply of such minerals, so our freedom from disease depends on good food grown on a healthy soil, eaten unspoilt by commercial processing and in as natural a state as possible.

In cancer the immune system will have taken a beating. The question is how to rebuild quickly. Our first job is to detoxify – to rid the body of its poisons. Our diet should therefore contain those things which raise natural immunity. These may include zinc, magnesium, selenium, and vitamins A, B, C, D, and K. Vitamin E is indicated for tumours where not found in the breast and womb.

Ideas on a non-meat whole foods diet are endless and many books are on sale. The first item would be wholemeal bread, the Doris Grant loaf springing to mind. Few breakfast foods are more sustaining than your own home-made muesli. Do not forget the many herb teas in place of tannin-packed teas of commerce. Brown rice is a must. The patient should learn to love raw green salads seasoned with a dressing made from two teaspoons of sunflower seed oil emulsified in one tablespoon of fresh lemon juice.

Let yoghurt and goat's milk take the place of cow's milk. If a place could be found for garlic, onions and a touch of sage, so much the better. Whatever is done, carefully avoid all those permitted colourings, additives and artificial flavourings of the supermarket.

Selenium

Scientists have discovered how selenium is linked with cancer-prevention. Where there is little in the soil there is a higher incidence of the disease. This fastest-growing food supplement is believed to offer a certain protection. It is used to prevent animals developing the condition.

Selenium is described as the world's rarest trace element. Our body's defences are vulnerable without it. Some experts in the field go as far as saying that selenium supplementation could save up to 80% of the world's breast cancers.

The National Cancer Institute of America reveals the interesting fact that populations subsisting on diets high in selenium have a lower incidence of cancer in the colon, stomach, lungs and bladder. Selenium-rich foods are wheat cereals, onions, garlic and cold-pressed vegetable oils.

A fascinating new science of 'mineral agriculture' has been born in which certain minerals are fed to plants by way of a mulch. A variety of barley grown by special methods contains a high content of selenium, magnesium and zinc, of value to the health-conscious and cancer-prone.

When it comes to longevity and freedom from disease it is all a question of the soil. Living on the selenium-rich land of north Norfolk, England, it is not surprising that many of the people there live to great ages.

Magnesium

As far as possible it would be wise for potassium salt supplements to be avoided. Your doctor may want to swing into action from the start, but they may prove gastric irritants. When magnesium is taken, the cell is enabled to take up potassium more easily.

The most popular magnesium supplement on sale is a combination of magnesium carbonate and calcium carbonate, marketed as dolomite tablets. The magnesium content of these tablets is too low for cancer patients who can easily double the dose, according to the condition.

Just as an old gypsy's preventive consisted of five almonds a day, so the old generation of homoeopaths often recommended a daily dose of magnesium phosphate for the same purpose.

It is a tendency among cancer practitioners to advise magnesium orotate where the bowel is distressed.

Zinc

More and more investigators look to human nutrition as the strongest influence upon cancer, leukaemia and tumour growth generally. The manipulation of trace elements in the diet, especially zinc, leads to more effective treatment, whether orthodox or unorthodox.

Zinc is an essential nutrient for tissue growth, cellular division and the synthesis of protein. If the cell has adequate zinc, the growth will be more vulnerable to chemotherapy and radiotherapy.

Cancer subjects may suffer an embarrassing body odour which is not always easy to mask. Zinc is equal to the task. But that is not the only embarrassment; their sense of taste and smell can go wrong. Zinc is likely to be the answer. Sunflower seeds are rich in zinc. Old-fashioned zinc and castor oil ointment is still at work in some surgeries for combating chronic discharging ulcers.

Those who are diabetic may know that their zinc levels are lower than average. Some may suffer ulceration of the foot for which zinc may be a consideration.

Carrot juice

A number of cures are on record in which the disease has been arrested by carotene – a precursor of vitamin A. Fresh carrot juice contains b-carotene, preferred by the practitioner because it is less toxic than the commercial vitamin A. The fresh is superior to the carotene of modern pharmacy, and three to five glasses a day may be drunk.

Ellis Barker, well-known homoeopath of the 1940s, records the case of Mrs S. who was sent home from hospital to die. A famous Edinburgh surgeon had diagnosed a hopeless case of cancer of the bowel and even went as far as to predict the actual time of death. Relatives were told that a week or two would see the end. But they were an independent family and wouldn't leave it at that. Carrot juice was made and they gave it to her experimentally. Listen to the results.

'The daily sickness ended on the second day of use of the carrot juice and did not return. On the sixth day, intestinal secretions were free from blood and pus. From that time a cleaner condition of the bowel was noticeable. Secretions and urine became normal. Ten pints weekly were given and as near as possible a non-acid diet was maintained.

Improvement in general health was apparent to all. In a few weeks all pain and discomfort had disappeared. The complexion improved and weight increased. So rapid was the improvement that six weeks and one day after the first glass of carrot juice the patient was able to go out for a walk with relatives.

An examination made by the doctor reported that no tumour could be traced, and the heart action was good. At this stage her weight was taken: it was found there had been a gain of nearly four stone. Thrilled at her good fortune, she had a new haircut and fully resumed interest in life.'

The story of Jason Winters

In the literature of green pharmacy there is scarcely a single herb which has not, at one time or another, been successfully used for the disease. From these, we will single out red clover, poke root, yellow dock root, golden seal root, thuja, mistletoe and clivers.

In the book *Killing Cancer*, Jason Winters recalls how he cured himself after being given only three months to live.[28] Refusing major surgery he travelled the world in search of a cure.

Jason had twenty adventurous years following his emigration from England to Canada. He did all those exciting things a boy ever dreamed of. He crossed the Canadian Rockies (and halfway across the Atlantic) in a balloon, travelled the great Mackenzie River by canoe down to the Arctic Ocean, hunted polar bears in Alaska and kangaroos (with the Aborigines) in

Australia. He crossed the Sahara Desert by camel, speared fish with the Maoris, and crashed cars through brick walls to safety test seatbelts for the New Zealand government.

You can imagine the kind of fight put up by this superman facing death from terminal cancer. His book is a revelation of a man determined to live at all costs, telling how he won through in the face of overwhelming odds with red clover, chaparral and a known spice.

Like other herbal remedies used for this purpose, all are great purifiers of the blood. The cancer cell cannot thrive in a healthy body.

Doubtless, the most controversial alternative to orthodox medicine for the disease is laetrile (*amygdalin*). This substance is made from apricot kernels with a history of many years folk medicine behind it. As a remedy for malignancy it again sprang to life in the 1950s when dramatic cures were reported. laetrile is taken together with additional vitamins and pancreatic enzymes. The purpose of the enzymes is to break down the muco-protein capsule which enables the cyanide in the remedy to penetrate the wall of the cancer cell and destroy its contents.

It was discovered by Dr Ernest Krebs who named it vitamin B17 and who cured many such patients. He claimed the body's own immune system broke down the cyanide content of apricot stones to produce a substance with the ability to destroy affected cells.

Does it work, or not? The answer seems to come from the surgeries of its proponents. Maybe we shall never know the truth. No one knows for sure how many people would have died had there been no laetrile therapy.

For this condition, there is no lack of people to come forward to testify of help received from acupuncture, homoeopathy, naturopathy and spiritual healing. But much work remains to be done in assessing and evaluating results on a rational basis.

The 'breakthrough' terminology has lost its meaning. Sometimes the answer to a question is not black or white, but grey. The solution to this most baffling of all health problems may not rest on the merits of any one particular therapy, but in a combination of what is the best of official medicine with the best of the alternative systems.

Both sides have convincing evidence to submit. At last, there is growing evidence of a new spirit and a closer co-operation between the two opposing schools.

Nobody can predict the course the disease may take. It is a condition beset by so many variables. Whatever decisions we make, one thing is certain: a large ration of courage will be necessary. This is where relatives and friends can help. Emotional attitudes have a positive influence upon survival.

To tell, or not to tell?

'I've been so worried – you must tell me the truth, I can't shake off things as easily as I used to.' Every doctor has heard these words.

Some say it is inhuman to tell a person he or she may have cancer. Others believe the telling may be responsible for an accelerated demise. There is a contrary view which believes that the unknown is often worse than the reality itself.

As one who has seen so many cases of a bitter 'let down' at the end, I would say that it is equally unkind not to tell. Not to do so violates that sacred area known as the doctor/patient relationship. We all have to die some day. But the sting can be taken out of it by the Christian faith.

An abundance of evidence is found in the Bible of the way 'He will give his angels charge over you' when problems are committed to the Good Physician. Stress is a major factor in the disease. Did you know that when your white-cell immune system suffers a violent emotional shock, as in prolonged anxiety or worry, it is much weakened? Emotional events have a physical impact.

To seek help from a spiritual dimension in an hour of need is no sign of weakness. Jesus said that faith could move mountains. Certainly it has enabled countless millions to scale pinnacles of suffering and soar into a clearer air where stress is unknown. Whatever our denomination or belief, it is good to know that the grace of God can bring real peace to a troubled mind. It is available to you – regardless of mental or physical condition if you humbly request it from One in whom we all 'live, move and have our being'. The sin and guilt problem is not very popular among psychiatrists, but all of us must one day face our Maker.

The sooner we make His acquaintance, the better. All He asks us to do is to commit ourselves wholly to Him, to believe that all things work together for good in the lives of all who believe in the existence of the Man of Nazareth. It is when we pray that His will be done in our lives that a power greater than our own takes over. At last we enjoy that peace which passes all understanding and which is superior to every mental state. There is no greater security for heart and mind against all things harmful.

I present these pages cautiously, not implying there is any one physical cure. Before you dismiss them as unscientific and experimental, remember they contain something you can do for yourself. They may favourably influence the sequence of events. I am not prescribing for the individual any specific treatment or product but, in a nutshell, present a few worthwhile ideas which may be of value in a moment of crisis.

Let us not leave everything to the over-worked hospital specialist. It is possible to augment his skills of chemotherapy, surgery and radiation in this way, though some practitioners claim that best results have followed where these alternatives are first employed. In our war against the most subtle enemy in the world we can't afford to ignore any chance – however unlikely it may appear – to renew hope and rekindle that most infinitely precious and sweetest gift of all – life.

When a person shows a zest for living and an inflexible will anchored and fixed in the certainty of God – he or she will never be disappointed.

Suggestions to minimize the risk of chronic blood disorder

'All cancer has its origin in the blood, later manifesting in body tissue sustained by the blood.'

Griffith Evans, *Operation Cancer*

With this in mind the following pages are concerned with cleansing the blood, in an effort to prevent chronic blood disorders. For instance, leukaemia is civil war between the immune system and the formation of the blood. Red cells carry oxygen, white cells fight infection, and platelets seal injured blood vessels by forming clots to arrest bleeding. Is it possible to prevent a decline in the quality of the blood brought about by today's pollution and dietetic deficiencies?

Welcome advances are being made all the time by conventional medicine. Are there alternatives?

A patient's X-ray history may be a significant cause of a deterioration in his blood condition. The average barium meal X-rays involve at least seven exposures.

'Leukaemia is an unwise iatrogenic result of unwise radiation.'

Dr Louis Hempelmann
University of Rochester Medical School, USA.

Is it possible to reduce the ill effects of radiation, chemotherapy and surgery? I believe it is possible to stimulate the immune system and maintain a positive quality of life.

We are all interested in foods that are said to minimize the cancer risk. Perhaps one of the most important things is a diet low in fats. Animals fed on high fat diets develop cancer.

Those who wish to note what the Bible has to say may consider the Old Testament Book of Leviticus.

'It shall be a perpetual statute for your generations throughout your dwellings, that you eat neither fat nor eat blood.'

Leviticus 3:v.17.

Milk and dairy products have long been under suspicion. Sugar is related to cancer of the breast and of the bowel, and should be replaced by honey. Never replace it with artificial sweeteners as many contain Aspartame, high levels of which are found in brain tumours when they are removed.

In many cases, cure is possible today by chemical and radiological medicine. In almost every case life can now be prolonged, but treatments are not wholly free from risk. Some patients may worsen. Are there less harmful alternatives?

In my opinion, a knowledge of traditional herbalism can assist body biochemistry for the perfect replication of blood cells. I believe the work of some of the outstanding herbalists of history (Hippocrates, Dioscorides etc.) together with today's medical research reflect a growing confidence in the use of herbal medicine without the necessity of bone marrow transplants and the transfusion of blood.

For sound blood cells, the heart of the bones (cancellous tissue) must be normal. Any injury to a bone is reflected into the cancellous tissue below the surface where it can affect the behaviour of the white cells.

Every bruise on a bone heightens the risk of haemolysis by shock or injury to the cancellous bed. For bruises affecting the bones, an older generation of herbalists used comfrey. Equally effective are Fenugreek seeds which, like comfrey, make strong and healthy bones.

For bruising of a bone or any body tissue consider homoeopathic arnica or calendula, internally.

We all need strong bones, which are not possible if we do not take advantage of the sun when it's shining. Vitamin D deficiency is becoming a major health problem, scientists linking it with diabetes and osteoporosis.

The appearance of boils, carbuncles, and external ulceration suggests there is taking place an elimination of morbid matter

continued

193

from the system. Such efforts of nature should be encouraged and not suppressed by drugs. Such action burdens the circulation with impurities, which may lead to serious blood disorder.

It goes without saying that diet is all important, and preference given to fresh raw fruit, dried fruits, green vegetables, nuts and seeds.

Prunes have been known to restore haemoglobin levels and red cell counts in cases of iron and copper deficiency.

Broccoli enshrines a whole galaxy of minerals, a small segment eaten raw in addition to the cooked vegetable.

Sunflower oil and seeds have a contribution to make towards healthy red blood cells. The seeds are high in calcium for robust muscle tone and firm bones. They contain phosphorus for strong teeth; iron, thiamin and natural fluorine for strong nerves.

Sesame seeds, as in sesame butter and tahini, contain vitamin T which enriches the blood and initiates a rise in blood platelet count.

Linseed or flaxseed is rich in essential fatty acids (EFAs) that have an important role in cell health and division. Haemoglobin deficiency requires EFAs (Dr Udo Erasmus).

Dates are rich in minerals and have much to offer the body.

Watercress has a long reputation as a potent blood purifier. The Crusaders are said to have valued it as a food to make up for blood lost through wounds of battle.

Vitamins B6, B12 and E are essential to an optimum diet. They are destroyed in chemicalized foods or excessive cooking.

Selenium appears to be essential to many people in this day and age. As a mineral it works well with vitamin E, their combined effort being greater than the sum of their action apart.

Marigold was a great favourite among the older herbalists. It was given to disperse congestion of the lymph system clogged with toxins, causing lymph glands to swell and harden. They believed that leukaemia patients were much benefited by the cleansing effect of measles. Children loved the rich golden tea made by pouring boiling water on the flowers.

Food colourings I've said it before and I'll say it again – be a good label reader. Avoid processed foods treated with nitrates, nitrosamines and certain hydrocarbons that heighten risk of disease of the brain, stomach and blood. Regard that vividly artificial red-coloured meat with suspicion.

Wine proves that alcohol is not all bad. If you really must have a little alcohol, consider Vermouth, made from the herb wormwood, a sovereign remedy to assist the cleansing work of the liver.

Red wine is known for its ability to increase the red cell population. A little each day helps to unstick platelets as well as lessen the risk of heart disease.

Honey is extremely beneficial to the body. Whatever the time during the day, take the opportunity to enjoy a teaspoonful of honey – but not if you're a diabetic.

Remedies contra-indicated in leukaemia: echinacea and tincture of myrrh. Though both are useful for infection, they increase production of white cells that clog the circulatory and lymph systems.

Apricot kernels (desiccated) were the basis of successful treatments in Mexico and America by Laetrile, a natural preparation from the kernels. They contain vitamin B17, responsible for the relief and cure of thousands of leukaemia patients before being suppressed by officials whose multi-million pound a year drug business was in danger of being eroded. The opposition claimed that laetrile contained cyanide, regarded by pharmacy as a poison, as indeed it is when prescribed apart from one of its natural contexts in apricots.

'To eliminate growths, the kernels of apricots should be crushed and mixed with your morning oats.'

Jacob Antworth, 1810

At the present stage of medical research, science has yet to discover that the innate body intelligence is quite capable of handling the cyanide. The Hunzas, among the healthiest people in the world, discovered it 1,000 years ago.

'The Hunzas breakfast consists almost entirely of a mixture of dried apricots, grain meal and their glacial water. To these they add freshly ground wholewheat, buckwheat, oats and barley meal.'

John Tobe, *Guideposts to Health*

A normal level of platelets is essential. Those subject to leukaemia should remember that garlic has an anti-platelet activity.

continued

Inner cleansing brings a sense of renewal, optimism and enthusiasm – maybe even joy in expectation of recovery. Our aim should be the healing of mind and body.

If health is ever on a 'down turn', the starting point of all recovery is personal discipline. We must be convinced that what we intend to do is right. We have to feel in control.

Sufferers from blood disorders should take heart. Many are the testimonies of those who have risen above a hopeless condition and fought back with a diet of natural foods and medicines and won. The immune system in everybody works towards a restoration of perfect health, whatever the risk of infection or injury. In 'Operation Leukaemia' (1965) Griffith Evans MA, FRCS wrote:

'This mechanism is activated by the Life Force which religion calls the Grace of God. This force was formerly recognized by academic medicine under the name *Vis Medicatrix Naturae*, the healing power of Nature.

'The Life Force not only creates molecules and cells, but provides the energy which binds them together . . . The crisis of our time is one of belief. Men have ceased to believe in the Author and Giver of Life . . .'

The Bartram Breakfast

7–8am.

1–2 cups of tea: any regular teas or herb teas (sweetened with honey if desired). Select from herb teas: green buckwheat, borage, nettles (for iron), lemon grass, mint or spearmint, sage, rosehip or chamomile.

3–5 almonds
1–2 Brazil nuts
1–2 teaspoons fenugreek seeds
1–2 teaspoons flaxseed (golden linseed)
1–2 dates

Method: Place the almonds and fenugreek seeds in boiling water and leave for a minute or two, after which the almond skins are easily removed and the fenugreek seeds softened (the skins of almonds are indigestible and constipating, so should always be removed). Grate the nuts if you desire. Mix all the ingredients into a generous plateful of oatmeal porridge, with a drizzle of honey. A wholegrain cereal with yoghurt and honey may be taken in lieu of porridge. Follow with one slice of whole meal bread, butter and honey, if desired. Your daily diet should include three to four servings of fresh fruits and one of raw green salad vegetables daily. Coffee should be avoided, being an antidote to many herbs. Dandelion coffee is one of many substitutes.

Tea for chronic blood disorders

Equal parts of the following:
Gotu kola
Red clover
Wild violet leaves

Method: Combine all of the ingredients together. Place one heaped teaspoon of the mixture per teacup into a non-aluminium teapot, and fill with boiling water. Allow to stand for 3–4 minutes. Drink one cupful or more, morning and evening – more frequently in desperate cases.

Gotu kola increases the number of platelets in the blood, and red clover increases the haemoglobin levels. Violet leaves detoxify the lymph system.

Eye health

Nutrition plays an important part in eye health. An intelligent diet should enable you to avoid a number of disorders including age-related degeneration (AMD).

If you eat a diet rich in carotenoids it would appear that you could bypass the risk of deterioration. Carotenoid-rich vegetables include kale, spinach (raw), collard greens, tomatoes, lettuce, carrots (raw), corn and green peas.

Research finds that free-radicals play an important role in the development of eye diseases including retinal disorders (conditions affecting blood vessels of the retina of the eye), and even damage to the retina caused by diabetes.

Antioxidants are indicated in prevention and treatment. Ginkgo biloba is found to improve circulation of fluids in the eye by dilating vessels and assisting in the blood flow.

Research into lycopene in tomatoes comes out strongly in favour of its use in eye strain, poor vision and fatigue.

Adopt a positive attitude to life. Visualize yourself with perfect eyesight. *See also* Bilberry (p. 220).

Heart problems

The average human heart beats seventy times a minute, 4,200 times an hour, 100,800 times a day, 36,792,000 times every year – about 2,575,000,000 times in a seventy-year lifetime. It is the most efficient pump ever created.

These are impressive figures, but there are times when this marvellous organ is taxed beyond its power and outside help is needed to put it right.

A news magazine observes: 'Beginning in the middle of the fourteenth century, the plague rampaged through Europe, killing a quarter of the population. But today, six centuries later, Europe and the West are facing a less dramatic but equally devastating and more insidious epidemic. Today's disease manifests itself in many forms, but all are rooted in the single poison: stress.' Dubbed a twenty-first century killer, stress puts an enormous strain on the heart of modern man. But there are other contestants for this role.

People who live in hard water areas, where the water is rich in calcium and magnesium, stand less chance of heart disease than those in soft water areas. Magnesium is required for the contraction of the heart muscle, while calcium is an important constituent of muscle tissue – the heart is one big muscle.

Studies at the London University Department of Nutrition by Professor John Yudkin convinced him that increased sugar consumption is also a common cause of heart trouble. Professors of other universities will tell you that salt is the concealed troublemaker.

Dr Yudkin's experiments revealed that refined white sugar as used in ice-cream, soft drinks and confectionery as a sweetener is a direct factor in coronary thrombosis. His comprehensive survey led to the unmistakable conclusion that the more sugar people eat the greater the risk of coronary disease.

But that is not all. Dr John Annand, a Scottish doctor, studied milk as a possible cause. For over thirty years he collected all the evidence available in medical journals and medical libraries. He has been able to prove that pasteurization by heating milk for half an hour considerably increased the incidence of coronary disease. He records: 'The increased consumption of milk protein that had been heated in this way was followed within one or two years by a significant increase in mortality from both brain and heart thrombosis.'

Dr Annand claims that milk proteins denatured in this way have an allergic effect. By placing patients on an egg-free and milk-free diet he has shown that, except in cases of advanced hardening of the arteries, they did not develop thrombosis.

Consider the great Finnish experiment. Finland was once Europe's black spot for heart attacks. The Government took firm action, introducing a five-year plan to wipe out cardiovascular disease by organizing a massive community programme. The net reduction of coronary cases through a simple dietetic approach startled observers.

The Finns, who had been the highest consumers of animal fats in the world made a dramatic switch to margarine made from vegetable oils, resulting in a spectacular fall in annual mortality rates. Now people of other nations share this knowledge by eating margarines made from corn oil, safflower oil, and especially sunflower oil, enabling those with a heart hazard to enjoy a healthier lifestyle.

Smoking must come high on the list of common causes of heart trouble. Tobacco smoke contains nicotine, an irritant, carbon monoxide, a toxic gas, hydrogen cyanide and other irritative substances. As the largest avoidable hazard to world health, cigarette smoking is responsible for more than 50,000 premature deaths in Britain alone. Eight times more people die each year from smoking than from road accidents. Seven times more working days are lost because of cigarette-induced disease than the total number lost in strikes. It takes a higher toll than alcohol.

It is generally agreed that alcoholism is a serious and growing problem all over the world. Where there is less agreement is in the quantity advised. Some people might never dream that the single alcoholic drink they had for lunch could be the cause of headache, insomnia and nervous irritability. Some have such a low tolerance threshold that a low intake may cause even more serious disorders, including irregular heartbeats and high blood pressure. Such symptoms can be difficult to cure.

If you can cut out alcohol from your new lifestyle so much the better. If not, make sure you imbibe well within your known tolerance level. It is lamentable the way in which films and TV often depict alcohol as a prop to turn to in times of stress.

Where the matter gets out of hand, facilities exist in most European and American towns under Alcoholics Anonymous. Their message is:

'Stay sober for the next 24 hours. Yesterday has gone, tomorrow never comes. You may be tempted to take a drink tomorrow – and perhaps you will. But don't take a drink today.'

If you have a sound heart – keep it that way. Should you ever have occasion to suspect your heart, see a competent practitioner. Do those things which lie within your power, such as to consider your intake of essential nutrients. Do you have sufficient vitamins C and E? How about the minerals calcium, magnesium and potassium? Each of these has something constructive to offer. All are good preventive medicine. In larger quantities they may be curative.

If your heart lacks propulsive power, vitamin E enables muscles and blood vessels to perform well on less oxygen. It is present in whole grains. Vitamin C (fresh fruits) and muesli for minerals preserve your blood vessels and help your heart derive maximum nutrition from the foods you eat. They help prevent blood clots and free blocked arteries.

If the heart ever becomes a problem – avoid drugs, except where absolutely essential. Instead, acupuncture, gentle exercise, yoga and spiritual healing may have something constructive to offer. On the herbal front a favourite combination consists of equal parts hawthorn and motherwort (heart muscle), prickly ash bark (conditions arising from early history of rheumatic fever) and cramp bark (angina – which is really cramp of the heart muscle).

Exercise, carefully managed, can be helpful for angina pectoris, the intense chest pain caused by a lack of blood supply to the heart muscle. Deep breathing has the effect of enlarging tiny coronary arteries, bringing more oxygen to the heart muscle. As a possible preventive of attacks a Minnesota doctor advises the person 'to inspire deeply, hold the breath for eight to ten seconds, and then exhale. Repeat the procedure about ten times.'

It is vital to get sufficient sleep which speeds up body repair and strengthens the heart muscle.

To prevent a heart attack make sure you exercise regularly. Avoid sugar, and add lecithin granules to your muesli. Include vitamins C and E in your diet and eat less meat and fewer eggs. Eat more fish and poultry and grill instead of frying. Select lean meat minus the fat. Use butter sparingly, preferring a soft margarine high in polyunsaturates, and avoid cream. Use corn oil, safflower oil or sunflower oil to cook with.

Charles Mayo said: 'Worry affects the circulation, especially the heart . . . I have never seen a man die from overwork, but many who died from worry.'

If you have heart problems, keep yourself cardiac fit and try to live as Nature intended. Hardening of the heart ages people more quickly than hardening of the arteries.

Hormone replacement therapy (HRT)

All over the world millions of working days are lost every day, in all grades of skills and employment, from pre-menstrual tension (PMT).

This may range from top supervisors who make hasty decisions to the office junior.

Although symptoms may vary from woman to woman, it is so easy to feel 'the odd girl out'. Terribly on edge, a wife or teenager gets crabby about the house, everything is too much trouble when she complains of being 'out of sorts'. Normally very efficient, a person may find herself making mistakes or becoming forgetful.

This complaint is now so distressing that women have been acquitted in the courts on the grounds of diminished responsibility. This has occasioned a great deal of research resulting in the administration of mass doses of (HRT). HRT is prescribed to restore the balance between the progesterone and oestrogen in the body. Progesterone and oestrogen play different roles in the phenomena of menstruation and pregnancy. PMT is believed to be due to a lack of progesterone. This is made up by giving injections, suppositories or tablets to redress the balance. HRT is the standard treatment, but many women look for an alternative. It is not generally known that the monthly recurrence of irritability, depression, breast tenderness and accident-proneness can yield to certain non-steroid preparations. The modern trend is to avoid tranquillizers and antidepressants in favour of a simple remedy such as Vitex Agnus Castus which initiates a response similar to that of HRT.

The brain plays an important part in starting menstruating by dispatching to the ovaries a chemical messenger called pyridoxine to initiate ovulation. The reader may recognize pyridoxine as none other than vitamin B6, supplements of which many women find helpful. Others find relief in vitamins C and E and ginseng, singly or in combination. Other favourites are the herbal teas of motherwort and raspberry leaves. None are known to increase mental dullness or depression and they have the advantage of acting without unwanted effects.

While any of these may be able to lift sufferers out of their monthly misery there is, of course, no one form of treatment or natural help that is effective for all.

Most therapies, including acupuncture, have their special techniques for releasing prisoners of this 'unrecognized syndrome'. Correction of displacements of the low spine and pelvis may remove abnormal pressure on the nerves, proving the answer in some cases. But none can make up for that kind of self-help which substitutes positive thinking for anger and irritation, and insists on those personal disciplines such as going to bed early and getting plenty of rest.

A change in the weekly routine can be well worthwhile. Important duties may be performed on days of lesser stress. Why should wash day not be switched from Monday to Wednesday? It is wise to cut down on drinking. Coffee can serve to aggravate. Salt, and salty foods all favour water-retention.

Yoga is a great tension reducer. Similar exercises and all natural measures are enhanced by a healthy lifestyle of wholesome foods, plenty of exercise and freedom from constipation. It is not necessary to eat less for fear of obesity, as a slight increase in weight is normal at this time because of fluid retention.

To many young women about to engage in exacting work this is a time which spells emotional upheaval and impaired concentration. They may be tempted to take tablets to reschedule their periods to suit themselves to leave them in the clear for exams, holidays, etc. Is it wise to attempt to deflect normal body rhythms to suit our convenience?

Do the benefits of HRT outweigh the risks? A woman may find it alleviates hot flushes and night sweats, yet scientific studies may be most revealing. Studies are now available to show how HRT increases the risk of breast cancer, heart disease, stroke and fractured bones.

An important American study was halted when it was revealed that a brand similar to that taken by millions of women throughout the world was not improving but damaging health. The trials found a 26% increase in breast cancer.

An Oxford University review in 1997 found that it increased the risk of breast cancer by 25%. Other studies discovered patients suffer 41% increase in the risk of stroke, and 25% of heart disease.

The above are but a few among a host of side effects including breast tenderness, headaches, high blood pressure, nausea and unhappy mood swings. Further researches reveal that the herbs black cohosh and don quai work as well as oestrogen products.

Oestrogen appears to cut the body's ability to use the insulin it produces by nearly one third.

A remedy once popular among our great-great grandmothers was sage tea made from one teaspoonful of dried garden sage (or two teaspoonfuls of the fresh plant) in a teacup of boiling water once or more daily.

Hormone-like substances are much weaker than HRT preparations. They may take longer to work. Such supplements include black cohosh, liquorice, don quai, kelp, red clover and vitex agnus castus. A selection from these is of value for change of life, frigidity, anaemia, general weakness and tiredness.

Homoeopathy, too, has its devotees who use sepia 30c (twice daily) for ten days. 'Selenium deficiency is very common and can cause a variety of hormone symptoms due to its effect upon the pituitary gland,' says Dr John Millward of Bournemouth.

For those looking for an alternative to HRT we would say: try to avoid strong tea, coffee and alcohol as they only worsen menopausal symptoms. Vitamin E also works well with some women, but it has to be taken in high doses (800–1000iu daily).

Foods that have a beneficial action on the hormone system are soya products (soya milk, tofu, soya), yoghurt and chickpeas.

Green leafy vegetables make a very real contribution towards relief: Brussels sprouts, broccoli, cauliflower and cabbage. A healthy diet and sensible exercise are essential around the time of the menopause when it is so important to feel good, and look good.

Emotional upsets fan the flame of a smouldering PMT. When tensions arise, there may be a strong impulse to take it out on boyfriend or husband. Patient forbearance of the average man is likely to be extremely limited when under attack from a woman temporarily at odds with the world.

It helps to have understanding parents and families. An affectionate hug can work wonders. It is a time when a husband's demonstration of affection means that somebody cares.

Prostate gland

As a man gets older he tends to lose his capacity to produce the male sexual hormone. This causes him a great deal of distress. He starts asking his doctor for some of those expensive steroid drugs to safeguard his virility. 'Why take artificial steroids,' asks Dr Devrient, physician, 'when there are pumpkin seeds for prostate troubles?'

Investigators researching countries of pumpkin seed eaters claim they can find no evidence of an enlarged prostate gland in men. They don't know exactly how these seeds work to rejuvenate, and suggest they contain elements which make up the male hormone.

Dr Devrient says: 'The plain people know the secret of pumpkin seeds – the secret which was handed down from father to son, for generations. The Hungarian gipsy, the mountain-dwelling Bulgarian, the Anatolian Turk, the Ukrainian, the Transylvanian German – all knew that pumpkin seeds promote prostate gland health. These people eat pumpkin seeds as the Russians eat sunflower seeds; as an inexhaustible source of vigour offered by Nature. They are rich in fatty acids.

'My assertion of the influence of pumpkin seeds is based on the positive judgement of old time doctors, also, no less upon my own personal observations throughout the years. The plant has scientifically determined effects on intermediary metabolism and diuresis [excessive urination]. But these latter are of secondary importance in relation to its regenerative, invigorating and vitalizing influences. There is involved in the pumpkin a native plant hormone; this affects our own hormone production in part by substitution, in part by production of new growth. Anyone who has studied this influence among peasant peoples has been again and again astonished at the beneficial effects of the plant.'

There are people who believe they know the secret of the pumpkin. The seeds are so rich in magnesium that no man with a suspicion of the trouble could afford to overlook them. To anybody on the hospital waiting list, a gram of such self-help can save many pounds of professional assistance. Who knows . . . when their time for admission arrives, it may be their good fortune to be greeted by the surgeon's expression of surprise: 'Well . . . that's funny! The trouble seems to have cleared up since you were here last!'

As the normal prostate gland contains more zinc than any other gland in the body, there is a case for zinc supplementation. Chlorophyll, vitamins A and C are also advised.

Rheumatism and arthritis

A registered nurse was plagued with an arthritic neck for seven years. Her employer, an ear, nose and throat surgeon, had the same problem. She also had a narrow disc in the lumbar area. She spent thousands for treatment without results. Then she read an article titled 'You Need More Calcium', and began taking nine to twelve calcium tablets daily and in one week was without pain!

A friend of hers had refused a total hip replacement for osteoarthritis and had been living on sixty aspirins daily. 'Within ten days (of taking calcium) she was totally free of pain – not one more aspirin!'

She then tackled the doctor who was naturally very sceptical. However, he started to take bone meal and within five days his pains were 50% better. By topping up blood calcium with bonemeal in powder or tablet form, others report results. It does not work every time, but the remedy is harmless and worth a trial.

It is true there are as many related causes of arthritis as there are cures. There must be a thousand different treatments which on occasion have proved successful for this crippling illness. Will there ever be a single cure?

Rheumatism remedies come and go. Each enjoys the limelight for a period before being superseded by another promise of a 'breakthrough'. A bewildering array of cures hovers between garden snails to green–lipped mussel extract, crude black molasses, honey and cider vinegar. All have something to offer. Over 300 different herbs have at some time been used for the relief of this baffling complaint. Somebody, somewhere, has experienced a 'miracle of nature' from any one of them. The problem is, correct selection of the one which fits your case.

The pharmaceutical profession rightly suspects any claim of a new spectacular cure. Some treatments are 'scientific', some hit and miss, and a few produce results. Advice can be as capricious as the wind.

Can you beat it? Mrs L. V. Phillips keeps hers under control with cabbage leaves. She pins a big leaf under her vest in the small of her back, replacing the leaves when dry. She knows she gets relief. Sometimes the leaf comes away almost black. Her husband tells her it's all her badness coming out!

Mrs B. M. Taylor, Bristol, had arthritis in her left knee owing to an accident. It was extremely painful. She had to use a stick. Enduring her misery for three months, she decided to take treatment into her own hands. She massaged the knee with hot olive oil and drank, in the early morning and last thing at night, two teaspoonfuls of cider vinegar and one teaspoonful of honey in a cup of warm water. After three months, she was cured.

Cyril Scott, a composer, practised homoeopathy and herbalism as a hobby and reported an earlier experience.[29] A lady had hip joints that were scarcely moveable, and not even her knees could be flexed. All she could do was have injections to ease the pain. Finally, her specialist advised a costly operation but could not promise success. Declining the operation she started taking crude black molasses (Two teaspoonfuls may be taken dissolved in warm water once or twice daily). After thirty-six drinks she could walk without her walking sticks and her knees became so flexible that she could even kick her backside with her heels.

Osteopathy and chiropractic have many devotees for joint troubles in which there is no active inflammation. Considerable improvement may be possible by spinal manipulation and work on the limbs.

Old bonesetters, after making sure the patella was free, would place their arm under a knee and circumduct – just a big word for saying that the leg is pushed around in a circle on a firmly anchored thigh. This was often followed by castor oil packs at night.

Arthritics are invariably cold mortals and are more comfortable in a warm atmosphere. A warm house in winter and exposure of affected limbs to direct sunlight in summer make for greater ease. Damp and cold exacerbate the condition as well as nervous strain and fatigue.

Epsom salt baths are recommended in certain cases, once or twice weekly. For hands, feet or knee aches, immerse them in a bowl or sink of hot water to which two tablespoonfuls of crude Epsom's salts have been added. Open or shut your fingers or toes slowly while they are in the water. Soak well. You may follow with a towel dipped in the hot Epsom's salt water, wrung out and wrapped round the joint. Dip again when cool, and repeat the process.

A three-day fast every two months on vegetable juices is helpful, and an occasional enema (if constipated) assists the cleansing process.

Some people benefit from a dry friction rub in the morning, on rising, and before going to bed. Two brushes, not too stiff, about 15cm (6in) long, are used to brush the skin all over the body. This stimulates the circulation and brings a rich supply of blood to the surface. Start off gently and slowly increase the pressure on the brush. An exhilaration of skin (and spirits) may follow. Soon you will not wish to start your day without a lively 'brush-down', which is one of the more gleeful aspects of keeping fit.

Remember that infected sinuses, tonsils, pyorrhoea or abscessed teeth and other focal infections may lie at the root of your trouble.

If you have arthritic hands you can still do a number of kitchen jobs. You can surprise your family by your ability to unscrew tight honey jars and apple-juice bottles. The secret? Put on a pair of rubber gloves.

Some folk swear by their copper bracelets, others bless their shopping trolleys; a woman with an arthritic spine reckons hers is a godsend. 'It means I can keep my independence a little longer – a thought that makes me feel my life is still worth living.'

Some people find relief by using castor oil packs. Dip a cloth or hand-towel in hot water and wring it out. Next, layer it with castor oil. Bind around the affected joint at night and remove it in the morning.

So many things spell lowered resistance, reduced vitality, poor glandular function and toxic build-up. They are a signal for the degenerative forces of the body to take over.

There is no universal diet for arthritics, but there are suitable foods. Experience has shown how a change from acid to alkaline-forming foods may be followed by definite well-being and often steady improvement.

As a general rule, it is wise for rheumatic sufferers to avoid 'berry' fruits (strawberries, bilberries, etc.). If you have rheumatic tendencies you should concentrate on uncooked grated raw vegetables, salad materials and other alkali-forming foods such as celery, carrots, celeriac, chives, cottage cheese, dandelion leaves, dates, figs, grapes, green peas, honey, kale, marrow, molasses, mustard-and-cress, olive oil, parsnips, peaches, pears, potatoes (baked in their jackets), runner beans, savoy, turnips and watermelon.

Where possible, avoid the acid-forming foods: cranberries, plums, rhubarb, chicken, game, jams, preserves, peanuts, all kinds of prepared meats, confectionery, walnuts and avoid white sugar as you would the plague.

Sparingly, use honey in place of sugar, soya or plant-milk, or goat's milk in place of cow's milk, dandelion coffee instead of coffee, wholewheat flour for white flour, and kelp powder or sea salt in place of table salt.

Avoid all acid fruits (citrus fruits), pickles, curry, spices, tinned foods, pork, bacon, ham, pastries and sweets. Where you can, try to avoid icy cold drinks or foodstuffs, piping-hot drinks and excessively hot food. It is wise to take alcoholic beverages in moderation.

Most joint troubles arise from a breakdown of the collagen connective tissue (or cushioning in the joints) due to inflammation or dietary mineral deficiency. All the above items lack precious vitamin C to keep your cushions free from rheumatism.

Some prefer celery seeds. Add one level teaspoonful of celery seeds to a teacupful of boiling water and steep until cold. Drink half a teacupful, morning and evening.

And so we could go on, indefinitely, with a host of herbal diuretics and alternatives, each with their reputation for relief: lignum vitae bark, poke root, etc., not to mention homoeopathic and vitamin therapies which can be effective. It is the work of the trained practitioner to be able to make a calculated selection from a vast number of remedies.

If you are troubled with the disorder, do not wait for the universal cure. Theories don't relieve pain. Sometimes we need to tackle the job ourselves after an intelligent reading up of the subject. Persistent morning stiffness with painful swollen joints need not appear if we rediscover Nature's way. A change of lifestyle can be your best prescription for preventing arthritis.

However, your life can still be well worth living, even if rheumatism insinuates its way into your body through no fault of your own.

Antioxidants

Antioxidants help protect the body cells and tissues against the damaging action of free radicals, which are toxic by-products of metabolism.

In a scientific study, it was found that high levels of antioxidants in the blood reduces the risk of heart disease. This is because antioxidants help protect body cells against the damaging action of free radicals.

The chief antioxidants: include alfalfa, fresh asparagus, beet tops, dandelion leaves, ginseng, gotu kola, goldenseal, parsley, walnuts and watercress. Perhaps the most effective is garlic.

Plenty of fresh fruit and vegetables are a ready source of antioxidants.

Corticosteroids

If possible we should try to avoid steroids. Why? Because they suppress symptoms of inflammation. There are rational objections to steroids. Bones and fibrous tissues are weakened. Water retention means there is a tendency to put on weight. Blood pressure rises and one might experience bruising of the skin with a known cause. If treatment has to drastically stop, the patient may have insufficient adrenal hormones from his/her own resources, thus creating a problem for the adrenal glands. Devil's claw is one remedy recognised as having a corticosteriod-like effect.

Free radicals

Free radicals are produced in the body by the breakdown of food to release energy in the presence of oxygen. They are oxidants. Oxidation is what causes a metal to rust, fats to go rancid and apples to go brown.

Free radicals are toxic to delicate mucous surfaces, enzymes and DNA. They are destructive in some degenerate conditions including arthritis and heart disease.

To combat these culprits requires adequate amounts of vitamin E (400iu daily) and carotenoid fruits and vegetables. Topline protection requires vitamins A, C and E against heart disease and cancer.

Devil's claw is a well-known anti-inflammatory.

Glucosamine

What is glucosamine? It is an amino acid formed in the body from glutamic acid and glucose – one of the building blocks of cartilage, ligaments and tendons. It is necessary for the repair of worn-out cells.

Testimonials enthuse over its important role in the maintenance of healthy joints. It is usually combined with chondroitin to enhance the effect of glucosamine sulphate. It may also be found in combination with other anti-inflammatory remedies: ginger, bromelain, oily fish and vitamin C. It is available in the form of tablets for internal use, and creams for external use to nourish cartilaginous tissues. Some creams are made more effective by the inclusion of soothing natural essential oils (aromatherapy) i.e., benzoin, sage, rosemary or chamomile. We should not overlook the use of ginger for relief of painful knees. Chondroitin sulphate imparts to cartilage its resilient quality, enabling a joint to 'take the strain'. It is a component of cartilage, tendons and ligaments and, like glucosamine, is a shock absorber and joint lubricant.

According to an Australian study of forty-six sufferers: 'Glucosamine seems to provide benefits to people who have knee pain that is likely due to cartilage damage, and these benefits are most noticed in daily activities, such as walking,' said lead author Dr Rebecca Braham of Monash University (*British Journal of Sports Medicine*).

Homoeopathy

Rhus toxicodendron
From the earliest homoeopathic times, *rhus* has been the great rheumatic remedy of the school, comparing only with bryonia, and the difference between these remedies must be repeated once more.

Rhus tox
For those with a restlessness and desire to move about continually, on account of the relief it brings to the aches and pains.

Suitable especially for rheumatism affecting fibrous tissues, sheaths of muscles, etc. It is also suitable for rheumatism which comes about from exposure to dampness when overheated and perspiring.

Bryonia alba
The sufferer has a disposition to keep still, since moving causes an aggravation of all aches and yet sometimes pain forces patient to move.

Suitable for rheumatism of the joints and of muscular tissue itself.

This is not especially the case with bryonia, though a bryonia rheumatism may occur from these causes.

Tinnitus

What is this thing called tinnitus? Specialists refer to it as hyperaesthesia of the auditory nerve and will tell you that even the faintest sounds may be heard with painful intensity. Paralysis of the stapedius muscle may also cause abnormal auditory sensation.

Noises in the ears are described as humming, buzzing, whistling, hissing or like thunder over the hills. It is common in people over forty years of age and can severely reduce the quality of life. It is usually linked with deafness, however slight the hearing loss is due to damage to the cochlea or inner ear.

Causes are legion. It may be due to genetic disorders, exposure to occupational noise or vascular lesions of the cerebral auditory centre. Trouble may arise when the lining of the eustachian tubes and parts of the inner ear become thickened and swollen by infection and catarrh, when adhesions may form.

Sodium salicylates have now been discontinued as a recognised medicine for rheumatism, yet the ears of many people over sixty may still be plagued with its persistent side-effects. Long distant effects of old-school drugs upon sensitive membranes are well documented in medical literature, aspirin and beta-blockers being offenders.

It is a symptom of Ménière's disorder where pressure of fluids in the middle ear affect the balancing mechanism. Chief cause would be a raised blood pressure. Other causes include the aftermath of a cold or flu for which a three-day fast is indicated with plenty of fluids and herb teas such as lemon balm, lemon verbena, elderflower, fennel, hibiscus, parsley, peppermint, rooibos (red bush), rosehip, sage, strawberry leaf, vervain and chamomile. In one severe case a free-lying hair was found on the ear drum.

It is believed there is a relationship between tinnitus and nutrition. A change in the diet to include more raw fresh fruits and vegetables is known to make a favourable change, especially in the presence of more vitamin E foods.

Scientists suspect a diet heavy in fats, sugar and white flour products, though others blame entry into the body of toxic heavy metals headed up by lead (lead water-carrying) pipes in old properties. Cadmium is known to cause dysfunction of the kidneys. Mercury (as in teeth-fillings) is known to have a toxic effect at capillary level.

Research has shown how patients with the disorder have reduced serum zinc levels, a deficiency of which can be restored by supplementation of 15mg daily.

If you find tinnitus difficult to live with, you may wish to try ginkgo which dilates peripheral vessels and ensures a good circulatory blood-flow within the ear.

Echinacea has a reputation for ear infections. Anxiety and tension worsen the disorder, calling for relaxing the body as opportunity permits.

Try listening to soothing music and avoid exposure to loud noises. Wearing a hearing aid has helped others. Cut back on coffee, alcohol, salt and smoking.

Are you sure your ears are not blocked up with wax? Your doctor or health consultant can check your ears for wax. Other agents which may prove helpful are rutin, chlorophyll and vitamin C. A standardized extract of ginkgo biloba, 120mg a day is known to maintain dilated blood vessels.

For more information contact the British Tinnitus Association on freephone 0800 018 0527.

8

Nature's Pharmacy:
A–Z of Beneficial Herbs

'Nature opened the first pharmacy', wrote Dr D. C. Jarvis. Primitive man and the animals depended on preventive use of its stock of plants and herbs to avoid disease and maintain health and vigour. Because man and the animals were constantly on the move, nature's drug store had branches everywhere. Wherever in the world you were sick, you would find in the field its medicine to cure you, its material for curative herbal teas and tizanes.'

The craft of healing by plants evolved from the hard-won experience of centuries. From time immemorial healing by herbs of the field have been offered as a relief from an open hand of a generous Creator for the ills of mankind. For ages it was the only form of medical treatment. Long before the Flood the Sumerian herbal was used by early physicians.

The Ebers Papyrus was a source of remedies used by the Temple physicians of Egypt for over 3,000 years. The ancient people of that land were an excessively clean people. Like the Jews, they were a 'washing' nation, with garlic high on their list of food supplements.

In the Bible we read that King Solomon knew all about the hyssop that grew on the wall. He tells us how he was acquainted with the diversities (virtues) of plants. It was a clump of figs clapped on King Hezekiah's ulcers, that cured. 'Give me some of your son's mandrakes,' demanded Rachel when seeking to give birth to a male child.

Do you remember how the Queen of Sheba brought spices, most precious, to Solomon? In those days, included among common spices were healing gums and resins, seeds and barks. 'Spices' were an important section of any primitive pharmacopoeia. She most certainly brought him cinnamon, turmeric, galangal, paprika, cloves and bay leaves – how these romantic names trip off the tongue!

Father of medicine

'Life is short, art is long, experiment uncertain, judgement difficult,' exclaimed the father of the art of healing, Hippocrates.

Hippocrates was born on the island of Cos, about 460 BC. He came from a long medical family and is believed to have lived to the age of ninety. He was one of Nature's botanist-physicians who used nothing but natural substances, selecting his materia-medica from the fields and forests of Asia Minor. His was the first scientific approach – associating plants with specific diseases.

Disciples of Hippocrates have come and gone. It was not until Paracelsus that their doctrine of 'nature cure' received a mortal blow. Perhaps the most enigmatic figure in medical history, this impetuous and turbulent genius was the first to introduce chemicals into the art of healing. Born into an era of alchemy and superstition, his use of mercury, arsenic and lead (all protoplasmic poisons) impressed the best scientific brains of his time and formed the foundations of modern chemical pharmacy.

To take a long and critical look at the treatments of Hippocrates is to reflect how little real progress we have made since he taught his pupils the basis of natural cure. His treatments were very sensible: fresh air, diet, rest, massage and herbs. His methods of treating spinal displacements were excellent, and would have delighted the heart of any osteopath.

But in the market square, people didn't think very much of Hippocrates' sober advice. They only partly followed him, quickly growing tired of his tedious routine when results were delayed. 'Can there be any virtue in wild thyme?' was a question raised by the militia when the common practice for battle wounds was searing with a red hot iron. The people craved something that smacked of the supernatural and spectacular.

A reappraisal and revaluation of Hippocrates' natural pharmacy at the present moment, when manufacturing chemists and druggists throughout the world flood the market with new synthetic drugs, would appear to be overdue. Some preparations coming into our doctors' surgeries contain aggregations of molecules which have never before been in this world, and whose long-term effects may never be known.

More members of the orthodox profession find themselves compelled to accept a an increasing weight of evidence surfacing in medical journals. There appears to be a growing tendency to accept truth from whatever source it may emerge. In the past, any medicine failing to see the light of day from the laboratory bench of a major drug foundation stood little chance of survival.

Since Thalidomide, drug-licensing regulations have been so stringent that five years could elapse before a new drug passes all the tests before being offered for sale in the shops. Blind and double-blind clinical trials may run into thousands of pounds. The question is often asked if it is reasonable to withhold from a sufferer from heart trouble the harmless traditional hawthorn berry until science has caught up with its *modus operandi*.

Folk medicines of known safety provide one quarter of the world's medical requirements. They are increasing at an impressive rate.

Thinking people everywhere eagerly seek effective alternatives to synthetic drugs by a return to the indigenous herbs of the East and the West. Major contributions come from modern China, India and Pakistan. Maybe we in the West can learn much from the old culture of the East, which married to our considerable wealth of expertise, could herald a new era in medicine.

Finns point the way
One by one, natural remedies are rediscovered and incorporated into ortho-dox medicine. Healing properties of seaweeds and lichens receive close scrutiny from research pharmacists seeking species to inhibit bacterial growth.

The Finns have been the first to exploit lichen antibiotics commercially. They extract an acid from reindeer mosses in Lapland and incorporate it in a salve. They say it is much more effective than penicillin salves for the treat-ment of external wounds and burns, and it has been used successfully to treat mastitis in cattle. A lichen acid in combination with streptomycin has been tested on tuberculosis patients with varying success.

In the handbook of the Smithsonian Institute, their official botanist, Dr M. E. Hale, Jnr reports how herbal extracts can act as potent antibiotics. 'During the Middle Ages, lichens held a high place in the pharmacopoeias of medical doctors. One was used to treat lung diseases because of its fancied resemblance to lung tissues.' The doctor is possibly referring to Iceland moss (*Cetraria islandica*) or polypody root (*Polypodium vulgare*). 'A widely used prescription for the treatment of rabies caused by rabid dogs called for half an ounce of one species of lichen mixed with black pepper. This mixture was taken for four consecutive days in a half-pint of warm milk. The Chinese and Seminole Indians use several kinds of lichens as medicines to this day.'

Today there is room for men and women using natural methods of healing, especially when fortified with a knowledge of herbs. A training course in the sciences is helpful, but not essential. Many proficient amateurs do not get as far as making it their profession, though the need is great. Some serve an apprenticeship with an established consulting herbalist.

What a wealth of vital information can be gleaned from health books today. Many contain facts which might prove useful when a family health crisis arises. Study of this engrossing subject can give life-long pleasure and interest. The list of favourite remedies in this chapter may be of help.

Back to nature

To do your best work you should feel secure about the remedies you use. Become an unashamed traditionalist. Think in terms of the 'comprehensive use of the whole plant'. Argue use of the 'whole' of the plant, with its complex of active components, minerals and vital properties enshrined in its structure. Be convinced that the best results are achieved when the remedy is used in its natural state.

Can we repudiate long traditional distinctions which have grown up around certain plants? Should herbs which have been in use for more than a millennia be on trial? You will find that after embarking along this path you, too, will be surprised at results achieved where drugs have failed.

Blood normalizers. All disease, sooner or later, reflects its presence in the blood. A deficiency of glandular secretion affects the behaviour of blood cells and lowers efficiency of the body's defence system. Over the course of time this places the body at risk.

An older generation of unregistered practitioners had a number of plants they called alteratives – because they 'altered the blood'. These blood tonics cover a wide range of remedies including blue flag root, red clover blossoms, barberry bark and yellow dock.

All alterative herbs influence the ductless glands such as the adrenals and thyroid. They also favourably affect the spleen. This is done by means of the chemicals they contain. They make a contribution to the body's nutrition, being rich in minerals absorbed into their structure from the soil in which they grow. In this way they act as an intermediary between animal life and man.

Though our knowledge of the first links in the chain of the ductless glands is far from complete, alterative herbs can be most powerful allies when things go wrong. Conveniently, they hasten renewal of tissues and endeavour to bring into harmony the function of the ductless glands.

It is known that much infection spreads via the lymphatic glands. These include a system of internal vessels through which toxins are eliminated. During this process the lymphatic nodes and vessels may become inflamed, as is so often seen in the case of a septic toe or finger when glands under the arm or in the groin are painfully swollen.

Though the spleen is seldom referred to as an organ of elimination it assists in removing by-products of inflammation. Herbal specifics for the spleen were in constant use among the older generation of practitioners.

Roots, such as yellow dock, are among the best remedies for the lymphatic system, when grown on the right soil. Success depends upon the quality of soil and the season harvested. Yellow dock restrains the onset of a number of chronic complaints, when the plant is right.

Dr N. G. Vassar, Ridgeway, Ohio, tells of a practitioner friend who had a blacksmith's shop near his property. This blacksmith cultivated docks for the doctor, pouring over them the washings from his cooling tank. At the end of the day a conglomerate of rust, iron, copper filings and the rest was tossed on the growing patch and left for the soil itself to sort out.

There never were yellow docks as flushed and up-standing as the ones carefully harvested by the doctor and made into concentrated fluid extracts. Vassar had a notion that this powerful blood purifier strengthened feeble constitutions, and slowed down the progress of degenerative disease.

How to use herbs

Herbs described in these pages are a very small selection of the large number available. Often, their best method of administration is by simple infusion (tea) or decoction. However, in the trained herbalist's dispensary will be found tinctures and extracts, etc.

Where preparation of the herb is not specified, the general rule is to place 25g (1oz) of herb in one pint (approx. 500ml) boiling water in a warmed vessel and allow to stand for fifteen minutes. This is strained and taken in divided doses throughout the day. Herbs used in this form of tea are of light structure, their constituents being soluble in water.[30]

The method of preparation for barks, roots and hard woody substances is by decoction. This is obtained by boiling, then simmering the herb in water. A decoction is usually made in the ratio of 25g (1oz) of the cut or crushed material simmered in one pint 500ml (1 pint) of water until the volume is reduced by one quarter. The whole is then cooled and strained and taken in divided doses according to the amount prescribed. Infusions and decoctions are not permanent preparations and should be prepared fresh daily.

Poultices are hot fomentations with the herb (marshmallow root, slippery elm bark, etc.) folded in linen or suitable material, as hot as can be borne. They are changed about every twenty minutes until relief is felt. To prevent scalding, the skin is wiped with a little olive oil.

Ointments are made by gently heating freshly ground herbs or spices (in a muslin bag) in fat or oil. The fat may be vegetarian cooking fat or lard. The herbal practitioner uses a cooking oil (olive or sunflower) with grated beeswax, the ratio being one part beeswax to ten parts oil. When all colour has been leeched out of the herbs, extraction is complete. The ointment can be strained and cooled and run into small pots or honey jars.

An interesting discovery[31]

Many people of the Western world suffer from peptic ulcers for which magnesium trisilicate and other chemical antacids are prescribed. Often referred to as gastric ulceration, treatments consist of reducing the level of stomach acidity. To achieve this, modern pharmacy enlists the aid of a multiplicity of drugs to help heal two million (mostly men) who, in Europe and the UK, suffer from this painful incubus. Conscientious, industrious and worthy citizens are its special victims. Doctors blame the stress of modern life.

If the peptic ulcer is the hallmark of today's busy executive, post–mortem figures are not reassuring. It is said that one in every ten has a healed or active lesion. Suffering is the word. For its victims, pain is almost continuous. (The past generation of doctors were clearly baffled by it). A Dutchman, Dr F. E. Revers, told of a lack of faith his ulcer patients had in his treatment, was surprised to see some of his most respected clients visiting a chemist's shop 'round the corner', to acquire some mysterious powder which seemed to bring a cure. His sense of curiosity was roused and, determined to discover reasons for the high level of cure, obtained some of the powder and had it analysed.

He was astonished to find it contained about 40% liquorice root. The laboratory report was most disconcerting. But he pursued the matter to its bitter end, and prescribed it for his ulcer patients.

More than a pain killer, results were startling. All made astonishing progress. Why hadn't this simple substance been used before? Wonder of wonders – his discovery met with the approval of colleagues and research authorities who confirmed its clinical efficacy.

Since Dr Revers made his discovery fewer stomach medicines have been flushed down the toilet – and all because of a legacy of days when great-grandma chewed black liquorice bootlaces on the way to school.

Theophrastus, (noted Greek physician, 332 BC), records how armies of the ancient world took it into battle with them for healing wounds. The quartermaster of Alexander the Great included it in the army's ration list. Soldiers chewed it to restrict temporarily the output of urine, preventing thirst and the necessity to drink.

Chinese records go back further. In the scrolls of Ts'ao medicine (3,000 BC), it 'preserved the life of men, keeping the body supple and enabling one to become old in years without causing ageing of the body.'

Mini-markets in the Middle Ages saw a steady sale of the root, before the days of sugar. Its important constituent 'glycyrrhizin' was not yet discovered, but it was as popular as the ginseng of the 1980s. Traders sold it as a salutary stimulant for the dried up glands of old men who found renewed youthful powers in their declining years. Little wonder it was once ascribed magical properties.

At the turn of the twentieth century, a number of Manchester physicians regarded it as a demulcent for sore throats. Mothers gave it to their children at bed-time to prevent bed-wetting. Before the days of Liquorice Allsorts confectionery liquorice tea was made from the shredded root.

Dr R. L. Sanders, physician, Prairie Point, Mississippi, reckons childhood's much-loved root is fifty times sweeter than cane sugar – yet it contains no sugar!

Dr Arthur Schramm, old-timer on the Canadian physio-medical scene, had a favourite prescription for 'acute' chests: 25g (1oz) each of – pleurisy root, marshmallow root, slippery elm bark and liquorice root. Placed in two pints of water, they were brought to the boil and simmered down to one pint. The dose: was one or two teaspoonfuls every half hour, taken warm.

It is still given as a 'sop' to hide the taste of nasty medicines. It is quite capable of acting on its own. One heaped teaspoonful of the shredded root in a teacupful of boiling water acting as a 'settler' for a queasy stomach. Tipplers still chew sticks to counteract effects of heavy drinking.

Shingles (*Herpes simplex*) can be exceedingly painful. Coming on suddenly, it may be related to chicken pox. It is possible for it to develop from a virus infection following contact with a child with chickenpox. At one time, liquorice root enjoyed a reputation in West Yorkshire for cutting short an attack of shingles. Now we know the reason. Dr Raffaelle Pompei and his colleagues at the University of Cagliari proved it inhibits growth of an impressive number of viruses.

Some people tire easily, having little stamina. Others endure temporary weakness of the adrenal glands. These glands regulate potassium use. If they are damaged the person feels weak, has flabby tissues, thick blood and poor circulation. He cannot eliminate the potassium taken in. Neither can he retain sodium and has to eat salt in heavy amounts. A recent study shows how effectively liquorice normalizes sodium/potassium levels of the body fluids.

The demand for sweets stimulates the liquorice Allsorts market. The world demand for liquorice is rising. Scandinavian countries and Finland have caught up with medical literature on the subject and offer supplies in a competitive market. In Russia it has always been an item of staunch pharmacy and national importance.

A–Z of beneficial herbs

Agnus castus *Vitex agnus castus, Linn*

This interesting alternative to drugs has been found to bear a special relationship to hormone imbalance in women. It rapidly acquires the reputation for relief of pre-menstrual tension, absence of monthly periods and pain in the breasts.

A particularly dramatic case concerned a woman of thirty-nine, whose marriage was at risk because she had not menstruated for over three years. This adversely affected her sex life. She lapsed into a personality change out of character with the disposition she once enjoyed.

One day, she visited her local doctor, not for this condition, but for simple acne vulgaris on the face – a cause of deep distress to many people. A herb, recently introduced into the UK and Northern Europe was recommended: *Agnus castus*. It was only with great difficulty that her husband persuaded her to take it.

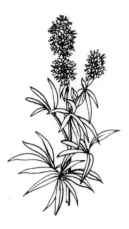

Agnus castus

She was told it acted as a 'precursor' – a catalyst which stimulates the body to produce its own hormones. Alkaloids of plants can provide a suitable stimulus to enable the body to synthesize its own enzymes. In short, they encourage the body to heal itself from its own resources.

A remarkable thing happened. The acne faded and disappeared. She began to feel better 'in herself'. Gradually, she found herself menstruating normally. Improvement continued until she regained her former vitality. Lively and full of energy, the subject of divorce was forgotten. 'A miracle has happened,' exclaimed her husband.

Vitex is prescribed by herbalists for gynaecological problems by helping balance hormone levels; a topline remedy in the world of alternative medicine for pre-menstrual tension. It is also an anti-depressant for mood-change and is useful for headache, bloating and breast fullness. Should not be taken together with progesterone preparations.

Cases are on record of the efficacy of Vitex for infertility and as an alternative to hormone replacement therapy.

Aloe vera *Aloe barbadensis*

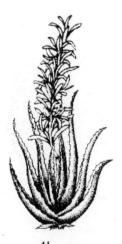

Aloe vera

Is a member of the lily family. Its juice contains important vitamins and minerals as well as enzymes and amino acids. It first appeared inscribed on the tombs of the Pharaohs where it was referred to as the miracle plant. Alexander the Great enjoyed the benefits of its leaves. Aloe vera has an impressive record for the successful treatment of acne, asthma, burns, scalds, indigestion, inflammatory bowel disease, bruises, colitis, and is a friend of the dentist. It brings relief to skin irritation in seconds.

Aloe is an antibiotic, astringent and anti-coagulant and may be used internally and externally. It also has a well-known record for haemorrhoids and bleeding piles, psoriasis, eczema, internal and external ulcers, stretchmarks of pregnancy, sore throat and scar removal.

As we grow older, 'brown liver spots may appear on hands and elsewhere. Some people claim the juice or gel of aloe applied two to three times daily removes them. A sixty-year-old lady on crutches with severe arthritis of the hip, found relief by taking 110g (4oz) of the gel every day. However, many people achieve good results on an ounce (25g (1oz) a day.

Cases are on record of the cure of rodent ulcer and prostate cancer. But it is in the care of the skin that aloe comes into its own. The wife of the writer had a skin cancer healed by aloe.

Aloe vera in combination with chamomile, peppermint and slippery elm offer a formidable solution of many digestive and intestinal problems. For constipation, one capsule of aloe latex a day for two weeks usually works the oracle.

Purchases should be cold-pressed and sorbital-free. Aloe can be easily grown in your own garden or conservatory. All you have to do is to cut off a piece and rub the juice over dry skin or a wound.

Artichokes *Cynara scolymus*

Were classified by a past generation of herbalists as a hepatic (liver remedy) to stimulate the flow of bile in chronic dyspepsia. It is a carminative (expulsion of wind); antispasmodic (relief of abdominal cramp); diuretic (increasing the flow of urine); and a liver restorative.

A number of studies confirm the benefits of artichokes for irritable bowel syndrome (IBS), whether manifesting as diarrhoea or constipation.

Helpful for dyspepsia, stomach cramps, nausea and gallbladder disorders. The artichoke is a healthful and appetising vegetable and adds variety to a meal.

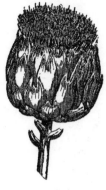

Artichoke

219

Artichokes are the diabetic's potato. They reduce fat in the blood and can be used with profit for gall bladder disorders, fluid retention, and high cholesterol levels. Rich in dietary fibre, they swell in the colon moving its contents in the right direction.

Artichokes have been used since biblical times and should not be confused with Jerusalem artichokes (*Helianthus tuberous*).

Dosage is usually one or two capsules of 300mg dried extract a day with meals. Patients with gallstones are advised to consult their doctor or health consultant before use.

Bearberry *Arctostaphylos uva-ursi*

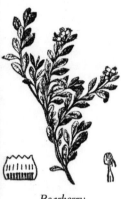

Known as bearberry because bears love the fruit. It has come to the fore as a diuretic and urinary antiseptic. Together with shepherd's purse it offers an effective haemostatic for the appearance of blood in the urine. Like cranberry it has become popular in recent years for bladder infection (cystitis).

Not to be taken in the presence of kidney disease or pregnancy.

Bearberry

Bilberry *Vaccinum myrtillus L.*

In the north of England and Scotland we can see bilberry bushes amongst the heather. Picking the juicy berries can be a very rewarding pastime, especially when gathered for bilberry pie.

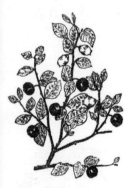

A grandfather said: 'Bilberries helped Grandma's arthritis,' containing properties that relieve muscular aches and pains, Grandpa didn't know why they helped, but he just knew they did!

Bilberries were a favourite food of those living in the Rocky Mountains and are now making their mark on the medical world.

'Bilberries may aid regeneration of the retina thereby dramatically increasing night vision,' says Michael McIntyre, Chairman of the European Herbal Practitioners Association.

Bilberry

Age-related macular degeneration (AMD) is the main cause of loss of sight. Bilberries can strengthen blood vessels. They are now linked with pycnogenol from the bark of the French maritime pine which is a powerful antioxidant and anti-inflammatory to protect capillary walls.

Paul Keogh, Herbalist, reported the following case: 'Frank, a farmer, who was nearly blind due to diabetic ophthalmic [eye] disease had his sight successfully restored after taking bilberry extract for three months. To the total amazement of the specialists he could resume the normal life on his farm. His blood sugar levels even significantly stabilized.'

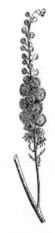

Black cohosh *Cimicifuga racemosa*

Said to be as effective as hormone replacement therapy for control of menopausal symptoms, black cohosh works powerfully upon the female reproductive system, reducing hormone-linked hot flushes and night sweats.

It is classified as anti-arthritic, anti-rheumatic, anti-inflammatory, spasmolytic and is believed to be of benefit in cases of brittle bones. Prescribed for cramps, lower back pain, and mood swings of the menopause.

Not advised during pregnancy, breast-feeding or for children.

Black cohosh

Blue flag *Iris versicolor*

Also called liver lily, and water flag, native American squaws collected it from the swamps of central North America for sick headaches. Dr E. Linnell reports cure of a sick headache of two years' standing which came on regularly after eating something sweet. Medieval European medicine knew the iris as the 'queen of flowers'. With it, no garden could look dull nor any apothecary's stillroom be without an effective liver remedy. Useful for swollen glands, cleanser of the lymph system and of value in right-sided shingles.

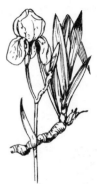

Iris is regarded as a detox remedy to accelerate elimination of body wastes, promoting a healthy flow of bile. It is a remedy for profuse saliva, tasteless belching, strong smelling sweat and rumbling in the bowels.

Blue flag

Borage *Borage officinalis L.*

Beekeepers cherish this plant which produces pollen-rich flowers from May until the early frosts. A past generation of farmers regarded it as a rich food for cattle in winter.

Borage seeds are high in linolenic acid (GLA) and are used as an anti-inflammatory, anti-fever and natural heart strengthener. Today its use as an anti-depressant is rediscovered.

As a regenerative anticoagulant, working without side-effects, it is given for cases of thrombosis and liver cleansing thus helping to banish melancholy.

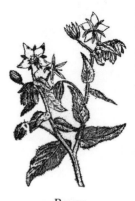

Borage

Romans infused the crushed leaf in their wine cups in the belief that it imparted courage.

In salads, tender young leaves exude a cucumber-like flavour. Tea made from fresh or dried leaves provide calcium, potassium and other vital minerals.

For a refreshing summer drink, infuse two to three fresh leaves and flowers in a jug of chilled homemade lemonade. Add honey if necessary.

Boswellia *Boswellia serrata*
An Indian plant resin used for rheumatic and arthritic conditions as it's an anti-inflammatory for aching joints and muscles. Popular as a cream (Boswellia Balm) used in massage for painful backs and joints offer a soothing comforting rub.

Bromelain *Ananassa sativa*
This enzyme, which comes from the stem of the pineapple plant, is a non-toxic aid to digestion and pain relief.

As an anti-coagulant it inhibits the clumping of blood cells, without side effects. Useful in many cases of inflammation, proving to be as effective as non-steroidal, anti-inflammatory drugs for soothing the discomforts of rheumatism and arthritis. It works well in combination with devil's claw. Usually taken as a dietary supplement.

Buchu *Agathosma betulina*
Often used as a urinary antiseptic or to relieve backache caused by tired, deficient kidney function. Buchu enjoys the confidence of the indigenous population of South Africa, being first used by the Hottentots who, besides using it for inflammation and irritability of the genito-urinary system, rubbed the oil on their bodies for preservation against ravages of the heat. Modern herbalism uses it for the relief of cystitis with pain, especially where caused by the organism E. Coli.

Calamus *Acorus calamus*
Sweet flag. An old favourite of the Dutch for gastritis and chronic dyspepsia. For colic and want of appetite. Maria Treben records the cure of a case of cancer of the stomach by placing a level teaspoonful of the root in a teacupful of cold water, to stand overnight, and to be drunk in sips throughout the following day.

Capsicum *Capsicum minimum*

Cayenne pepper plays an important part in natural medicine. You may recognize it as one of the peppers (African chillies). Dried pods are powdered and used to prepare a tincture for professional use. It is a favourite culinary item, used in exotic dishes and curries. For digestive organs debilitated by abuse or old age.

Use in medicine was discovered by Dr Samuel Thomson, son of a New Hampshire farmer, and founder of the Physio-Medical School of Natural Medicine in the USA at the beginning of the last century. Its use was recommended to his 3,000,000 faithful followers who regarded it as the purest and most natural stimulant known. Some say it is better than whisky.

Even a mere sprinkling of this fascinating spice in your favourite beverage or food sets red blood corpuscles racing; speeding up the interchange of oxygen and nourishment through the cell walls.

The older generation of herbalists believe cayenne to be a heart stimulant without parallel. After its initial action has passed off, it leaves no suspicious side-effects or depression. It reduces a rapid pulse by increasing the flow of blood to the surface of the body. For icy cold hands and feet in winter, a few grains in a favourite beverage generate a feeling of warmth and improve the circulation.

There are practitioners who prescribe it for its iron content, while others advise it to stimulate metabolism and increase resistance against disease.

One natural way of reducing a high body temperature is to 'sweat it out'. A cayenne-induced perspiration has something to commend it for getting rid of impurities.

A few shakes from the red-pepper pot aids digestion of eggs and dairy products. It makes a lively seasoning for winter soups, pasta and rice savouries. Fine flavours of herbs and spices give local cheese their distinctive character. Cayenne is still used in soft, bland cottage cheeses to which it imparts its own unique flavour.

A snip off one of those fiery little chillies in the teapot keeps out the cold, imparting a warm glow on a cold winter's day. Red pepper is for the diner who loves a bit of pungency.

Capsicum

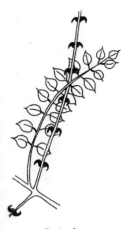

Cat's claw

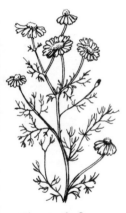

*Chamomile flowers
(German)*

Cat's claw *Uncaria tomentosa*
A powerful antioxidant, anti-tumoral, anti-inflammatory, anti-viral, and which is being used with some effect for treatment of cancer alongside other agents, but which is now a threatened species of the Peruvian rainforest.

Has been adopted with some enthusiasm for joint mobility and for the immune system. It is generally blended with ginger, cinnamon and cardamom, available as a powder in standardized doses but should be taken under the supervision of a qualified medical herbalist.

Chamomile flowers (German) *Matricaria recutita L.*
This is among the oldest of garden plants. Chamomile goes back to Roman times when it was recognized for stomach troubles. It is one of the gentlest sedatives we have, relaxing the central nervous system. It is ideal for nervous excitability, and has a special reference to the female reproductive system. It influences the ovaries, having been successful in cases of infertility.

The flower heads are plentiful, containing a volatile oil widely used in the healing art of aromatherapy. It is popular in Europe for restlessness and insomnia from stress conditions. An alternative to the teabags is to drink the fresh flower. Place three to five flower heads in a teapot and pour on boiling water. It is necessary to cover with a lid, when infusing, to prevent escape of the precious volatile oils into the atmosphere. A cup of chamomile tea is excellent for travel sickness.

It would be no exaggeration to say that on the European continent over a million cups are consumed every day. Has an affinity for the fifth cranial nerve, is of value for facial neuralgia. Its versatility relieves pre-menstrual tension (PMT) and hyperactivity in children.

Chickweed *Stellaria media*
Abbe Kneipp, nineteenth century German herbalist, also called 'the father of hydrotherapy' told his followers this was one of the best medicines for the chest. It has since proved to be a cooling agent as a diaphoretic for sweaty conditions. It is in use as an ointment for foetid ulcers and nasty painful eruptions. Also known as starweed, chickweed has come down to us through the great herbals from Grecian times. It is rich in

potassium, vitamin C and healing mucilage. It is helpful for the granulation of ulcers that refuse to heal, as a poultice of the fresh leaves. In *Grace* magazine, Miss Ann Bentley, writes of her experience of the dog, Kem, with an intolerable itch and eczema: 'Kem was a big dog, stripped of fur from chin to tail, underparts, thighs and lower back. After various treatments the vet advised them to have Kem put to sleep. However, I persuaded the owners to wash the dog in a brew of chickweed. They did so. In two weeks there was no sign of the trouble.

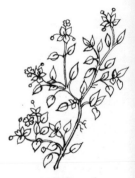

Chickweed

'I also told another owner, who had spent hundreds of pounds on veterinary surgeons, to use it on his dog, who was suffering from the same skin disease. Again, it cleared up in good time.'

According to Mrs Grieve, herbalist, the young leaves when boiled can hardly be distinguished from spring spinach and are equally wholesome.

It is a favourite for birds in cages when they go off their seed, and chickens also adore it.

Chlorella

This green food of single-celled algae is said to be richer in vitamins and minerals than many foods. As a supplement it contains all the naturally occurring amino acids and is complete in itself. It would appear that if there was one supplement alone that should be taken, chlorella would satisfy the body's daily requirements.

Chlorella is particularly rich in RNA and DNA, which are involved in body metabolism, growth and hormones for reproduction. It has the strange feature of being able to reproduce the plant within twenty-four hours.

As a detox remedy it is employed in nature cure homes, and sometimes advised for its chelating effect in binding with plant poisons and heavy metals prior to their expulsion from the body. It goes without saying it is a nutrient for the immune system.

Comfrey *Symphytum officinale*

'I called in to see a girl with gastric ulcer, haematemesis (vomiting of blood) and severe vomiting, and treated the case in the usual orthodox manner,' wrote a Lancashire physician. 'In three weeks the patient was able to return to the mill. When congratulating me on the girl's speedy recovery her mother said to me: "Do you mind me telling you something, Doctor?"

"No," I said.

"Well," she continued, "my girl has never had a drop of your medicine. All she has supped is pints of strong comfrey tea".'

He might have been intensely annoyed and denied the patient further consideration. But he was not that kind of man. With a certain sense of humility he confided his experience to a friend who was a distinguished consulting physician on the staff of the Liverpool Royal Infirmary. 'Since the occasion,' he admitted, 'I have found comfrey tea an excellent sedative for the gastric mucosa.'

The consultant was impressed. Conducting research at the hospital he was able to confirm the doctor's experience and used it for his own gastric ulcer cases. Though not the first to discover it, he found that the plant contained allantoin, which was known to stimulate tissue formation and speed up the healing of wounds. It has even cleaned up areas eroded with necrotic tissue followed by healthy tissue granulation.

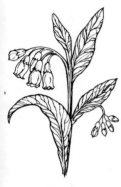

Comfrey

I, myself, used this many-sided healer most days in my forty years active practice and it is no exaggeration to repeat that it was one of the herbalists' sheet-anchors of the past. I was taught to use it by that fine old East Midlands herbalist, Edgar G. Jones, whose busy surgery attracted people from all over the UK.

My first experience was the case of a Sheffield saw-doctor whose power-driven saw, in a split second, severed three fingers from his hand. The remaining little finger hung on by a thread. The miracle was that Jones was able, not only to attain first-degree healing, but to save the little finger so that in future years the patient had the use of thumb and little finger to handle weights and carry on his job. The news spread. Edgar Jones was able to help the healing of bones which refused to 'knit', considerably shortening patients' attendance at the local Fracture Clinic.

One of the old country names for comfrey is 'knit-bone'. It was given this name because it promoted formation of a 'callus', which is an exudate deposited around fragments of a broken bone and which accomplishes the work of repair. A deficiency of calcium in the body can delay formation of a callus. It is the purpose of allantoin in comfrey to mobilize body calcium reserves and hasten healing.

It is a true nature-remedy, increasing the speed at which cells divide (mitosis). I have had many cases of chronic leg ulcers which, failing to respond to other forms of treatment, have skated away when comfrey tea has been drunk freely and the crushed root applied externally as a poultice. Very fine work on delicate tissues can respond well to this 'woundwort'. Symphytum means 'I cause to grow together'. Officinale means it was regarded as 'official' medicine as prescribed by doctors and apothecaries of the past.

Operations to rejoin a severed arm or leg to the body after accidents, which years ago would have maimed a victim for life, are one of the modern marvels of micro-surgery. Operations involve rejoining the bones of a severed limb, reconnecting the blood vessels and nerves, bringing the lacerated muscles together and stitching the skin. Powerful microscopes are needed for the operation and surgeons are trained in new techniques.

And yet, there are cases where healing is tardy and complete union delayed because tissues fail to granulate. It is due, among other things, to a lack of essential minerals in the blood. This is where comfrey can be of untold assistance because of its rich mineral complex. Add to this, the invaluable allantoin it contains, and the success rate of microsurgery could be high.

Miss Wicksteed of Berkshire, a reader of *Grace* magazine, sustained a severe injury to her knee, with a break across the tibia plateau condyle. The bone was severely crushed and the joint cracked. Consultants were amazed that it knitted so quickly. They expected to have to 'pin' the bone. The day after the accident she commenced the comfrey treatment, taking a double dose of the remedy three times daily. She continued until the bone was mended.

The tea may be made by placing three or four heaped teaspoonfuls of comfrey leaves into a teapot and pouring on boiling water. It needs a good stir and will be ready after fifteen minutes.

Dr Charles MacAlister MD, FRCP, had his own method of preparation which he described in his book: 'Use a liquidizer or other juicer. Take about four large leaves plus half a teacup of water, liquidize and put through a sieve – it will make a glass of bright green fluid without very much taste which can be drunk easily. This is comfrey without its fibre, containing most of its proteins and vitamins, with the bulk of its nutritionally useful minerals.

'It should always be made fresh, for it ferments rapidly In Britain it is available from March to early November. Plants for drinking should be picked in turn, and those which run to stem must be cut down to ground level so that they grow more leaves to maintain the supply. Because it is rich in vitamin C it is excellent for colds, and allantoin appears effective in relieving throat irritation and huskiness.'

For fractured limbs a poultice may be made from the crushed root and applied externally.

Claims that comfrey is a toxic plant are unsubstantiated by a mass of clinical evidence to the contrary. Attempts to equate the effects of its isolated constituents apart from the whole plant yield conflicting results.

For thousands of years the plant has been used by ancient and modern civilizations for healing purposes. Risks must be balanced with benefits.

Experiments reveal that in sufficient doses comfrey can cause liver disease in laboratory animals. Its risk to humans has been a subject of serious debate since the 1960s, and is still unresolved. Although the overall risk is very low, a restriction has been placed on the plant as a precautionary measure.

Fresh comfrey leaves should not be used as a vegetable, which is believed to be a health risk. It is believed that no toxicity has been found in common comfrey. No restriction has been placed on the use of dried comfrey leaves as a tea.

It would appear that use of the root of Symphytum officinale may be justified in the treatment of severe bone diseases, for which it has achieved a measure of success throughout medical history, such as rickets, Paget's disease, fractured bones, tuberculosis etc., its benefits outweighing risks. Few other medicinal plants replenish wasted bone cells with the speed of this plant.

There is a growing body of opinion to support the belief that a herb which has without ill effects been used for centuries and capable of producing convincing results is to be recognized as safe and effective.

For over forty years I have used the officinale in a busy herbal practice with no known toxicity.

Cramp bark *Viburnum opulus*
Also known as snowball tree and high cranberry. As its name suggests it is used for cramps and spasms. Angina pectoris is a cramp-

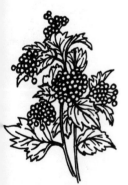

Cramp bark

like pain of the heart muscle which may yield to this spasmolytic nervine. It is used for lower-back pain as supportive treatment by some osteopaths and chiropractors. Helpful for pain in the calves on walking and writer's cramp. The present-day herbalist prescribes it for palpitation and clutching pains around the heart, which get worse on exertion. It works well with hawthorn for cardio-vascular conditions.

Cranberries *Vaccinium macrocarpon*

Traditionally related to roast turkey, especially in America on Thanksgiving Day, we are now discovering how this little berry is an effective natural ally against E. Coli infection present in cystitis.

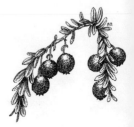

Cranberries

Cranberries contain Vitamins A and C, iron and potassium. They are crammed with other useful nutritional assets and are believed to reduce the risk of cancer, particularly of the stomach. They are today advised also for heart and circulatory disorders.

These small brilliantly red berries are also high in antioxidants. Some researchers claim them of value for dental plaque.

The pure juice is rather bitter and unpalatable and is usually diluted to about 25% juice. For cystitis the Cranberry Information Bureau recommends 300ml (10fl oz) per day for an active urinary infection, and 200ml (7fl oz) per day for maintenance of urinary health and comfort.

You should find cranberries in the dried fruit department of your supermarket. Sometimes they are heavily sugared, so make sure you check the nutrition label. Also check for undesirable chemical sweeteners.

In alternative medicine the berries are sometimes combined with Uva ursi, another valuable anti-bacterial herb with antiseptic properties for the urinary tract. More men take the juice for prostate outflow problems.

Sir Kenneth Calman has warned about overdosing with antibiotics for cystitis. Perhaps we should consider the humble cranberry?

Cranesbill *Geranium maculatum*

Cranesbill or the dried rhizome is a perennial herb indigenous to Canada and the United States. An anti-haemorrhagic, styptic astringent, it is used for internal bleeding of the genito-urinary

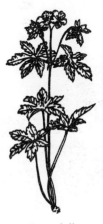

Cranesbill

organs and upper alimentary canal as well as peptic ulceration, melaena, piles, diarrhoea and heavy menses. The decoction may be used as a douche for leucorrhoea (vaginal discharge); as a wash for external ulcers which refuse to heal; or as a gargle for quinsy and mouth ulcers. Combines well with comfrey. Its chief use is for frequency of urine in the incontinent, and bed-wetting in children.

Damiana *Turnera diffusa*
Mexican aphrodisiac for men.

Dandelion *Taraxacum officinale*

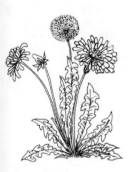

Country folk will tell you dandelion is a medicine chest in itself. It is a mild laxative for habitual constipation, strengthens feeble arteries, promotes sweating (for those of dry skin), and is an effective expectorant for congestive chest conditions. Old gardeners were in the habit of chewing the root for temporary kidney hold-ups.

Being a cholagogue, it is helpful to counteract any tendency to form gallstones. It is a fine digestive and liver tonic. It acted successfully on liver damage caused by carbon tetrachloride poisoning. Its special job seems to be to keep the liver sweet and clean, that organ being the largest gland and general cesspool in the body.

Dandelion

I use dandelion to assist the liver in the formation of bile. As a bitter tonic, it stimulates action of the pancreas. That is why dandelion root is often found in prescriptions for troubles of that organ. Most people know that it is a first-class diuretic. Helpful for the early stages of cirrhosis of the liver, it is also used for jaundice and inflammation of the gall bladder.

A wealth of anecdotal evidence of its efficacy has grown up around this ubiquitous and far-from-useless plant.

There are no chemicals or preservatives in dandelion coffee, which is caffeine free. Dandelion leaves can be cooked the same as for spinach in very little water before mixing with a little seasoning and butter. They add a piquant flavour to salads.

Devil's claw *Harpagophytum procumbens*
Devil's claw has been used for centuries by the indigenous population of Central Africa. It grows naturally in the Kalahari Desert on red sandy soil, its shape resembling a large scrawny

spider with barbed hooks that get caught in the hide of animals, especially on the wool of sheep. It is known as grappleplant and wood spider. After rainfall, water is stored in fat tubers for survival during times of drought.

The root system of this extraordinary plant penetrates the soil to a great depth, enabling the plant to 'pull up' a whole complex of minerals from far below the surface.

For some curious reason the plant failed to bloom for a number of years. When flowering eventually returned, the occasion created such a stir that attention of the local inhabitants was again focused on its healing properties. Today it is classified as an anti-rheumatic, analgesic (mild), diuretic, detoxicant, digestive and lymphatic. It is also a cholagogue for gallstone disorders, liver congestion and itchy skin conditions.

At one time it was used for malaria before the discovery of quinine. But it is for arthritis, stiff joints, polymyalgia and inflammation of the veins that it is now used worldwide.

As an anti-inflammatory, it is capable of reducing pain and swelling as in lumbago and gout. Today, it is one of the most popular supplements for lower-back pain and fibromyalgia, others being glucosamine and chondroitin.

Devil's claw has been used with success for osteoarthritis, which largely affects the shoulders, hips and knees, and for rheumatoid arthritis which may attack smaller joints. Decrease of pain is reported, together with improved mobility within a few weeks of treatment. After five weeks some patients were able to reduce their dosage. The conclusion is the remedy is both safe and effective.

The discovery of this versatile plant brought to the world a new anti-inflammatory and healer of great power. But the welcome outcome is that in all the many hundreds of tests carried out by research workers, little evidence has been found of toxicity. This means if you have an arthritic condition, it has no injurious side effects and you can go ahead with confidence.

Dose: two 480mg standardized extract tablets daily. Avoid in pregnancy, breast-feeding and gallstones.

Echinacea *Echinacea angustifolia. E. pallida, E. Purpurea*
Also known as black sampson and cone flower. There are so many powerful, yet harmless, healing plants that one may be guilty of excessive enthusiasm. This stimulating blood tonic is a great

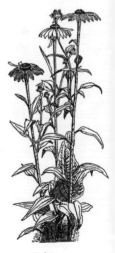

Echinacea

'purifier'. A badly ulcered leg of twenty years standing, healed rapidly after it was treated with this. Once used by the 'outback' doctors who attended the first settlers beyond the prairies (it grows freely from Minnesota to Texas). It is now seen as an antibiotic increasing the white corpuscles of the blood. In doing so, it builds up the body's immune system for the destruction of harmful bacteria.

When other agents have failed echinacea has been known to be helpful for chronic sinusitis, urethritis, dermatitis and nasty irritative skin rashes, endometritis (inflammation of the lining of the womb), mastitis, discharging ears, laryngitis and ill-effects from vaccination, and varicose ulcer.

Echinacea should not be taken for such progressive diseases as multiple sclerosis, tuberculosis, HIV infection or leukaemia. Dose: 250–300mg standardized extract, three times daily.

Echinacea is one of the polycrests of the herbal world, its versatility increasingly recognized.

Elderflowers *Sambucus nigra*

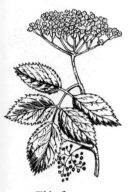

Elderflowers of black elder is common in open woods and hedgerows. To make you sweat-out a fever and effect a reduction of temperature in influenza and colds. The elder combination of elderflowers and peppermint herb are a well-known recipe, taken as a tea, for winter's chills. It may be used as a gargle for tonsillitis and stomatitis (inflammation of the mouth) as well as for catarrh. It works well when taken with yarrow.

Elderflowers

Evening primrose oil *Oenothera biennis*

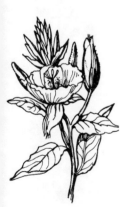

To watch the beautifully shaped buds of this plant open is like observing a butterfly emerge from its pupal chrysalis. Lovely and fragile petals reveal a heart of the purest yellow, as incandescent as the moon itself.

The name is derived from *iones* (wine) and *thera* (hunt) and was given to it by Theophrastus for over-indulgence on the bottle.

Primrose attracts attention in the medical journals for its ability to reduce blood-clotting time as an anti-coagulant, which is of value for thrombosis, and to stop platelet-clumping. Rich in linolenic acid, it is a fatty acid essential for the production of prostaglandins which are necessary for cholesterol control, regulation of blood pressure and of the menstrual

Evening primrose oil

cycle. Has been given with success for Raynaud's disease, pre-menstrual tension and breast pain. It is said to delay the progress of multiple sclerosis. Primrose helps regulate cell growth and maintains a balance of the hormone system. The average dose is 500mg, twice or three times daily.

The whole plant may be used as a demulcent and nutritive, the roots 'put down' into pickle or together with tomatoes into chutney.

Doctors at Bristol Royal Infirmary reported significant improvement in cases of eczema in their study of the plant.

Eyebright *Euphrasia officinale*

Eyebright is an intriguing plant growing half hidden in long grass in meadows and moist verges. It doesn't grow readily in gardens, and depends upon the protection of its host plant.

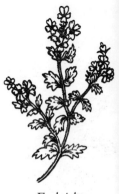

Eyebright

Some of our most effective remedies are parasites. Mistletoe, for high blood pressure, enjoys the company of its host which might be oak, poplar or apple. Eyebright is no exception, relying on the roots of grass for its nutrition.

How expressive can be the local names of plants! This elegant little healer wears a necklace of charming synonyms: eye-comfort, 'casse-lunette', augentrost, and bright-eye. It flowers from June to August.

The Greeks called it Euphrosyne, one of the three graces of their mythology meaning 'gladness', the preservation of eyesight in old age bringing gladness. Villanovanus, living in the thirteenth century, recorded how 'Euphrasie makes a precious water (eye lotion) to clear man's sight.'

Early physicians believed that plants bore certain symbolic marks which gave an indication of the disease for which nature intended them as special remedies. Although this doctrine brings us into a wide region of surmise and divination between the plant and its image, there may appear to be a case for science to investigate.

Many names witness to a belief in the doctrine of signatures. A mandrake root bears a crude resemblance to the body of a man (as does ginseng!); kidneywort is shaped like a kidney. Because of a black pupil-like spot on its flowers, eyebright is supposed to be good for the eyes.

Scores of examples can be advanced for this primitive belief. Yellow turmeric was thought to be good for yellow jaundice.

We wonder how far the use of milkwort for nursing mothers was due to the udder-like shape of its flowers, or because it really did work – assisting the body in laying down calcium and other salts in the developing foetus and ensuring a smooth easy delivery. Birthwort looks like a womb.

It is necessary to repeat eyebright eye baths daily for conjunctivitis, corneal opacity, thickening or white patches on the cornea. Eyebright lotion once enjoyed a wide use among practitioners looking for alternatives to boracic and the mercury of golden-eye ointment. It is available from health stores and herbalists.

Those who wish to prepare by the simple home method should place one teaspoonful of the dried herb into a teacup and fill with boiling water. Allow to cool. Strain when cold. This may be taken in wineglassful doses before meals, three times daily, internally. To use as a lotion, half fill an eye bath and use as a douche, warm or cold according to preference.

Eyebright is not at its best as a compress, a warm compress of chamomile flowers often bringing a treatment to a successful conclusion.

It might be called to mind where visual acuity is poor due to overstrain or from metabolic disorders. Think of diabetes!

The infusion (tisane) may be drunk by the wineglassful, two or three times daily before meals, for children and adults with a history of runny eyes, sneezing, catarrh and hay fever.

The busy practitioner will see scores of cases whose eye troubles have been caused by an attack of measles. You, too, will have seen people with a thick red rim around their eyes, and an absence of eyelashes. You'd be surprised how many of them would turn out to have had measles.

This gift from the ancient world may be used internally for measles with strong eye symptoms. It makes a useful protective for children and others when the complaint is in the neighbourhood.

'I have been credited with working magic,' said Maurice Mességué, the natural healer from France (1880–1978) who perhaps had a bigger following than any other through his practice and his published books. 'But I use only my natural medicines.' With his herbs, Mességué stimulated the natural health movement.

Feverfew *Chrysanthemum parthenium*

It was in his famous Herball (1597) that John Gerard, early herbalist first drew attention to this garden weed of white daisy-like flowers with yellow centres. Feverfew, also known as nose-bleed, bachelor's buttons and headache plant, was found by Gerard to be growing on a rubbish dump, spreading profusely without any encouragement. He writes of its use in dizziness:

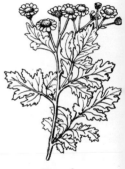

Feverfew

'Feverfew dried and made into powder, and two drams of it taken with honey or sweet wine dispels melancholy and phlegm; there it is good for those that are "giddy in the head", or who have the turning called vertigo – that is, a swimming in the head.'

Two hundred years later, Dr John Hill, an apothecary of Covent Garden, London, again took up the theme: 'In the worst headache, this herb exceeds whatever else is known.'

But it was another 200 years when the wife of a Cardiff doctor overcame a lifelong migraine with this strong-smelling perennial plant. Through television and radio the cure was soon taken up by other sufferers who expressed enthusiasm. Soon, a number of laboratories took up the challenge and a lot of anec-dotal evidence amassed. Seven out of ten patients claimed their migraine was less frequent and less painful.

Throughout history the herb has been used for fevers hence its name. A decoction, with honey, is a traditional remedy for colds, especially those which 'go down on the chest'. A cold infusion was taken as a tonic.

The diverse activities of this plant are believed to be due to prostaglandins responsible for the constriction and dilation of blood vessels of the brain, which occurs in many attacks of migraine. It encourages anti–platelet activity, thus reducing the risk of coagulation of blood. Among other healing components are those of a phospho–lipase inhibitor which is responsible for its anti–fever activity.

By eating two or more leaves of the fresh plant in a sandwich, sufferers from chronic headache claim relief. Others prefer to drink it in teacupful doses as a simple herb tea – two to six leaves in a special teapot kept for this purpose because its action is viti-ated by deposits of brown tannin on the inside of the average teapot.

It does not yield the same results where water is boiled in aluminium vessels or where aluminium teapots are used. Its

235

preparation should be kept as simple as possible, its power being lost in the presence of strong chemicals.

Daily dose of tablets is up to 200mg. Continue for at least a month for results.

In the days of Dr Hill, it was used to antidote the effects of mercury which was an ingredient of some medicines. Mercury is no longer used in medicine, but is today an environmental poison. Could it be that feverfew will prove effective in dealing with this menace, after appropriate experimental work?

Garlic *Allium sativum*

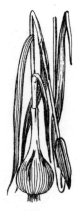

Garlic

Garlic is an excellent spasmolytic (for relief of spasm and tension) and expectorant, for loosening phlegm. It can be used as an anthelmintic, for expulsion of worms and an anti-viral, to act as an antiseptic for bacterial invasion. Garlic prevents a cholesterol build-up in the blood, and is therefore good for thrombosis and high blood pressure. May drastically reduce the level of sugar in the blood, which should assist insulin in the treatment of diabetes. The purifying power of garlic has been known since its use by the builders of the Cheops pyramid.

Dr Kristine Nolfi mentions that in Yugoslavia and Bulgaria garlic is used in almost every household every day. She draws attention to the fact that in those countries many individuals live to over 100 years, and are still able to do a good day's work. 'Garlic,' she says, 'has a strengthening effect, lowering too high blood pressure and raising one that is too low.' Of its 5,000 years of history, its use in paroxysmal sneezing is quite recent. During the plague, no sickness was found in houses in which this vegetable was consumed. The usual objection to its use may be removed by chewing a sprig of parsley which soon erases the smell from the breath.

Researchers led by Dr Ron Cutler, the University of East London, confirmed that allicin in garlic is highly effective against MRSA, the antibiotic 'superbug' which brought some hospitals to a standstill. It could save many lives.

This remedy is a welcome alternative to aspirin, reducing platelet clumping and improving blood flow by relaxing smooth muscle cells in the walls of blood vessels. Heating destroys some of its biological activity.

A man aged fifty-one, 100% disabled, with myocardial infarction (heart lesion) was due to enter hospital for thirty-two days. He was told he could do no more work for the rest of his life – he had about six to eight years left. After ten years he can now climb five flights of stairs, and has gone back to work. Instead of hospital treatment, he settled for garlic, mild exercise and elimination of salt.

Dose: 500–600mg daily or fresh bulb at table. Not to be taken with other anti-coagulants or aspirin.

The Mediterranean diet is reputed to be among the healthiest in Europe, particularly for heart health. One of its chief ingredients is garlic.

Gentian *Gentiana lutea*

Gentian has always been used as a tonic for indigestion and lack of appetite. It is popular in Germany where it is known as Gelberenzian. Country names are bitterwort, bald money, yellow gentian, fillwort, and *Gentiane jaune* (France) and *Genziana gialla* (Italy).

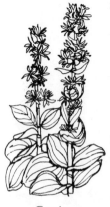

Gentian

It enters into wine-making in Europe where it is used as an aperitif. The Swiss ferment is for such wines as enzieu to impart stamina on mountain travel. The Chinese use ginseng for the same purpose – to allay effects of severe physical exhaustion. Gentian lacks the aphrodisiacal properties of ginseng.

The plant was named after Gentius, King of Illyria, (second century BC), who had a passion for botany and who 'proved' this one on himself.

It would appear that Hungary owes a special indebtedness to this legendary invigorator. It was there that King Ladislaus Gentian prayed to be divinely guided to a forest medicine he could use against the spread of plague. Throughout the year the pestilence raged. Firing an arrow into the air he requested guidance and heavenly intervention. Courtiers cried aloud when the arrow pierced a root of gentian. Legend has it that from that hour the city was saved.

Unlike many medicinal plants gentian has no virtue in its leaves – it is all in the intensely bitter root. It has been given with success in cases of anorexia nervosa, which some believe is largely a psychological condition. It is still given for achlorhydria (want of stomach acid), nausea, bitter taste in the mouth, dry mouth, for recuperating from debilitating attacks of influenza and other illnesses, and to accelerate recovery from surgical operations.

Being a powerful gastric stimulant it was not overlooked by the Elizabethan nobility. A knob of the root sucked before a banquet was regarded as a suitable preparation for the night's excesses in which one was likely to consume not less than twenty eggs, hunks of meat and bread washed down by liberal draughts of English mead.

This is one of the few roots to be steeped in cold water before use. One teaspoonful is placed in a teacup and filled with cold water at night. It can be strained and drunk the following day before meals in wineglassful doses. A nugget of liquorice chewed afterwards offsets the bitterness.

A homemade tincture may be prepared by macerating the root in vodka for eight days, shaking vigorously each day. It is then filtered, and twenty to thirty drops in water taken to ensure your gastric juices get the message.

Ginger *Zingiber officinalis*

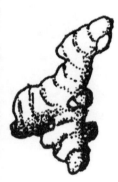

Ginger

Of the family Zingiberaceae is an exotic plant from the East. Like ginkgo, it is a peripheral vasodilator opening up the veins in the extremities. The circulation is thus improved and the heart stimulated, strengthened in its beat, with improvement in the bloodflow.

A Japanese study found that while blood pressure was reduced, ginger slowed down the heartbeat, giving it greater force.

We think first of garlic or onions as anti–coagulants, but it has now been discovered that ginger is equally effective for thinning the blood and reducing cholesterol levels. It is not indicated for those on doctor's prescriptions for the heart or ginger for blood thinning.

Ginger is of value in pregnancy and there are no unpleasant side-effects when taken for morning sickness; oral dose: 250mg before meals and at bedtime.

Ginger stimulates digestion by increasing bile secretion and springs to mind for flatulence and stomach cramps, but for young children chamomile is recommended.

In recent years it has been recognized as a remedy for the prevention of travel sickness, when a knob of crystallized ginger brings relief.

Ginger is a useful expectorant for a productive cough. Though not as potent as myrrh, it is a useful antiseptic against streptococcus and certain other bacteria.

Marked improvement has been found by a number of scientific investigators in that it can reduce joint pain in arthritic subjects. It is an anti-inflammatory for osteo and rheumatoid arthritis.

A cup of ginger tea and a warm ginger compress comprising a hand towel saturated with ginger tea, wrung out before application, can take the dull-ache out of period pains.

For old age in winter there are few things as effective as ginger tea to give the body added warmth and a comfortable feeling. It should not be taken in heavy doses. Place ¼–½ teaspoon powdered ginger into a warmed teapot and pour on freshly boiled water; replace the lid to prevent the escape the vapour of its essential oil into the atmosphere.

Other conditions in which it has proved helpful are: the common cold for which it is a useful diaphoretic to promote sweating and to replace the initial chill with a glowing warmth; in diabetes it reduces blood sugar.

Many conditions related to a poor circulation feel its benefit, such as Raynaud's syndrome (scleroderma) where it has been known to reduce the numbness.

As a massage oil place five drops of ginger essential oil into an eggcup of almond oil. Gently mix. This is sufficient for one massage session for aches and pains in muscles and joints.

Ginger is a first-class remedy but is contra-indicated in patients presenting with gall bladder disorders and gallstones. It should never be taken in excess when it might interfere with a doctor's treatment for diabetes, heart troubles and thrombosis, burning skin diseases, peptic ulcer or high temperatures.

It should not be taken with aspirin or other anti-coagulants. If you are taking medicines for nausea or sickness, first check with your doctor or health consultant.

Ayurveda, the traditional healing system of India records the virtues of over 700 plants of which ginger is an important medicine. Today 50% of all Chinese medicine contains Ginger.

Ginger beer still has a brisk sale in some of our northern cities. Crystallized ginger makes delicious confectionery. Its use in the kitchen adds zing to a number of foods.

Ginger covers a wide range of ailments including: sinusitis, hiccups, varicose veins, period pains, hypothermia with increase in body heat for cold hands and feet.

So you see, ginger has a real wealth of benefits to offer.

Ginkgo *Ginkgo biloba*

Maidenhair tree or ginko is one of the oldest trees on the planet.

As we grow older our memories deteriorate through living in these stressful days. This is a herb to remember.

In Germany, ginkgo is one of their highest sellers for heart and circulation. In that country it is known for anti-ageing, headache and impairment of brain function. It is a powerful antioxidant, anti-inflammatory and anti-depressant. It has restored hearing in cases of temporary deafness, reduced 'head noises' of tinnitus and alleviated dizziness. Is also prescribed for asthma, fibromyalgia, carpal tunnel syndrome, varicose veins and as a tonic to enhance well-being.

Average dose: 40mg three times daily. Should not be taken with anti-coagulants or aspirin.

Ginkgo is a fillip to the over-nineties for sharpness.

Ginseng *Panax Ginseng*

Asian Ginseng meaning 'cure-all', is widely known in the Far East by a number of names lauding its exceptional properties. 'Herb of eternal life' and 'king plant' may be sufficient to convey to the uninitiated the deep regard with which it is held by rich and poor.

A mystery plant to the West until quite recently, ginseng has always excited the curiosity of travellers who recorded the fascinating characteristic of its root: that it is similar to the shape of a man, hence its name 'man's root'.

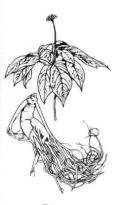

Ginseng

This elixir of life to the early mandarins is a member of the Araliaceae family with an attractive green foliage, white flowers, and intensely crimson fruit which appears at maturity.

Ginseng is the most temperamental of plants, but because it is such a money-spinner its growers can pardon its idiosyncrasies. It grows in the mountain woods of Asia, preferring to be in the dark or feeblest light. That is why, in its wild state, it flourishes in sensitive colonies within the shade of dark, damp woods.[32]

It has grown wild for untold centuries in China and Siberia. At the present point of history, it is also very successfully cultivated on the green hills of Korea where conditions and climate are uniquely right.

Ginseng is so precious to the Chinese that there were times

in the past when it was almost literally worth its weight in gold. In today's plantations a regular 'look-out' is seated on a platform in every compound, alert for thieves. It was not so very long ago that a purse full of stolen ginseng could be exchanged as currency in payment of goods or services.

Ginseng reaches maturity six years, though it may live from forty to sixty years. Some plants are reputed to be as old as 200 years, but they are very scarce. The young ginseng plant is the object of watchful attention, and it should be treated with the care you would give a child. This is especially true as governments realize its value as a fertile source of revenue.

In China, Korea and Russia every ginseng plantation has to be registered and the crop, without exception, is sold to the government. This precious asset is not just dug up out of the earth; it is handled with the utmost care, washed, brushed with a soft brush and subjected to a painstaking curing process by drying and steaming.

Standards of excellence are achieved by skills handed down in families for generations. The best roots – 'Imperial Ginseng' – fetch a fabulous price and in China were once seized for the Emperor's pleasure.

The Koreans run an efficient state-run industry, in the charge of highly qualified scientists and pharmacists. Something about the ginseng explosion galvanized the Korean nation into a consciousness of its key position as a supplier of the international markets for this new beverage and medicine.

A wave of enthusiasm has hit the West, confirmed by articles on ginseng in scientific journals. Authoritative works on Far Eastern pharmacy now appear regularly in the medical bookshops as China impresses the world with its astounding marriage between the orthodox and the unorthodox. No longer are medical practitioners contemptuous of the efforts of native healers but, taking them into their confidence, have come to terms with an unexpected number of one-time killers. This is the more remarkable when we consider their formidable history of cholera, smallpox, plague and venereal disease. Now, for the first time for untold centuries these afflictions are not merely being suffered, but are being fought. Some with the aid of ginseng.

A writer records a thrilling bit of history. 'The latest discovery from China is ginseng, the rejuvenation herb, considered by the Chinese as a panacea of all diseases. It is believed by its enthusiasts that ginseng overcomes disease by building up general vitality and resistance and especially by strengthening the endocrine glands, which control all basic physiological processes, including the metabolism of minerals and vitamins.

Chinese ginseng users consider as infantile Western attempts at rejuvenation by gland operations and treatment. Centuries of experience among millions of people have convinced them that in ginseng exists a natural method of rejuvenation, of restoring vitality to depleted glandular organs by feeding them the mysterious radioactive elements that ginseng has proven to contain.

Whatever happens on the world scene ginseng is likely to be the subject of worldwide research for a long time to come, especially for stress, heart and circulation. Stress causes more illness than is generally recognized. It is something we have to learn to live with in the modern world. This is an aspect in which the Russians are most interested – the anti-stress factor which they were able to harness and incorporate into their astronauts' daily regime.

There's more to ginseng than its aphrodisiac qualities. While not entirely sure how the root works, scientists agree on its general nerve tonic properties and salutary effect upon the central nervous system. For this purpose it can be found on sale in combination with bee pollen and vitamin E. Siberian ginseng has linked up with guarana, a Brazilian cocoa vine, the roasted seeds of which have been used by the Amazon Indians for centuries.

Siberian ginseng *Eleutherococcus senticosus*
Another ginseng occupies the scene. Siberian ginseng, once a poor relation of the popular ginseng, is poor no longer. Although a different species, the close relationship was discovered by Russian scientists who now claim: 'In all respects it is better than ginseng.'

Eleutherococcus is a shrub of considerable charm with deep green leaves like ginseng but with this difference – the flowers are violet for male and yellow for female. In autumn its berries are not crimson but a deep purple.

World pharmacy will doubtless be hearing more about it

in future as scientific investigation reveals its protective action against the effects of radiation.

Radiation sickness may sometimes interfere with a patient's course of deep-ray therapy by causing sickness and other symptoms. The Russian plant rapidly gains a reputation for preventing the dizziness and sickness following undue exposure to the rays.

Like ginseng, this plant enables blood donors quickly to make up their haemoglobin levels after transfusion. Few agents have the ability to restore to normality a high or a low blood pressure. Another paradox.

Eleutherococcus-fed bees so stimulated hive performance that the bees foraged more pollen and nectar than the normal hive, heaping up 40% more honey.

American ginseng *Panax quinquefolium*
This is one of the most prized American plants since its discovery 300 years ago. It has been referred to as a 'cure-all' or panacea by the Seneca Indians for infertility, fatigue and promoting longevity.

Though largely used as an aphrodisiac, it has been shown to be a stimulating nervine, anti-tumour and protective against radioactivity. Today it is valued as an adaptogen, a substance to assist maintenance of the immune system.

Korean ginseng is considered the most potent as a general health tonic. Studies suggest its radioactive content helps the body to adapt to environmental stress. Like all ginsengs it has a positive effect upon the pituitary gland in maintaining immune defence.

Ginseng should not be taken in the presence of diabetes without your doctor's supervision because it can increase blood sugar. It should not be taken by those with high blood pressure.

Ginseng is available in tablets or easy-to-swallow capsules. Dose: 500mg, but not more than 600mg daily for a short length of time.

Goat's rue *Galega officinale*
Galega is the Greek word for 'milk'. The plant acquired its name for increasing the flow of milk in women and animals. French peasants discovered long ago how the output of cows could be increased by as much as 40%. Since that time French physicians have prescribed it for their patients.

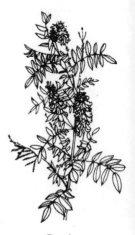

Goat's rue

243

Goat's rue tea is made by pouring boiling water on the dried or fresh herb. It has been used with success to reduce levels of sugar in the blood, and for this reason is in demand among natural therapists for diabetes. In their circles it is known as a 'hypoglycaemic'. It bears attractive mauve and pink pea flowers, and is no relation of garden rue (herb o'grace o'Sundays).

Goldenseal *Hydrastis Canadensis*

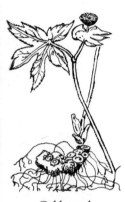

Goldenseal

Is a small perennial growing in North America and Canada on sites where trees have been recently felled. It loves shady woods, a rich soil and damp meadows.

It is an antiseptic, haemostatic, diuretic, laxative, antibacterial and has an affinity for the liver.

It is used for inflammation of mucous membrane, haemorrhoids, digestive disorders, peptic and duodenal ulcers, tinnitus (humming noises in the ears).

The Cherokee Americans used it for cancer. Dr Hale (*The Homoeopathic World*) says: 'This is important as showing that the traditional reputation of the plant agrees with results of the latest experience. For though by no means a specific in all cases, it is in cancer cases that Hydrastis has won its chief fame. I think it may fairly be said that more cases of the disease have been cured with it than any other single remedy.'

It is used by the herbal practitioner for duodenal and peptic ulceration, liver congestion and all forms of catarrh (nasal, vaginal and bowel). It is effective for mouth ulcers, sore gums and thrush. Used externally for wounds, acne and ringworm.

Gotu kola *Hydrocotyle asiatica*

Also known as Indian pennywort and *Centella asiatica*, the oldest man recorded in Chinese history was a renowned herbalist: Li Chung Yun who, according to legend, lived to 256 years (*Guinness Book of Records*).

Professor Li Chung Yun was born in 1677 and in 1923 the *New York Times* announced the death of this remarkable man. He outlived twenty-three wives and was living with the twenty-fourth when he died.

Gotu Kola is a fruit rich in B vitamins, which is good for the brain. In addition to its tonic effect upon the blood, it is known to benefit the memory and promote mental alertness. Today it is prescribed for stress, especially for students studying for examinations. It is being adopted by psychiatry for mentally retarded children, increasing ability to concentrate. Double-blind clinical trials support its reputation as an anxiety reducer.

It is well known in Ayurvedic medicine as the 'fountain of youth'.

This is a remedy for the busy executive or worn-out carer with a heavy workload and no time to relax. It is a very versatile agent, having been successful in cases of arthritis, Raynaud's disease and emphysema. Tumours have been known to stop growing, even shrink. It should not be confused with kola nuts, which are high in caffeine.

Grape seed

The medicinal use of grapes has always been recognized. We hear of people who have lost weight on a grape diet, which is also a helpful protection against coronary heart disease. The important role played by the seed in restoring a sick body to health fascinates the scientists.

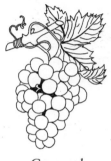

A powerful antioxidant, it is a member of the group known as the procyanidolics (PCOs) the activity of which is said to be fifty times greater than vitamin E and twenty times greater than vitamin C. Grape seeds are shown to be rich in PCOs capable of disposing of free-radicals entering the body from pollution.

Grape seed

Anti-inflammatory and anti-cancer properties of the seeds are today given priority in the laboratories of researchers.

Hawthorn *Crataegus oxyacanthoides*

The botanical name for this thorny tree or shrub is *kratos*, meaning strength, referring to the stony-hardness of its wood, and *akantha*, meaning a thorn. It was not long before primitive man associated the strength of the hawthorn to man's heart, the red berries being used in heart weakness.

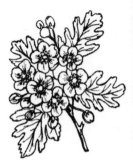

According to records, an old Irish doctor in the last century obtained excellent results administering an unknown remedy to his heart patients. Years afterwards it was discovered he was using the 'haws' (berries) of the hawthorn tree.

Dr T. J. Lyle, Professor of Therapeutics and Pharmacy at the

Hawthorn

Chicago Physio-Medical College, wrote: 'The fruit of this hawthorn shrub, or small tree, is highly recommended as a heart tonic. By some, it is thought to be superior to cactus for angina, oedema, regurgitation, enlargement of the heart, fatty degeneration, palpitation.' (Cactus flowers are another effective heart remedy used by herbalists.)

Hawthorn is a vasodilator and can prove helpful in lowering high blood pressure by increasing the 'bore' or dilation of the vessels. Its special field of application is in coronary thrombosis where it improves blood flow, especially where the heart muscle is weak.[33]

Marked improvement has been noted in heart disease of old age.

A Dr Jennings reports: 'Mr B., who suffered from a weak heart, was found gasping for breath with a pulse rate of 158 and very feeble. There was considerable collection of fluid (oedema) in the lower limbs and abdomen. A more desperate case could scarcely be found. The doctor gave him fifteen drops of crataegus extract (hawthorn) in half a glass of water. Within fifteen minutes the pulse rate was 126 and stronger, breathing was not so laboured. In twenty-five minutes the pulse beat was 110, and still improving.'

Millions of people are afflicted with some form of disease of the heart and circulatory system. Hawthorn is essentially a mild cardiac tonic. It is perfectly safe and has no toxic effect. Jennings continues: 'It can do no harm . . . the entire nervous system seems to be favourably influenced by its use; appetite increases, assimilation and nutrition improve, showing an influence over the sympathetic and solar plexus. Also a sense of quietude rests on the patient. He who before its use was cross, melancholic and irritable, after a few days shows marked signs of improvement in his mental state.'

Strange as this last statement may appear, from actual experience Jennings was able to verify the marked sedative effect of hawthorn on the general system. Good as it is, we cannot see how it can take the place of that king of the heart, digitalis, as a universal heart tonic – but it runs it second!

Hawthorn has been used with success for cardiac arrest, preventing sudden death. One day its advance may see it in general use in chronic stroke therapy.

Henna *Lawsonia alba*

Henna has been used to beautify women's hair since Cleopatra ensnared Anthony. No one of the Hundred and One Arabian Nights was perfect without it. The Chinese used it internally as an astringent for simple congestive headache.

Horsetail *Equisitum arvense*

You are not likely to miss this perennial in the field. Also known as scouring rush, shavegrass, pewterwort. It has a prehistoric look about it. If any plant has not evolved since the primeval forests of the early ages – this is it. It has a flinty 'feel'. This is because of its silicic water-soluble compounds. Silicea (siliceous earth or flint) is of no service to the physician till trituration has released its curative virtue. Horsetail offers an ideal alternative and will put up much the same performance as the 'Silicea' of the homoeopaths and tissue-salt therapists.

Horsetail

Today, its asparagus-like heads are used to promote the flow of urine and expel gravel. John Gerard, sixteenth-century herbalist, records its use for the healing of wounds when pounded in a mortar and applied to the affected parts. It is popular for irritation of the bladder, especially in women with frequent desire to urinate and with pain as from distension.

It has been used where surgery might have put the patient at risk, being a gentle diuretic, promoting function of the kidneys. Preparation is by simple herbal infusion, pouring boiling water on dried herbs in a covered vessel, e.g. a teapot. Care should be taken to see that the teapot is free from old tannin deposits left over from use with ordinary teas.

The impression of this leafless plant may sometimes be seen on the surface of a piece of coal. All plants absorb minerals. There are particles of gold in almost every soil, even in Britain and Eastern Europe, but not enough to make commercial recovery possible.

Horsetail rhizomes will take it up along with other metals. Scientists have proved this by burning large quantities of the weed and extracting minute traces of gold from the ashes.

Iceland moss *Cetraria islandica*

An expectorant to loosen sputum in bronchitis and for use as a nutrient in wasting disease and cachexia. For susceptibility to winter's chest hazards.

Ispaghula *Plantago ovata*

Native of the Indian sub-continent. Also related to fleawort spogel and flea seed. Ispaghula provides a natural source of fibre and is regarded as a lubricant for the intestines, without griping.

It has been used successfully for stubborn bowel conditions, which are often a taboo subject.

Ispaghula is a popular help for anything intestinal, from attacks of flatulence, spasm, gastritis, ulcerative colitis and other acute inflammatory conditions.

It is recommended for chronic constipation in the elderly and for irritable bowel syndrome (IBS). Known to reduce cholesterol levels, aiding detox and absorption of iron. Useful in pregnancy, it also assists slimming in obesity.

Dose: Two to four teaspoons (children one teaspoon) after each meal.

Jojoba *Simmondsia chinensis*

Also called deer nut and coffeeberry. The sperm whale is not far from extinction. The jojoba bean may prove to be its salvation. The plant extract has been found to be an efficient lubricant for machinery, high precision instruments and is essential for the production of antibiotics, all of which were provided by spermwhale oil. Jojoba has become an important element in today's economy.

Early settlers made a coffee from the nuts after the custom of the Apache Americans. Pronounced *hoh-hoh-bah*, its nut-like seeds are one of the important food plants for wildlife and domestic livestock on the Indian reservations of Arizona. The Apaches used it as a hair oil; their women to dress their braids and tresses.

Jojoba is a rich natural moisturiser for hair and skin. Used for massage and as a salve for wounds. A few drops of the oil on the face preserve a healthy complexion. It enriches the skin on any part of the body. Of special value for sports people as a skin protective in winter and a suntan lotion in summer.

Shampoos and conditioners are available for dry or chapped skin, warts and for over-active sebaceous glands which are responsible for acne and dandruff.

The plants thrive for about 100 years. Some have been claimed to survive to 200 years.

Lemon balm or sweet balm *Melissa officinalis*
John Evelyn wrote: 'Balm is sovereign for the brain. It strengthens the memory and powerfully chases away melancholy (depression).' Combined with nutmeg it has a great reputation for nervous headache and neuralgia.

This garden weed has been found to promote calmness and improvement of memory and may even help sufferers of Alzheimer's disease.

Edwardians knew it as the scholar's remedy given to those who spend their lives studying 'to clear the head and sharpen the memory.'

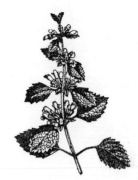

Lemon balm

Melissa has the same properties as lavender in its ability to soothe and heal. As an antiseptic it may be used on dressings for the treatment of wounds and ulceration.

John Hussey, Kent, UK, lived to be 116 years, drinking balm lemon grass tea daily. To make the tea, place a few fresh leaves (or one heaped teaspoon dried) into a teapot and infuse for five to fifteen minutes. Drink freely. For daily use, set aside a special teapot for its preparation.

Lemon grass *Cymbopogen citratus DC*
A remedy with a long traditional history as hypertensive, anti-inflammatory, antipyretic, anxiolytic and carminative.

Today, its use is in the form of tea, tincture or one of the essential oils of aromatherapy. Its oil has an inhibitory effect upon E. Coli, Staph aureus, Salmonella species, B. Cereus and certain other bacteria. Its potent anti-microbial action is completely lost when the oil is extensively oxidized by faulty storage.

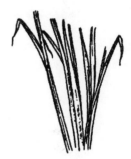

Lemon grass

It is effective against Candida albicans and Aspergillus fumigatus. It is one of the weaker remedies for high blood pressure, while it gains in popularity for the control of cholesterol. It is said to have an anti-tumour action.

The oil of lemon grass is an effective insecticide and repellent.

(Bob Harris and Rhiannon Lewis, *International Journal of Alternative and Complementary Medicine*, July 1994).

Liquorice *Glycyrrhiza glabra L. (see page 216–18)*

Lobelia *Lobelia inflata*
Also called Indian tobacco and pukeweed. A broncho-relaxant to clear the lungs of sticky mucus, lobelia can be used to ease bronchitis, difficult breathing, a blocked nose and nasal obstruction, laryngitis, tonsillitis, hay fever and hacking cough. Useful for those seeking to break dependence on aerosols and to increase breathing capacity.

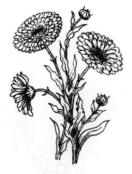

Lobelia

Marigold *Calendula officinalis*
Since the dalliance days of Elizabethan England, this gentle vulnerary has been cherished in every garden of herbs. Internally, it aids local healing of damage to the skin and prevents infection. The flowers, chewed, make an admirable dressing to relieve pain and swelling caused by the sting of a wasp or bee. Pressed on a cut finger, they can arrest bleeding, as many an old–time gardener knows. The near planting of marigolds assists the fruiting of tomatoes.

A plant often regarded as a garden weed has been found to prevent pain and suppuration in wounds and sores, healing without formation of a scar. Its vivid orange hue lights up the garden in summer.

Marigold offers valuable volatile oils and flavonoids, being anti–inflammatory, anti–haemorrhage and is sometimes given after surgical operations.

It is used for wounds where the skin has been broken and bleeding. Part of its action resembles arnica, which is used for unbroken skin.

Herbalist's friend; One part tincture calendula to four parts witch hazel, for phlebitis and painful varicose veins.

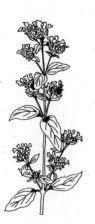

Marigold

Marjoram *Sweet marjoram, Origanum vulgare*
Gastrointestinal stimulant, mild antiseptic, anti–viral, anti–stress, and an aphrodisiac, marjoram is also used to promote menstrual flow suppressed by cold, to relieve tension headache, and to control convulsions.

Externally, it is an antiseptic. Mrs Hilda Leyel, of London, consulting medical herbalist, fell over a wall in Troy, sustaining a serious injury to her knee. A doctor rushed for the iodine bottle, but this fine old–time herbalist gathered some of the marjoram growing nearby and used the juice. The wound healed in record time much to the amazement of the doctor.

Marjoram

Marjoram is related to oregano but is sweeter and milder. Avoid during pregnancy and breast-feeding.

Marshmallow *Althaea officinalis*

Hot fomentations and poultices are used for allaying the pain of inflammatory swellings and for drawing to the surface the contents of a boil, before squeezing out the 'core'. The ground root is brought to the boil in milk, adding a little powdered slippery elm bark. When reaching a doughy consistency, the poultice is spread thickly on linen or other form of dressing and applied as hot as can be borne. It is renewed when dry. It can also be used for abscesses, ulcers and septic wounds that refuse to heal.

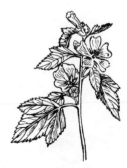

Marshmallow

Marshmallow is a well-known diuretic and at one time was a popular remedy for respiratory disorders, including bronchitis and stubborn coughs. Known as the 'mortification root', it can be used as a cleansing wash for offensive skin ulceration.

Milk thistle *Silybum marianum L.*

For many years herbalists have been using milk thistle seeds in their treatment of liver disorders and as a gall bladder stimulant.

In Germany, physicians have been aware of its properties as long as can be remembered. It is given for chronic hepatitis and to prevent toxins from penetrating liver cells.

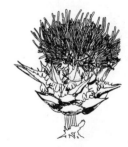

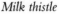

Today, it is recognized as valuable in preventing liver damage, even having an inhibitory effect upon alcohol liver erosion. Known as a scavenger for free radicals, it is believed to prevent cirrhosis and to stimulate regrowth of liver cells and new tissue.

Milk thistle

It is a first-line remedy for fatty degeneration of the liver. Some studies exist to show that it can prevent – and even cure it.

Mistletoe *Viscum album*

In 1930, more than forty papers were published in highly respected medical journals in the US and in France, in which men of international standing commended mistletoe for lowering blood pressure, especially where accompanied by pain at the back of the head, dizziness and buzzing in the ears.

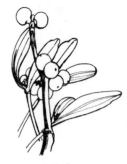

Injections of iscador (mistletoe) are used extensively on the continent in the treatment of cancer. Dr Rudolph Steiner, physician and scientist, made a life-long study of mistletoe and

Mistletoe

reached the conclusion that the efficacy of the remedy depended upon the 'time' when it was gathered, according to the moon and planets. Dr Agnes Fyfe of the Arlesrein Society for Cancer Research, Switzerland, contributed much valuable work in this field. She showed how an important new knowledge of the life of plants and their association with the heavenly bodies had been won. Incidentally, mistletoe is a familiar remedy for shingles.

Nettles *Urtica dioica*

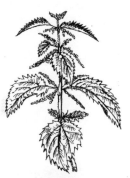

Nettles

Also called stinging nettle. Women of diminutive breasts may find a new hope in nettle tea. Nettles increase the secretion of milk, as also does caraway and aniseed. Dr Compton Burnett, one of the shrewdest medical sleuths of his day, refers to this and also to its gravel-expelling power. Those taking nettle tea often pass small quantities of gravel, sometimes for the first time in their lives. Nettle tea is useful for high blood pressure, nervous eczema and nosebleeds. Mrs Hilda Leyel said: 'No plant is more useful in domestic medicine.' Nettle rash caused by eating lobster, cheese and strawberries often yields to nettle tea.

Pellitory of the wall *Parietaria diffusa*

Pellitory of the wall

Pellitory belongs to 'pellitory of the wall' the family of nettles, a humble, inconspicuous plant. Its name 'parietaria' is derived from the Latin *paries*, meaning a wall. It needs well-riddled earth and plenty of lime.

Being found on old ruins, its presence has a small part to play in the disintegration of stonework. This property may well bear some relationship to its success in dissolving stone in the bladder or for expelling gravel. All parts of the plant contain nitre (*saltpetre*) which shows up in the ashes of the incinerated plant.

William Fox, MD, conducted what must have been the largest botanical practice in the country in the 1920s. This was one of his favourites. His experience proved it to be a gentle diuretic for stimulating the flow of urine; he used it also with some success for stones. It is indicated for a sensation of pellitory of the wall distension of the bladder, with pain.

Pellitory works best in a simple infusion as tea: one heaped teaspoonful to a teacupful of boiling water, three times daily. It is sometimes combined with wild carrot and parsley piert for kidney troubles failing to respond to other methods of treatment.

Peppercorns *Piper nigrum L.*

Who would have thought that black pepper, a condiment, would be so useful as a gastrointestinal stimulant? Our forebears, including sailors on Nelson's men-o'War carried them in a twist of paper, holding their ration for many days at sea when foodstuffs perished.

It is a remedy for flatulence and indigestion – even for dreaded intermittent fevers of the tropics!

Of recent years it has regained popularity for the relief of breathlessness and to clear excess mucus from throat and chest. The dosage for powdered peppercorns is up to to one teaspoon.

Peppermint *Mentha piperita*

What is more comforting than a cup of hot mint tea? All readers will be aware of the digestive uses of the mints – especially peppermint. One teaspoonful of the dried herb, or a sachet on sale in the shops, can bring instant relief from an attack of the collywobbles.

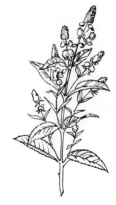

Peppermint

Mints established themselves wild in Britain and Europe at the coming of the Romans. How they flourish in a rainy climate! English oil of peppermint is the finest in the world, commanding a high price. The plants love damp places. If set in the shade they grow too lanky.

Peppermint is the star performer of the group of labiates of which all the mints are members. Dioscorides found it so refreshing that even wearing a spray on his garment helped raise his depressed spirits.

Pungent oil of peppermint is a powerful invigorator. It has found a new lease of life since the advent of aromatherapy. Aromatherapists see no inflexible dividing line between medical and cosmetic treatments. They believe the stimulating effects of this oil on the skin will impart tone to the whole body. They regard the skin as a vital organ, suggesting that care in its maintenance never goes unrewarded.

Unlike mineral oils, essential oils from plants are easily absorbed by the skin. Filtering through to the circulation, their remedial influences are soon felt throughout the entire body.

As an inhalant, peppermint oil is still used for asthma, colds, influenza, shock, fainting and mental fatigue.

It is one of the few essential oils taken internally, even then, only in one-drop doses in water when it is especially helpful for uncontrollable hiccups, wind, headache, irritable bowel syndrome, nausea, travel sickness, sinusitis and toothache. It simply refuses to allow milk to curdle in the stomach.

Peppermint should not be taken with antacids. Those with long-term existing bowel conditions should check with their doctor or health consultant before use.

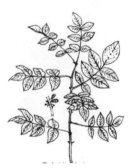

Pilewort

Pilewort *Ranunculus ficaria*
Has been used since the days of Dioscorides for piles and itchy conditions.

Prickly ash bark *Zanthoxylum americanum*
Also called toothache bark. Its chief use among drugless healers is for cramp-like pains of the leg on walking, rheumatism and for those of arthritic tendency. Helpful in Raynaud's disease as a 'supportive' to a doctor's treatment, it combines well with hawthorn and motherwort to strengthen a weak heart and reduce the beat.

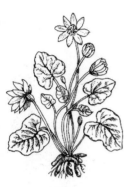

Prickly ash bark

Propolis
One of nature's powerful antibiotics. It is one of the bees' building materials. It is the chief cement they use for structural repairs and sealing cracks to keep out draughts and the cold.

All the world over, one of the chief topics of conversation among the medical fraternity is that of viruses, the cause of so many infections. This is an area into which propolis is moving, with a promise of being able to arrest the remorseless advance of these deadly microbes. It has proven successful in the treatment of chest infections that have in the past not responded to modern drugs.

Sister Carole, St Joseph's Home, Newcastle, had a hunch that propolis may be beneficial to sufferers of Alzheimer's disease. Giving it to one of the residents, she observed results.

After a few days she noticed the woman had become more

alert and confident about herself. Heartened by this, Sister Carole read up current literature on the subject and gave the resin to other residents. The response was noticeable.

One woman, no longer able to eat because of her brain disorder was fed liquidized form of the resin through a syringe. Weeks later, she was feeding herself and more conscious of what was going on around her.

Raspberry leaves *Rubus idaeus*

A growing number of specialists tell their antenatal patients to drink raspberry leaf tea to allay labour pains and prevent sickness.

'Raspberry has a relaxing action on the human pregnant uterus,' Sir Beckwith Whitehouse: *BMJ*, 1941, 2,370.

Raspberry leaves are an astringent uterine tonic taken as a tea – one heaped teaspoon to one teacupful of boiling water (or tablets) during the last three or four months of pregnancy. They have a reputation for painless and easy delivery. During labour a little ginger may be added with a teaspoonful of honey.

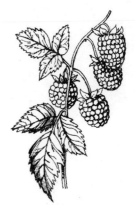

Raspberry Leaves

Raspberry is a great favourite among alternative practitioners for uterine haemorrhage, catarrh, leucorrhoea, peptic ulcer and chronic irritable bowel syndrome (IBS).

They are so fantastically beneficial in pregnancy and a number of female problems that every expectant mother should get acquainted with them.

Raspberry can prevent miscarriages, increase milk flow and reduce labour pains. The agent is safe – never has a case of toxicity been attributed to its use.

Red clover *Trifolium pratense*

Loves to grow in most parts of the UK. It is happiest in meadowland of a light sandy nature. It is not the clover worked by the honeybee – which is the white clover – a favourite ingredient of hay as a valuable animal food.

To the herbalist, red clover is an alternative of considerable power, influencing the glandular system by its catalysing enzymes.

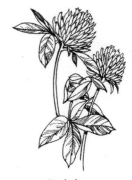

Red clover

In red clover, as in other herbs, the Creator has given us a vitalized context of minerals prepared by the chemistry of Nature.

Modern science now sustains herbal practice of the past, especially that of an older generation whose craft now shows red clover to have a sounder base than many people would wish to admit. Red clover is a great detox remedy, eliminating from the body accumulated poisons that may have been locked up in tissue for years. In the case of cancer, Nature has a chance to eliminate those effete materials through the intestinal canal or kidneys. Such elimination is enhanced by judicious fasting which enables the body to unload (*see also* Fasting, pp 155–57).

Successful treatment in many cases of inoperable carcinoma have been recorded.

Hyde quotes a member of the National Institute of Medical Herbalists (NIMH) who wrote, 'If symptoms indicate a malignant diathesis it is "undoubtedly of value".'

At least it proves of some help in delaying the process of malignancy.

It has been used successfully in gastric carcinoma in conjunction with wood betony, wormwood and violet odorata: prescribed locally and *per se*.

In the same article another member of the NIMH is recorded: 'Valuable in the treatment of rodent ulcers. It is an anti-tumour agent.' April 1979.

'We have known people cured of cancer by washing the breasts in red clover infusion and by drinking the herb tea.' Dr Melville Keith, Professor, Indiana Physio-Medical College, USA.

Coffee and strong tea antidotes vitiate the beneficial effect of red clover and many other gentle-acting herbs.

Red clover has a special reference to women at menopause by its phyto-oestrogens that prove to be a near-approach to the body's own oestrogen. When produced in the female body it protects against certain disorders that may follow the menopause. Research has discovered this remarkable remedy to have the same effect and is regarded as a naturally produced hormone.

Night sweats and hot flushes have been reduced to less than half after taking capsules of the remedy. The findings of a study carried out at the New York University Medical Centre came as a welcome surprise. Red clover in its synthetic form can be responsible for decreasing the risk of cancer of the womb and its lining (endometriosis). One tablet a day containing 40mg of red clover natural isoflavones is the average dosage.

Red clover flowers should contain the seeds. The practitioner is aware of a strong infusion bringing relief for whooping cough. For stubborn dry coughs it acts as an anti-spasmodic and demulcent.

Rosemary *Rosmarinus officinalis*

'As for Rosemary, I let it run all over my garden, not only because the bees love it, but because it is the herb sacred to remembrance and friendship . . . hence a sprig of it has silent speech,' wrote Sir Thomas More.

This delicately scented and much loved herb is one of our favourite old-time remedies.

Mr F. Fletcher-Hyde, distinguished consulting medical herbalist, Leicester, writes: 'Rosemary is effective for flatulent distension of the gastro-intestinal tract. Salivation is increased and digestion improved. It is an anti-depressant useful for migraine and hysteria.' William Meyrick concurs that rosemary 'is excellent for headache, dizziness and trembling of the limbs.' *Herbal Review*, Summer 1984.

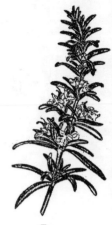

Rosemary

Rosemary is one of the favourite old-time remedies for falling hair, applied externally as a wash or rinse to strengthen and nourish, helping the hair to a better 'set'.

Rosemary essential oil, as used externally in massage by aromatherapists, is in wide use today. They refer to it as a diuretic, muscle relaxant, anti-catarrhal and prescribe it for intermittent claudication and candida albicans. It should not be used in pregnancy, breast-feeding, liver disorders or given to children.

Sage *Salvia officinalis L.*

At one time wealthy Chinese merchants failed to understand why we in this country went to such trouble to import from the East large cargoes of China and Indian tea, when the most valuable of all teas grew in our own gardens!

You haven't a sage bush in your garden? To make a simple infusion place a heaped teaspoonful of dried herb into a teacup and pour on boiling water. Allow to cool. Drink a wineglassful (or more) every morning for general health. Just the daily lifesaver for preserving the quality of the gastric juices in old age. Cover the cup to prevent the escape of volatile properties whilst cooling. Drink a wineglassful after meals three times daily for sore throats, ulcers on mouth or tongue, soft or spongy gums, for increasing appetite, allaying flatulence and unpleasant breath. Once referred to as 'woman's friend'.

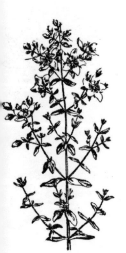

St John's wort

St John's wort *Hypericum perforatum*

Also referred to as 'the sunshine herb' and 'nature's prozac'. Recent discoveries promote this flowering herb to one of the top herbal anti-depressants. Favourable articles in the medical press relate it to the neurotransmitters, noradrenaline and serotonin. Studies from a number of universities confirm its efficacy for mild to moderate depression, regarding it as effective as conventional anti-depressants.

Its cost of production is below that of potent drugs from which some people suffer distressing side effects. Others have no desire to expose delicate tissue of the brain to powerful chemicals. Herbalists of British history regarded it as a relaxing nervine and anti-spasmodic. St John's wort is concerned with our 'feelings' – that low feeling from stress, overwork, unexplained fatigue and a sense of being unappreciated.

The herb is taken for loss of energy, sadness, lethargy and hopelessness. For the depression of liver origin, milk thistle is more effective. Physicians of a past generation used it to inhibit growth of Koch's bacillus in tuberculosis. Hypericum wounds are very sensitive to the touch – parts rich in nerves: coccyx, brain and the spine after concussion from falls by the elderly. It is a traditional remedy for rabies.

Daily dose varies from 500–1000mcg of hypericin, the active ingredient. Clinical research confirms it to be well tolerated by patients, with extremely few adverse reactions. Often overlooked, it helps insomnia.

Unfortunately for orthodox medicine, St John's wort can interact with certain drugs: blood-thinning warfarin, the birth control pill and cyclosporin – an immune system suppression drug used in kidney and other major operations. In Germany, St John's wort is prescribed eight times as often as prozac.

For years my wife and I gathered the herb in the New Forest to make tinctures from the fresh flowers and leaf tops for patients' medicines, and as a healing lotion. Herbalists gathered it on St John's Day, midsummer.

Steep flowers in olive oil to make St John's red oil for bruises, burns, neuralgia and general purposes.

Do not take with drugs to which it acts as an antidote. The Department of Health advises patients to consult their doctor before use because it makes some drugs ineffective.

Sarsaparilla *Smilax officinalis*
Contains the male hormone, testosterone, and progesterone for the function of the sex organs. Progesterone is produced by the ovaries and is necessary for uterine health. Cortin is secreted by the adrenal glands upon which it exerts a positive influence.

Sarsaparilla was much prized by the Eclectic School of Medicine in America at the beginning of the twentieth century. Doctors of the eclectic persuasion left impressive records of its efficacy for rheumatism, gout, arthritis and the skin disorders eczema and psoriasis. It promotes the healing of ulceration, internal and external. Has a reputation for use in bacterial dysentery and mercurial poisoning. Since its arrival into Europe from Jamaica and Mexico it has become one of the most popular of blood purifiers.

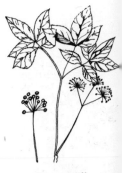

Sarsaparilla

Saw palmetto *Serenoa repens* or *Sabal serrulata*
This North American plant has been used in the treatment of male problems of the prostate gland and urinary tract for many years. It is indicated for benign prostate hypertrophy due to an enlarged prostate gland compressing the urethra, thus arresting a smooth unhindered flow of urine.

Urologists became increasingly interested in a natural remedy which helps relieve the gland's discomfort, reducing night-time urination, and at the same time improving the flow.

A double-blind trial in Germany revealed its efficacy in BPH, when 160mg of palmetto extract was taken morning and evening, with no side-effects and loss of libido.

Sometimes described as a plant catheter, it is well tolerated and there is no increase in blood pressure. However, it may be wise to discuss any case with your doctor or health consultant before use.

Dosage in the early stages is 160mg standardized extract twice daily, or as a tea made with 5–6g of dried berry powder.

Scullcap *Scutellaria lateriflora*
A stimulating relaxing nervine for headaches. A sedative of value in hysteria, nervous excitability and prolonged physical strain. Helpful for workaholics compelled to put in long hours with ensuing mental exhaustion. For over-study, weakness after long sickness, nightmares and brain-storms in children.

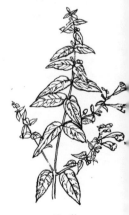

Scullcap

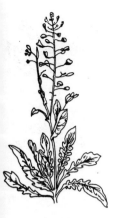

Shepherd's purse *Capsella bursa-pastoris*
A urinary antiseptic and for control of excessive bleeding from the womb. For the elderly, chronic disorders of the genito-urinary system.

Slippery elm *Ulmus Fulva*
The powdered inner bark makes a wonderfully strengthening and soothing porridge for complaints of the stomach and intestines. Before travel, it helps to allay travel sickness. Before festivities, it may reduce 'hangover' embarrassment from too hearty feeding. Used as a poultice for inflamed skin, ulcers and chilblains, and for drawing to the surface matter as a preliminary to expulsion from the body, as in boils.

Shepherd's purse

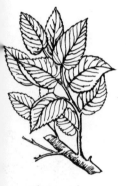

Spirulina
Studies at the Norwich Institute of Food show that beta-carotene, as found especially in carrots, actually boosts part of the immune system which helps target and destroy unhealthy cells. Spirulina is rich in beta-carotene – richer even than carrots!

Spirulina is an algae vegetarians can adopt because it is rich in chlorophyll which has a chelating effect in the removal of mercury and other heavy metals from the body. It is also believed to repair damage by radiation.

Its effect upon the body is of a cleansing nature, also a detox. Rich in B vitamins, enzymes and trace elements it is an ideal form of protein for digestive and intestinal disorders in an easily assimilable form. It provides beneficial nourishment when unable to partake of a sit-down meal.

With a protein content of 60% it offers a substantial cholesterol-free item of diet. World suppliers, Hawaiian Pacific Spirulina write: 'This miniature floating plant was highly cherished by ancient civilizations, such as the Aztecs, due to its health–enhancing qualities. It provides a remarkable combination of protein, vitamins and minerals and a host of other nutrients.'

It is said to be a whole food source, rich in iron, chlorophyll, calcium and GLA – richer than mother's milk! Available as a powder or tablet.

Slippery elm

Turmeric *Curcuma domestica* or *C. longa*

One of the basic ingredients of curry and a member of the ginger family. One of the important Ayurvedic medicines with a long history for uncomfortable stomach pain, calming the intestines and increasing the flow of bile, which is very often the solution of a number of abdominal disorders. Of value for irritable bowel syndrome with bloating and flatulence.

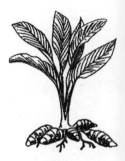

Turmeric

Turmeric has a cortisone-like effect and is therefore of value for polymyalgia and rheumatoid arthritis. It covers a wide range of diseases.

Turmeric is a potent antioxidant which appears to block the growth of breast and prostate cancer cells and defective DNA in colon cancer cells. It is an aid to digestion and in one study stomach and duodenal ulcers disappeared in nearly half of twenty-five volunteers who took 300mg five times a day for a month. However it may irritate the stomach. It is anti-inflammatory and a potent natural antibiotic. (American Herb Association 2002, 18(2):3. *Green Files.*

Valerian *Valeriana officinalis L.*

One of life's rewarding practices is to know how to 'let go'. That is what relaxation really means. Yet, how many of us attain it?

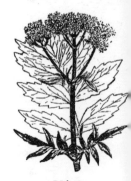

Valerian

For those who find it difficult, valerian, regarded as the safest mild sedative, may help. It offers a good night's sleep without that drugged feeling. It has acquired a reputation to relieve muscular spasm and menstrual cramps. The spikenard of the New Testament is believed to be valerian, which grows in the Holy Land. More physicians are returning to valerian, once a foundation medicine for nerve tension. It has proved of benefit for nocturnal bed-wetting in adults and children.

Cats are attracted to its roots due to its perfume and become ecstatic in their preset. It is well tolerated, dosage up to 500mg or up to one teaspoonful of the tincture for restlessness. Dosage may have to be doubled during the day. Its effect is cumulative and it may have to be taken over several days, but it is not known to have a toxic effect, being regarded as one of the safest sleep-inducers on the market.

Violet *Viola odorata*

Whatever we call this modest perennial, whether love-in-idleness or kiss-me-in-the-kitchen, it has an appeal of her own. It

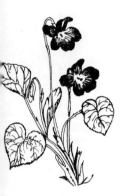

Violet

is the cleansing property of the tea which is used as an expectorant for chest troubles – especially bronchitis.

Violet leaves (dried or fresh) make a palatable cup of tea for a cough or for a distressing catarrhal discharge. It was once used as a soothing gargle for irritative sore throats. The leaves are slightly laxative. Indian hakims making their home in Europe bring with them knowledge of its uses for certain kinds of headache and for dizziness.

From leaves steeped in boiling water a 'drawing' poultice may be prepared to ripen and bring-to-a-head lesions about to erupt to expel morbid matter through the skin. The dried leaves are one of the ingredients of a number of herbal beverages drunk as alternatives to ordinary tea, including the leaves of agrimony, lemon balm, raspberry, dandelion, peppermint and great burnet. Such combinations have a reputation for cooling the blood and relieving indigestion.

Violet leaf tea assuaged the pains of terminal cancer suffered by Dame Evangeline Booth, wife of the founder of the Salvation Army. Members of that vigorous organization scoured railway embankments and local woodlands for wild violet leaves to be dispatched post-haste to her home for making the tea which gave her so much relief.

We have yet to plumb the secret depths of the active principle – ionine – the mysterious essence which imparts to this gracious, tiny plant the keen, sweet fragrance we know so well.

Wild yam *Dioscorea villosa*

Also known as rheumatism root, colic root and wild yam root. A common perennial growing in the USA and Canada. It has been used for many years in Mexico for pain in the womb and ovaries, and for infertility.

Dr C. Asada, USA, said: 'There is no known remedy that equals wild yam for the relief of appendicitis.'

Other eclectic physicians report successful treatment for diverticulitis, muscular rheumatism, intermittent claudication, cramps, inflammation of the gall bladder and painful colic.

Wild yam is one of those natural remedies for correcting hormone imbalance by its precursor effect by stimulation of the production of oestrogen. When administered, it enables the patient to produce oestrogen from her own resources. A tradi-

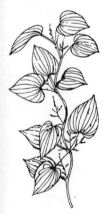

Wild yam

tional remedy for bilious colic used by southern Indian natives of the USA.

Willow bark *Salix alba L.*
Also called white willow. Discovery of the healing potential of the white willow tree has led medical scientists to uncover some of the most vital secrets of nature. It was this tree that opened the door to aspirin (acetyl-salicylic acid).

Although aspirin is now produced in synthetic form, preparations from the tree bark are still used in alternative medicine.

Willow is a fever-lowering agent used to reduce high body temperatures. But it is because of its action as a depressant on the central nervous system that it has become a pain-reliever.

Other uses include: influenza, headache, malaria, dyspepsia and backache. Rheumatism and arthritis are known to respond to its anti-inflammatory action.

Witch hazel *Hamamelis virginiana L.*
In our analysis of living plants we must be careful not to destroy the centuries old confidence which has grown up around their use.

Witch hazel is a well-known lotion which has been in the European pharmacopoeias for as long as can be remembered. It is a local astringent and haemostatic for cuts and bruises, but it finds its fullest expression in day-to-day skin care by bringing a welcome refreshment to tired flesh.

An older generation of doctors at the turn of the twentieth century would have been hard put to find its equal for troublesome nosebleeds. Many famous cosmetic brandnames have grown out of its bark, usually collected from this well-known garden ornamental in the spring. Though a native of the US and Canada it lives happily in almost any English garden. One part of the tincture to ten parts boiled water was once a common injection for cases of severe piles.

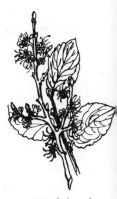

Witch hazel

As an alternative to hazel twigs, forked witch hazel branches, may be used for the ancient art of dowsing or water-divining. Dowsers do not seek scientific proof of their powers, it is enough if water is found and flows. No one has succeeded in rationalizing the process and, until someone does, there are old-timers with a personal preference for witch hazel.

The word *hamamelis* comes from the Greek 'together apple',

and some people claim its scent is suggestive of that fruit. An effective eye lotion may be prepared by diluting one of the many good brands of distilled extract on the market.

Mr Adcock was a boiler-scaler who discovered long ago how to assuage red-eyed irritation with a swab of cotton wool saturated with the watery extract. Wiping over closed lids and corners of the eyes makes an easy-to-apply face-freshener after a long day at the office or shopping centre.

Wormwood *Artemisia absinthium L.*

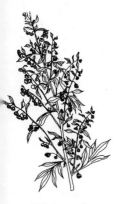

Wormwood

It was the Greek Hippocrates, father of medicine, who discovered the medicinal use of wormwood. It became one of his indispensable remedies prepared as a tincture, which was in reality vermouth, the wine that attracts today's millions of wine buffs.

Wormwood is almost unknown among the sophisticated, yet it is when we refer to it as vermouth that it merits respect. Pliny, the Roman historian, wrote: 'Wormwood stimulates the appetite and gladdens the spirit.'

Wormwood was well-known to the apothecaries of the Middle Ages who prescribed a tea made from its leaves and flowers for patients going into a decline with loss of strength and 'change of colour' – as well as foul-smelling breath.

Father Kneipp writes: 'A patient's jaundiced complexion will rapidly give place to a healthy colour.' Wormwood was never one of the 'great' wines but it can do marvellously for the sickly liver and delicate stomach.

Wine drinking in moderation is a pleasant pastime but excess may cause acidity, sore heads, sickness, dangerous driving, corpulence and short tempers. Call for wormwood the morning after a big night out.

No germs, it is claimed, live in wine, especially with wormwood. Over the years a number of imbibers have claimed it promotes long life. Wormwood powder may be sprinkled over food like salt and pepper.

'Artemisinin, a derivative of wormwood, is highly toxic to cancer cells, but has a marginal effect on healthy cells. This is because cancer cells contain levels of iron sometimes 1,000 times higher than healthy cells. Artemisinin combines with iron to form free radicals inside the cancer cells. The free radicals attack the cell membranes and kill the cancer cell.

'In this study, after eight hours 75% of the leukaemia cells had been killed. After sixteen hours all were dead. In another study it took only eight hours to kill all leukaemia cells.' *Holistic Health* 1.3.02. P39.

Yarrow *Achillea millefolium L.*
Known also as, milfoil, the sacred herb. and soldier's wound-wort. Look for this perennial in fields and hedgerows. You will find it belongs to the daisy family. Look at the cluster of flowers terminal at the end of the stiff woody stem. They are just a collection of tiny white daisies. Yarrow is an anti-inflammatory, diaphoretic, anti-rheumatic, anthelmintic (for expulsion of worms). As a haemostatic it can staunch bleeding.

As an infusion, hot or cold, yarrow is drunk for stomach unrest, lack of appetite, flatulence, diarrhoea, piles, painful and delayed periods. It can also reduce high blood pressure and reduce fever.

Place one heaped teaspoonful into a teacup and pour on boiling water. Or you may wish to take it the traditional way: 30g to 500ml (1oz to 1 pint) of boiling water.

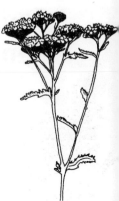

Yarrow

'When I or my husband, the Admiral, are ill,' said Lady Meade Fetherstonhaugh, 'we take yarrow recommended by Mrs Hilda Leyel, and which is well-nigh infallible. By the next morning the cold is gone. I haven't needed to go to a doctor for years.'

Further information
Further information on herbal medicines in this book may be found in *Bartram's Encyclopedia of Herbal Medicine*.

Some of My Favourite Remedies

Abortion, Threatened
Agnus Castus, Ladiesmantle,
Raspberry leaves.

Abscesses, boils
Echinacea, Slippery elm powder
compress.

Accidents, bruises
Echinacea, Comfrey compress. *See
also* Wounds (p. 280).

Acne
Blue flag root, Red clover, Locally:
Calendula cream or ointment, Tea
tree oil: dab oil on face.

Adrenal gland stimulants
Liquorice, Ginseng, Wild yam,
Borage.

Ageing
Hawthorn, Red clover, Ginkgo,
Ginseng, Vitamin E, Honey,
Ginger.

Alcoholism
Blue flag root, Dandelion.

Allergies
Echinacea, Pulsatilla, Garlic, Honey,
Grapeseed, Vitamin B6.

Alzheimer's disease
Ginkgo biloba is said to ameliorate
symptoms, Ginseng, Ginger.

Amenorrhoea
Motherwort, Agnus castus.

Angina pectoris
Hawthorn, Motherwort, Vitamin
E, Garlic.

Anorexia nervosa
Papaya, Wild yam.

Antibiotic alternatives
Echinacea, Wild thyme, Cloves,
Myrrh, Goldenseal.

Anti-histamine alternatives
Nettles.

Anus, itching
Pilewort, Witch-hazel extract
(local).

Anxiety states
Mild to moderate: Lemon balm tea, Ginseng, St John's Wort.

Apoplexy
Lavender, Mistletoe, Marjoram, Hawthorn, Vitamin E.

Appendicitis
Wild yam, Echinacea, Myrrh.

Appetite, loss of
Papaya, Apples, Wormwood, Sorrel, Peppermint.

Arteriosclerosis
Hawthorn, Motherwort, Vitamin E, Garlic, Vitamin C.

Arthritis
Garlic, Prickly ash bark, Devil's Claw.

Aspirin poisoning
Papaya, Blue flag root, Garlic.

Asthma
Iceland moss, Lobelia, Elecampane, Hyssop, Golden linseed.

Atherosclerosis
Garlic, Vitamin E, Flaxseed.

Athlete's foot
Echinacea, Comfrey cream or ointment.

Autism
'It's all in the gut!' Gluten-free diet. No milk or dairy products. Supplement: vitamin B12. Oily fish, Bacillus coli, Papaya, Peppermint.

Backache
St John's wort, Balm, Rosemary.

Backache (from urinary disorders)
Buchu, Dandelion coffee.

Backache, muscle pain
Wild yam, Devil's claw.

Backache
Old spinal injuries: Prickly ash bark, St John's Wort.

Backache and womb disorders
Wild yam, Agnus castus.

Back passage disorders
Pilewort, Figwort, Wild yam.

Bad breath
Papaya, Milk thistle, Diluted Tea tree oil.

Bed sores
Local Comfrey cream, ointment or lotion.

Bed-wetting
Cranesbill.

Belchings, sour
Chamomile, Aniseed, Wormwood.

Bell's palsy
Valerian, Chamomile, Echinacea, Sage, Black Cohosh.

Bile, to stimulate secretion of
Milk thistle, Blue flag root, Wild yam, Barberry, Sarsaparilla, Dandelion coffee.

Some of My Favourite Remedies

Biliousness
Milk thistle, Artichoke, Seaweed
and Sarsaparilla, Artichoke.

Bladder, pain on passing water
Cranesbill, Shepherd's purse,
Slippery elm powder, Cranberry,
Bearberry.

Bleeding, to stop
Comfrey, Marigold, Nettles,
Tormentil, Witch hazel.

Blood-platelet-clumping-reducer
Grapeseed, Oily fish.

Blood, expectoration of
Cranesbill, Comfrey, Marigold.

Blood, impure
Echinacea, Blue flag root, Yellow
Dock, Burdock.

Blood pressure, high
Garlic, Mother wort, Vitamin E,
not megadoses, Oily fish for
Omega-3-fatty oils, Potassium-rich
foods, Green buckwheat tea,
Avoid Ginseng.

Blood pressure, low
Prickly ash bark, Ginger, Cayenne,
Echinacea.

Body odour
Wild yam, Thuja, Sage tea.

Boils
Echinacea, Poke root,
Marshmallow, Slippery elm
poultice.

Bowel inflammation
Slippery elm, Agrimony, Aloe vera,
Marshmallow.

Brain booster
Ginkgo Biloba, Rosemary, Oats,
Echinacea, Skullcap.

Breasts, painful
Poke root, Red clover.

Breasts, sense of fullness
Poke root.

Breasts, discomfort
Evening primrose, Starflower oil.

Breasts, to reduce
Poke root.

Breasts, to stimulate secretion of milk.
Fenugreek seeds, Milkwort,
Borage, Fennel, Goat's rue,
Raspberry leaves.

Breath, offensive
See Halitosis (p. 272).

Breathlessness
Hawthorn, Lily of the valley, Garlic.

Broken bones
Fenugreek seed tea, Comfrey
poultice.

Bronchitis
Lobelia, Iceland moss, Echinacea
(acute), Olive oil (one teaspoonful
daily), Flaxseeds.

Buerger's disease
Motherwort, Wild yam, Hawthorn,
Vitamin E.

Bunions
Local: Comfrey cream, ointment or lotion.

Burns (see your doctor)
Local dressing: Honey, Comfrey, Houseleek. Aloe vera, Almond oil, Chickweed.

Bursitis (house-maid's knee, etc.)
Local: Comfrey cream, ointment or lotion.

Caffeine syndrome
Papaya, Valerian, Chamomile.

Calculus, urinary
Pellitory-of-the-wall, Cornsilk, Stoneroot, Gravelroot.

Calmer-downer
Valerian, Lemon balm, St John's wort, Chamomile, Lavender, Passion flower.

Candida albicans vaginal infections
Agnus castus, Cider vinegar, Garlic.

Candidiasis, monilia, infection of the vagina.
Avoid yeasts. Goldenseal.

Carbuncles
Echinacea, Blue flag root, poultice. Cloves, Wormwood, Slippery elm poultice.

Cartilage injuries
Comfrey cream, ointment or lotion. Glucosamine.

Catarrh
Goldenseal, Hyssop, Garlic.

Change of life
Agnus castus, Helonias, Evening primrose, Black cohosh, Dong qual, Red clover.

Chestiness
Iceland Moss, Lobelia, Slippery elm, Flaxseed.

Chickenpox
Poke root, Agrimony, Chamomile, Echinacea, Marigold (*Calendula*) cream locally. External: Dilute Tea Tree oil to take irritation out of spots.

Chilblains
Prickly ash bark, Cider vinegar, Vitamin E. Rub with raw onion.

Cholecystitis (inflammation of the gall bladder)
Milk thistle, Wild yam, Barberry, Blue flag root. Carrot, beet and cucumber juice.

Cholesterol, to reduce
Artichoke, Garlic.

Chronic Fatigue Syndrome (ME)
Liquorice root, Ginseng, St John's wort. Supplement: Magnesium. Brewer's yeast, Cider vinegar.

Circulation, poor
Prickly ash bark, Hawthorn, Ginger

Cirrhosis of the liver
Wild yam, Milk thistle, Blue flag root, Aloe vera.

Claudication, intermittent
Hawthorn, Vitamin E., Garlic

Coeliac disease
Wild yam, Gluten-free diet,
Tomatoes.

Cold hands
Ginger, Cayenne pepper.

Colds, the common cold
Echinacea, Eucalyptus inhalant,
Liquorice, Tea Tree oil as an
inhalant, Chicken broth.

Colic, intestinal
Ginger, Chamomile, Wild yam,
Peppermint, Fennel.

Colic, kidney
Buchu, Cramp bark,
Gravelroot.

Colic, liver
Wild yam, Milk thistle, Fennel,
Agrimony, Lemon balm,
Dandelion, Wormwood.

Colitis, ulcerative.
Echinacea, Wild yam, Peppermint,
Ginger.

Constipation
Senna, Ginger, Flaxseeds, Psyllium
seeds.

*Convalescence, recovery from illness or
operation*
Ginseng, Honey, Fenugreek seeds,
Molasses, Cider vinegar, Brewer's
yeast.

Corns local
Comfrey. Apply crushed Garlic.

Coronary heart disease
Garlic, not with anti-clotting drugs
or aspirin, Vitamin E.

Cough, dry
Iceland moss, Angelica, Elecampane,
Flaxseeds.

Cough, moist
Lobelia.

Cramp
Cramp bark, Prickly ash bark,
Lavender, Ginger, Butcher's broom.

Crohn's disease
Wild yam, Chamomile tea,
Echinacea, Marshmallow,
Goldenseal, Slippery elm.

Cuts
Local treatment: Echinacea,
Comfrey, Calendula, Honey.

Cystitis
Buchu, Uva ursi.

Dandruff
Rosemary lotion, Cook with olive
oil.

Debility
Agnus castus, Red clover, Ginseng,
Ginger.

Dementia
Ginkgo biloba appears to slow
down the stroke-related symptoms
in mild and moderate cases.

Depression
St John's wort, Valerian, Lemon balm, Ginkgo biloba, Ginseng (not anxiety disorder, heart palpitations, manic-depressive illness or asthma).

Dermatitis
Echinacea. Local: Marshmallow and Slippery elm cream, Comfrey lotion or cream.

Detox
Cleansing of the system with Castor oil packs, colonics and massage, Flaxseeds, Dandelion coffee, Celery seeds, Milk thistle, Red clover, Cat's claw, Schizandra.

Diarrhoea
Wild yam, Peppermint, Aloe vera juice, Ginger.

Digestion
Chamomile, Artichoke, Ginger, Peppermint.

Dizziness
Rutin, Hawthorn.

Diverticulitis
Wild yam, Goldenseal, Fresh Ginger tea. To reduce flatulence: Slippery elm, Goldenseal.

Dog bites
Wipe with Tincture Calendula, Tincture Myrrh, or Tincture St John's wort. Follow with Slippery elm poultice.

Dropsy
Buchu, Dandelion, Chamomile.

Duodenal disorders
Papaya, Goldenseal.

Dysentery
Wild yam.

Dyslexia
Starflower oil, Evening primrose, Flaxseeds, Fish oils.

Dyspepsia
Papaya, Chamomile, Peppermint.

Ear noises
See Tinnitus (p. 279).

Earache
Echinacea, Valerian, Oil of Mullein.

Eczema, dry
Echinacea.

Eczema, moist
Red clover.

Energy booster
Ginseng, Ginger.

Epistaxis, nosebleed
Cranesbill. Local: plug with witch hazel on cotton wool.

Erysipelas
Echinacea.

Eruptions
Red clover, Echinacea.

Eyes, inflamed
Echinacea, Bilberries.

Eyes, styes
Echinacea.

Eyes, swollen lids
Buchu.

Fainting
Lemon balm.

Fevers
Yarrow, Elderflowers, Echinacea.

Fibrositis
Black Cohosh, Devil's Claw. Local:
Comfrey,

Finger nails splitting
Echinacea, Almond nuts.

Flatulence
Fennel, Caraway, Papaya, Wild
yam, Ginger, Peppermint.

Furuncles
Echinacea, Blue flag root.

Gall stone diathesis, tendency to form stone
Wild yam.

Gall bladder inflammation
Wild yam, Milk thistle, Blue flag
root. Consult your doctor for
gallstones and hepatitis.

Ganglion, cystic tumour on a tendon
Prickly ash bark.

Gastric ulcer
Papaya, Slippery elm powder,
Liquorice, Wild yam.

Gastritis
Papaya, Chamomile, Mint,
Dandelion.

Gastro-enteritis
Papaya, Chamomile, Slippery elm.

Gingivitis, gum disorders
Slippery elm powder, Poke root.
Gargle with Goldenseal

'Gone all to pieces' syndrome
Valerian, Wild yam, Chamomile,
Comfrey tea.

Gravel in urine
Buchu, Apples, Slippery elm (to
facilitate passage of gravel),
Apricots, Parsley, Nettles.

Greasy skin
Milk thistle, Dandelion coffee,
Artichoke.

Haemochromatosis
Bronzed diabetes, Milk thistle.

Haemorrhoids (piles)
Pilewort, Figwort. Chickweed,
Plantain.

Halitosis, bad breath
Wild yam. Gargle: dilute Tea tree
oil.

Hay fever
Honey in the comb.

Head lice
External: Tea tree oil.

Headache
Betony, Lemon balm, Valerian,
Vervain, Fever few, Butcher's broom.

Head noises
See Tinnitus (p. 279).

Heart and circulation
Garlic, Hawthorn, Artichoke,
Honey, Starflower oil, Evening
primrose oil, Ginkgo, Ginseng,
Soya isoflavones, Oily fish for
Omega-3-fatty oils.

Hepatitis
See your doctor. Wild yam, Milk
thistle, Dandelion.

Hepatitis C
Castor oil packs over liver area,
three days in succession on a
weekly basis. Milk thistle.

Hernia, hiatus
Papaya, Goldenseal.

Herpes zoster
See Shingles (p. 278).

Hiccough
Papaya, Onion juice, Chamomile.

Hoarseness of speech
Echinacea, Poke root, Iceland moss,
Honey and Lemon.

*Hormones, including pre-menstrual
symptoms*
Evening primrose oil, Starflower
oil, St John's wort, Agnus castus,
Black cohosh.

Hormone replacement therapy alternative
Black cohosh.

Hormone system: to sustain balance
Starflower oil (borage), Hydrocele,
Pulsatilla, Poke root.

Hypoglycaemia
Echinacea.

Hysteria
Valerian, Passion flower.

Immune system, to stimulate
Echinacea, Garlic, Ginseng
(Siberian).

Impetigo
Echinacea, Blue flag root. External:
Wipe with dilute Tea tree oil or
Calendula lotion.

Impotence
Agnus castus, Turnera, Siberian
ginseng, Saw palmetto.

Incontinence of urine
Cranesbill, Bearberry, Horsetail.

Indigestion
Papaya, Artichoke, Peppermint.

Infertility
Agnus castus.

Inflammatory condition
Grapeseed.

Influenza
Echinacea, Chicken broth. Tea tree
oil as an inhalant: two drops to
bowl of hot water.

Insomnia
Valerian, Hops, Lettuce.

Intermittent claudication
Ginkgo biloba, Vitamin E.

Intestinal colic, abdominal cramp
Papaya, Wild yam.

Some of My Favourite Remedies

Irritable bowel syndrome
Peppermint.

Irritability, nervous
Valerian, Lemon balm tea.

Ischaemic Heart Disease
Hawthorn, Lily of the Valley,
vitamin E.

Itching of skin
Echinacea, Wild yam. External: Tea
tree oil.

Jaundice
Agrimony, Milk thistle, Dandelion.

Jet lag
Ginseng, Gota kola, Capsicum,
Garlic, Kola.

Joints swollen and painful
Devil's claw.

Joint mobility
Devil's claw, Ginger.

Kidney stone, tendency to form stone
Buchu.

Kidney weakness (see your doctor)
Buchu, Parsley, Juniper.

Labour pains, to assist
Agnus castus, Helonias.

Lacerated wounds
See Wounds (p. 280).

Lactation, to stimulate
Fenugreek seed tea.
See Breasts (p. 268).

Laryngitis
Poke Root, Lobelia, Echinacea.

Lassitude
Hawthorn, Cider vinegar, Brewer's
yeast.

Legs, aching
Hawthorn, Motherwort, Vitamin E.

Legs, locking at the knee
Prickly ash bark.

Leg ulcer
Echinacea, Blue flag root, Honey
dressing.

Legs, pins and needles
Cramp bark, Vitamin E.

Legs, giving way sensation in ankles
Cramp bark, Calcium and
Magnesium supplement.

Leucorrhoea, vaginal discharge
Agnus castus, Helonias, Cranesbill,
Echinacea, Goldenseal.

Lichen planus
Echinacea.

Lips, sore
Slippery elm powder, Poke root,
Honey. Dilute Tea tree oil and
apply to lips.

Liver, disorders.
Wild yam, Milk thistle, Agrimony,
Cynara artichoke.

Long life
Ginkgo, Watercress, Broccoli.

Low mood
St John's wort.

Lumbago
Buchu, Black cohosh, Devil's Claw.

Lymphadenoid disorders
Red clover, Poke root, Violet.

Marasmus, wasting, emaciation
Echinacea, Flaxseeds, Fenugreek
seeds.

Mastitis
Red clover, Poke root, Echinacea.

Masturbation, help break the habit
Agnus castus, Thuja, Marjoram,
Black willow.

Maternity aid
Agnus castus, Motherwort,
Raspberry leaves.

Measles
Marigold petals, Saffron, Agrimony,
Thyme, Chamomile.

Memory and concentration
Ginkgo biloba, Gotu kola.

Meniere's disease
Valerian, Feverfew.

Menopause
Agnus castus, Black cohosh, St
John's wort, Sage.

Men's disorders
See Prostate gland (p. 277).

Menstruation, painful
Agnus castus, Lavender, Black
cohosh.

Menstruation, excessive bleeding
Cranesbill, Beth root, Yarrow.

Menstruation, irregular
Motherwort, Lavender, Feverfew.

Mental confusion
Ginkgo biloba.

Mental performance, enhance
Ginkgo biloba, Ginseng, Flaxseeds.

Metabolism, to stimulate
Ginseng, Nettles, Ginger.

Migraine, nerve origin
Valerian.

Migraine, sick headache
Feverfew (not in presence of aspirin
or Nonsteroidal Anti-inflammatory
Drugs).

Migraine, hormone imbalance
Agnus castus, Black cohosh.

Migraine, kidney malfunction
Buchu.

Migraine, congested liver
Milk thistle, Dandelion, Wild yam.

Morning sickness
Ginger, Raspberry leaves.

Morning stiffness
Devil's claw.

Motion sickness
Ginger, Papaya.

Mouth ulcers
Echinacea, Poke root, Goldenseal.

Some of My Favourite Remedies

Mucous colitis
Wild yam, Peppermint, Goldenseal.

Muscle, aches and pains
Devil's claw, Prickly ash bark.
External: Tea tree oil.

Nails
Paint: Tea tree oil or Tincture
Myrrh. Eat five almonds a day.

Nappy rash
External: dilute Tea tree oil,
Comfrey oil

Nerve tensions
Valerian, St John's wort.

Nerve tonic
St John's wort, Ginseng.

Nettle rash, hives
Red clover, Echinacea,
Chamomile.

Neuralgia
Chamomile.

Neurasthenia
Valerian, Cider vinegar, Brewer's
yeast.

Neuritis
Cramp Bark, Chamomile tea,
Devil's claw.

Nosebleed
Cranesbill, Marigold.

Numbness
Lavender, Wormwood, Sage.

Nymphomania
Agnus castus, Black willow, Hops.

Osteoarthritis
Black Cohosh, Devil's Claw,
Guaiacum.

Osteoporosis
Black Cohosh, Calcium and
vitamin D, 1000mg daily, Horsetail,
Fenugreek seeds.

Ovaralgia, pain in an ovary
Agnus castus, Echinacea, Castor oil
packs.

Palpitation
Hawthorn, Balm, Lavender,
Vitamin E.

Peptic ulcer
Papaya, Goldenseal, Echinacea,
Slippery elm, Goldenseal.

Personality unstable
Valerian, St John's wort.

Phlebitis
See your doctor. Hawthorn,
Echinacea, Butcher's Broom,
Vitamin E.

Physical performance decreased
Ginkgo biloba, Ginseng, Brewer's
yeast, Cider vinegar.

Piles
See Haemorrhoids
(p. 272).

Pleurisy
See your doctor. Iceland Moss,
Angelica, Sage, Marshmallow,
Pleurisy root.

Pregnancy, vomiting
Agnus castus, Helonias, Raspberry leaf tea.

Pregnancy, nervous restlessness
Raspberry leaf tea, Chamomile.

Pre-menstrual tension (PMT)
Agnus castus, Valerian, Evening primrose oil, Starflower oil, St John's wort. The liver needs B vitamins and magnesium to metabolise oestrogen properly.

Prostate gland
Benign prostatic hyperplasia (BPH), Saw palmetto, Soya isoflavones, Garlic.

Pruritis, intense itching
Echinacea, Wild yam, Dandelion, Red clover.

Psoriasis
Echinacea, Thuja, Yellow dock, Dandelion.

Pyorrhoea, purulent disease of the gums
Echinacea, Myrrh, Goldenseal.

Quinsy, acute suppurative tonsillitis
Poke root, Cinquefoil, Cudweed, Wormwood, Sage.

Rashes, dry skin
Blue flag root, Yellow dock, Seaweed and Sarsaparilla, Comfrey lotion.

Rashes or moist skin
Echinacea, Red clover. Topical: Jojoba oil.

Raynaud's disease
Ginkgo biloba, Hawthorn, Ginger, Valerian, Vitamin E, Garlic.

Relaxation, to promote
Valerian.

Respiratory ailments
Iceland moss, Garlic. *See* Bronchitis (p. 268) and Asthma (p. 267).

Restlessness
Lemon balm tea, Chamomile, Valerian.

Rheumatic fever
Black cohosh, Echinacea, Devil's claw.

Rheumatism, acute
Black cohosh.

Rheumatoid arthritis
Devil's claw, Ginger.

Rickets
Dock root, Horsetail, Comfrey tea, Nettle tea, Calcium/Magnesium supplements, Fenugreek seeds.

Sciatica
Black cohosh, Devil's claw.

Seasonal Affective Disorder (SAD)
St John's wort, Valerian, Gota kola, Hops, Liquorice, Siberian ginseng.

Sexual debility
Damiana, Ginseng, Ginkgo biloba, Ginger.

Some of My Favourite Remedies

Shellshock and explosive shocks (as in airraids of wartime)
Valerian, St John's wort.

Shingles
Valerian. Alternatively, wipe over affected area with pear juice.

Sickness
Ginger, particularly during chemotherapy or after anaesthesia.

Sickness (altitude)
Ginkgo, Ginger.

Sinus disorders
Garlic, Poke root.

Skin complaints
Echinacea, Starflower oil, Evening primrose oil.

Sleep problems
Valerian, or a milky drink with honey. Chamomile, St John's wort, Hops, Passion flower.

Smell, loss of sense of
Papaya, Zinc supplement.

Smelly feet
External: Tea tree oil. Treat liver (p. 274) and kidneys (p. 274).

Sneezing, uncontrollable
Chamomile tea, Lobelia.

Sore throat
Chamomile, Echinacea, Poke root, Chicken broth.

Spina bifida, neural-tube birth defects
For women at risk: Folic acid supplement.

Sprains, local
Comfrey.

Sterility
Agnus castus, Wild yam.

Stomach, sour
Chamomile, Balm, Agrimony, Meadowsweet.

Stomatitis, inflammation of the mouth
Echinacea, Honey.

Stress, nervous effects of
Valerian, Black cohosh, Ginseng, Lemon balm, St John's wort, Passion Flower.

Stroke, to reduce incidence
Garlic, Honey, Hawthorn.

Stye
Echinacea.

'Superbug' (methicillin-resistant staphylococcus aureus)
Tea tree oil, Myrrh, Boswellia.

Swollen ankles
Buchu (if due to kidneys), Hawthorn (if due to heart), Juniper.

Synovitis
Devil's claw.

Tachycardia, rapid heart beat
Hawthorn, Passion flower, Valerian, Motherwort.

Thrombosis
Hawthorn, Motherwort, Vitamin E.

Thrush, vaginal
Goldenseal, Pulsatilla. External:
Dilute Tea tree oil. Also, yoghurt
inhibits infection.

Thyroid gland, underactive
Kelp, Brewer's Yeast, Blue flag,
Parsley, Gotu kola.

Tinnitus, ringing in the ears
Parsley tea, Plantain, Ginkgo
biloba, Sage.

'Tired-all-the-time' syndrome
St John's wort, Ginseng, Ginger.

Tonic, general
Echinacea, Ginseng, Ginger.

Tonsillitis
Echinacea, Poke root.

Toothache
Suck a clove.

Travel Sickness
See Motion sickness (p. 275).

Trench mouth, bacterial infection of the gums
Echinacea.

Trichomonas, vaginal infection
Agnus castus, Goldenseal, Thuja,
Garlic.

Tuberculosis
Iceland moss, Elecampane,
Liquorice.

Tuberculosis, ill-effects of BCG vaccine
Echinacea.

Ulcers of the mouth
Echinacea.
Gargle with Tincture of Myrrh.

Ulcers of the legs
See Leg Ulcers (p. 274).

Ulcerative colitis
Slippery elm powder, Wild yam.

Under-weight
Agnus castus, Fenugreek seeds,
Brewer's yeat.

Uric acid diathesis
Black cohosh, Nettles, Celery
seeds, Wild carrot.

Urinary infections, general
Buchu, Cranberry, Echinacea.

Urinary disorders, pain on passing urine
Buchu, Goldenseal.

Urinary disorders, incontinence
Cranesbill, Cranberry.

Urinary disorders – always passing urine
Uva ursi, Shepherd's purse.

Urinary disorders, retention of urine
See your doctor. Magnesium,
360mg daily for two months.

Urticaria
See Nettle rash (p. 276).

Uterine cramp
Agnus castus, Cramp bark, Black
cohosh.

Uterine haemorrhage
Shepherd's purse, Cranesbill.

Vaccination, ill-effect of
Wild yam, Thuja.

Vaginosis
External: Dilute Tea tree oil.
Yoghurt in diet.

Varicose ulcer
See Leg ulcer (p. 274).

Varicose veins
Hawthorn, Motherwort,
Horse-chestnut, Vitamin E,
Butcher's Broom.

Vegetarian and Vegan health hazards
Vitamin B12, Calcium, Zinc.

Venous disorders
Hawthorn, Horse-chestnut,
Vitamin E.

Vertigo, giddiness
Ginkgo, Green buckwheat tea.

Vincent's disease
Echinacea, Tincture Myrrh,
Tincture Goldenseal.

Vitality
Ginseng, B vitamins.

Vitamin deficiency
Multivitamin supplement.

Vitiligo
External: Black pepper extract.

Vomiting
Papaya, Onions, Fennel.

Vulva, inflammation of
Agnus castus, Yoghurt.

Warts
Dandelion or Celandine: juice of
the fresh plant.

Whooping cough
Red clover, Lobelia, Iceland moss,
Chicken soup.

Wind, to expel
Ginger.

Womb, catarrh of
See Leucorrhoea (p. 274).

Womb, pain in
Agnus castus, Black cohosh.

Womb, change of life
Agnus castus.

Worms
Garlic, Wormwood, Sage,
Anthelmintics.

Wounds, bruises
Where skin is broken: Marigold
(Calendula). Where skin is
unbroken: (Arnica) Comfrey
compress.

Wounds, suppurating
Echinacea, Comfrey or Slippery
elm powder poultice, Honey
dressing.

Wounds, broken bones
Echinacea and Goldenseal to avoid
infection, Comfrey poultice.

Aromatherapy

Aromatherapy was an art practised by the ancient Egyptians and older civilizations for healing the body. Of later years it has been rediscovered by a French chemist (in 1928) – René-Maurice Gattefosse – when he recalled an episode in his life in which he sustained a burn on his hand.

On the spur of the moment he plunged the hand into a vessel of lavender oil. To his amazement it healed within hours with little evidence of a scar. Using the same technique, some medical officers during the Second World War treated the wounds of soldiers with success.

Essential oils are not usually taken internally, but as a mix in a massage oil with a carrier oil – usually almond oil. They may be added to a bath. As an inhalant, a tissue or clean linen may be impregnated with a few drops to use as a compress. For a refreshing footbath five to ten drops of your selection (say, clary sage) may be welcome at the end of a busy day.

For a massage oil, place one drop of your selection of two or three oils into a teaspoonful of carrier oil, in an egg cup, mix and use. A 10ml dropper bottle ensures an accurate number of drops.

Aromatherapy oils should not be used in pregnancy, given to children, or used neat. A patch test may sometimes be necessary, as some oils have an allergic action which varies according to the individual.

'Being in an intensive care unit can be extremely frightening to some patients,' said a senior nurse. 'Just being here is anxiety-provoking, and on top of that is all the discomfort associated with being severely ill. Aromatherapy calms them, reduces anxiety levels and helps them to sleep.'

A number of hospitals prescribe essential oils of aromatherapy instead of drugs to get elderly mentally ill patients to sleep.

Aromatic lavender oil was placed in a wall heater at night, with the nursing staff monitoring patients' sleeping patterns. After a six-week trial it was confirmed that patients slept as well, and in some cases better, than with drugs.

Some oils may be taken into the body as tea– one heaped teaspoonful lemon balm infused in a teacup of boiling water provides a tea made more beneficial by the small amount of essential oil of the plant being liberated by the water. The same applies to a cup of tea made with chamomile, fennel and peppermint, etc.

Oils are useful as inhalants: a few drops on a tissue can relieve catarrh, colds, etc. Fragrant burners and electronic diffusers are available for vapour inhalation. Bring to the boil two litres of water and allow to stand for three to four minutes; sprinkle five to ten drops of oil (say eucalyptus) on the surface and inhale steam with a towel over head for influenza and respiratory troubles.

Nature's Pharmacy

Condition	*Essential oil*
Acne	Geranium, Sandalwood
Anxiety states	Chamomile, Neroli, Jasmin
Arthritis	Ginger, Juniper, Rosemary, Tea tree
Arthritis *(joints)*	Benzoin, Chamomile, Rosemary, Sage, Ginger, Black pepper
Asthma	Eucalyptus, Lavender, Marjoram
Athlete's foot	Tea tree, Lavender
Blood pressure *(high)*	Ylang-ylang, Lavender, Marjoram, Nutmeg, Lemon balm, Clary sage
Blood pressure *(low)*	Ginger, Clove, Thyme, Cinnamon
Backache	Benzoin, Chamomile, Ginger, Sage, Basil
Breasts *(painful)*	Lavender, Geranium
Breast *(cyst)*	Cypress
Breasts *(discomfort)*	Evening primrose, Starflower
Breasts *(increase and firm)*	Clary sage
Breasts *(to reduce)*	Lemongrass
Bronchitis	Hyssop, Sandalwood
Bruises	Lavender, Marjoram
Bunions	Chamomile, Cedarwood
Burns	Chamomile, Yarrow, Lavender
Bursitis *(House-maid's knee)*	Juniper, Ginger, Cypress
Calmer-downer	Cedarwood, Cypress, Roman Chamomile
Carbuncles	Cinnamon
Catarrh	Eucalyptus, Cajeput, Cedarwood
Cellulite	Geranium, Fennel, Juniper, Sage
Chestiness	Eucalyptus, Tea tree, Lavender
Chickenpox	German Chamomile
Chilblains	Cypress, Lemon, Lavender
Circulation, poor	Rosemary
Chronic Fatigue Syndrome *(ME)*	Rosemary, Cypress, Peppermint
Cold hands	Ginger, Benzoin
Colds	Cajeput, Basil, Eucalyptus, Peppermint
Constipation	Fennel, Ginger, Rosemary
Corns, local	Tagetes
Cough	Benzoin, Eucalyptus, Hyssop, Black Pepper
Cramp	Cypress, Lavender, Basil, Marjoram

Condition	Essential oil
Cystitis	Basil, Bergamot, Juniper, Rosemary
Dandruff	Rosemary, Lavender, Lemon Sage
Depression	Neroli, Geranium, Nutmeg, Clary sage
Dermatitis	Benzoin, Clary sage, Juniper, Lavender
Diabetes	Ginger, Cypress, Geranium
Diarrhoea	Ginger, Sandalwood, Roman Chamomile
Dog bites	Calendula, Myrrh
Ear-ache	Tea tree, Lavender
Eczema	Lavender, Juniper, Bergamot, Sandalwood
Endometriosis	Clary sage
Eruptions	Lavender, Tea tree
Fainting	Geranium, Lavender
Feet perspiring	Clary sage
Fevers *(cooling sponge-down)*	Lavender, Eucalyptus
Foot care	Benzion, Rosemary, Geranium
Fibrositis	Clove, Lavender, Rosemary
Finger nails, splitting	Tea tree, Myrrh
Gingivitis *(gum disorders)*	Peppermint, Eucalyptus
Gout	Birch, Basil
Greasy skin	Clary sage, Lavender, Roman Chamomile
Hair disorders	Cedarwood, Rosemary, Juniper
Hangover	Lavender
Hay fever	Lavender, Chamomile
Headache	Peppermint, Lavender
Head lice	Tea tree
Heart and Circulation	Bergamot, Rosemary, Peppermint
Hepatitis C	Castor oil packs over liver area
Hernia, Hiatus	Fennel, Ginger
Herpes zoster	Lavender, Lemon, Geranium
Hydrocele	Hyssop, Lemon, Juniper
Impetigo	Tea tree
Indigestion	Basil, Melissa, Fennel, Peppermint
Infertility	Clary sage, Nutmeg
Insect repellent	Eucalyptus, Cedarwood, Citronella
Insomnia	Valerian, Chamomile, Roman, Marjoram
Irritability	Valerian, Lemon, Melissa
Itching	Peppermint, Eucalyptus
Jet lag	Peppermint, Eucalyptus
Joints *(swollen & painful)*	Rosemary, Ginger, Black pepper, Sage, Chamomile, Benzoin

Some of My Favourite Remedies

Condition	Essential oil
Laryngitis	Sage, Sandalwood
Leg ulcers	Castor oil (and Zinc)
Leucorrhoea	Clary sage, Juniper
Lips, sore	Calendula, Tea tree, German Chamomile
Liver disorders	Lavender, Rose
Low mood	St John's wort
Lumbago	Ginger, Benzoin, Sage, Basil, Chamomile
Memory and concentration	Basil, Rosemary
Menopause	Clary sage, Bergamot, Nutmeg, Sage
Menstruation, painful	Sage, Lavender
Menstruation, irregular	Chamomile, Melissa
Mental confusion	Basil
Mental performance *(to enhance)*	Rosemary, Lavender, Basil
Migraine	Valerian, Lavender, Chamomile
Morning sickness, of pregnancy	Ginger, Spearmint
Mouth ulcers	Geranium, Thyme, Chamomile, Myrrh
Mumps	Tea tree, Lavender
Muscles *(aches and pains)*	Rosemary, Sage, Eucalyptus
Myalgic encephalitis *(ME)*	Cypress, Rosemary, Peppermint
Nappy rash	Dilute Tea tree
Nerve tension	Sandalwood, Fennel, Black Pepper, Juniper, Bergamot, Rosemary
Neuralgia	Chamomile
Neuritis	cramp, Bark
Numbness	Sage, Lavender
Osteo-arthritis	*See*: Arthritis (joints)
Osteoporosis,	Ginger, Nutmeg, Roman Chamomile
Ovaralgia *(pain in an ovary)*	Clary sage, Fennel, Geranium
Parkinson's Disease *(for muscle stiffness)*	Basil, Nutmeg, Lavender, Valerian, Rosemary
Pelvic, Inflammatory Disease	Lavender, German Chamomile
Pre-menstrual tension	Clary sage
Pre-menstrual cramp	Cypress, Lavender, Eucalyptus
Raynaud's Disorder	Nutmeg, Lavender
Restlessness	Valerian
Rheumatic fever	Eucalyptus, Thyme, Sage
Rheumatism *(acute)*	Melissa, Marjoram, Lavender

Condition	Essential oil
Rheumatoid arthritis	Juniper, Rosemary, Marjoram, Lavender, Ginger
Sickness *(nausea)*	Peppermint
Sinus disorders	Basil, Eucalyptus, Lavender, Peppermint
Skin complaints	Chamomile, Roman and German
Slipped Disc	Ginger, Rosemary, Black Pepper, Fennel, Juniper
Sore throat	Sage throat wipe
Sportsmen's oils	Lemon, Lavender, Chamomile, Rosemary
Sport's runner's oils	Basil, Rosemary, Bergamot
Sprains	Lavender, Marjoram
Stress	Valerian, Melissa, Chamomile, Ylang-ylang, Rose otto, Juniper
Tired-all-the-time	Orange, Peppermint, Rosemary, Geranium
Trichomonas *(vaginal infection)*	Tea tree, Oregano, Bergamot
Urinary disorders	Juniper, Rosemary
Vaginosis *(external)*	Dilute Tea tree
Varicose ulcer	Eucalyptus, Tea tree
Varicose veins	Lemon, Geranium
Warts	Lavender, Cypress
Whooping cough sponge-down	Thyme, Lavender, Hyssop
Worms	Lavender, Lemon, Eucalyptus

The Bartrams

I have always had a profound admiration for my namesake, John Bartram (1699–1777), who, in the true scientific spirit opened-up the American wilderness in search of plants – medicinal and ornamental. Records of the epic travels of John and his son, William, in the early eighteenth century, are now part of the botanical heritage of the United States.[34]

John's grandfather had emigrated to America from Derbyshire, England, in 1682, 'before there was a single house in Philadelphia'. After surviving many hardships they settled in Pennsylvania as farmers.

It all started the day farmer John stepped on a daisy when ploughing his field. Halting the horses to reflect on what he had done, he reached down, taking it thoughtfully in his hands. Pulling the flower to pieces he was smitten by the knowledge that for untold centuries men have tilled the earth, destroying countless millions of flowers 'without ever being acquainted with their structure and uses'.

Little did he realize from that transforming moment that he would blaze a trail over dangerous American territory that was to thrill Europe and inspire such poets as Wordsworth, Southey and Coleridge with a new awareness of the world about us.

John became the first botanist to develop hybridization, thus opening up to the world a wide range of different species. He formed the first botanical garden in America, unique for its cultivation of rare native plants. Incidentally, he was the first to record the presence of ginseng.

Early in life he had a passion for the study of physics and surgery. His knowledge of healing by natural remedies enabled him to bring welcome relief to sick neighbours and native Indian Americans he met on his travels. Though not a trained doctor or apothecary, his medicines were all derived from the botanical kingdom, and his knowledge empirical.

John's versatility earned him the respect of all he met. Not only was his farm a model of advanced agricultural planning of the time, but his knowledge of medicinal plants impressed all, including the celebrated Swedish naturalist, Peter Kahn, who sometimes travelled with him.

We often wonder if his interest in herbal healing stemmed from the tragic event of his wife's death in a raging epidemic of unknown cause only four years after his marriage. I believe his activities would have been devoted exclusively to healing had he not received a commission from King George III to explore and report upon the natural history of the country. This offered the exciting prospect of living the life of a robust adventurer in an age when a brave New World promised undreamed of opportunities.

Bartram's amazing talents for using medicinal plants so impressed Kahn that his own journal is studded with remedies collected from the Bartrams during their friendship.

Kahn learnt that a decoction of alder bark made an antiseptic dressing for wounds. As lacerations were all part of hazards along the way, we can understand why many recipes were for the relief of pain and bleeding. These included the 'life everlasting' plant. For a bruise there were few things better than a leaf from the poke root plant (*phytolacca*). Native Indian Americans prepared a tasty sweetmeat from wake robin by boiling the spadix and leaves.

It was discovered that sassafras flowers were good for making tea. Sassafras berries were boiled and the oil skimmed off the surface to be saved for use as a rubbing-oil for rheumatic joints. When kicked by a horse, John boiled a plant described by Kahn as *Sarothra gentianoides*, which was said to 'appease' the pain.

When at home the Bartrams kept an open table for all visitors where their own servants were free to sit down in an atmosphere of simple Quaker piety. Benjamin Franklin would sit with John in his garden, drinking cider brewed on the farm. Famous names of the contemporary world of botany visited and corresponded, calling John 'the greatest natural botanist in the world'.

William, his son, was destined for even greater fame. Sharing his father's passion for natural history, he began sketching plants from the age of ten. His exquisitely executed drawings are now highly prized. He gathered around him dedicated botanists who organized study of the science in the New World and saved many rare plants from extinction. They were forerunners of the thriving present-day Bartram Society.

We wonder how many flowers and trees that enchant us on European estates are descendants of seeds and seedlings gathered 250 years ago by those intrepid men.

A wise man has said:

'In medicine there is both a science and an art. they are closely allied, but they are, at base, different from each other. One can learn science, even those possessing moderate talent can do this. But art is a gift from heaven. Therefore, do not consider yourself a great physician because you have a great stock of scientific knowledge.

The learned man is merely an unceasing receiver of material. The artist creates new thought associations. The former is suffocated by his mass of knowledge, the latter is ever receiving new inspirations. Thus, learn as much as you can, but your knowledge should not be for yourself, but only material for your art.'

Conclusion – Prescription for Living

It may seem strange in a book on Nature's plan for your health to have a chapter on art, music, gardening and other forms of recreation. Yet in a very real way these are all part of the whole person. 'All work and no play makes Jack a dull boy' goes the adage. 'Play' may take many forms, but the mind and the spirit need their own nourishment as much as the body does. Art, music, literature and all forms of culture are, so to say, the constituents of this diet.

Art and the full man

To the average person a picture in a gallery is a conglomeration of colour for our enjoyment. The elevating influence of a good picture – its emotional content – is often hidden from them. So they remain strangely unmoved by its magic power.

But I would like you to be aware of that vast reservoir of rich emotional experience to be found in the world of pictures. Is it possible to acquire a 'new eye' for the visual pleasures of Renoir? There can be sheer delight in the poetry of paint. Your choice in art can decide what heights you can attain, and what help you can get.

The figure of a labourer, sheaves in a harvest field, a breathless hush in a Provencal rose-garden can be so beautiful that we want to know more about the fascination of colour.

We cannot stand speechless before some great picture without letting into our lives more emotional wealth. Pictures, like travel, not only broaden our outlook, they widen our sensibilities.

This is an age of superb reproductions. Most galleries and art shops sell excellent prints of the great paintings. There is an old master for every home. You can transform your walls into vivid magic.

An understanding of pictures can be immensely rewarding. We are likely to become better acquainted with art, and the refreshment it brings, if we are not looking solely for intellectual satisfaction. As soon as the theme of a picture becomes a mental exercise, its value as recreation is destroyed. It is when our new interest becomes a focus for close concentration that advantages will be strictly limited.

You may be tempted to look at art in intellectual terms. If you don't, you'll be dubbed as a sentimentalist. Since emotional enrichment is our principal object, entry into a famous gallery will be like passing the threshold into a new world. We are taken out of ourselves. We become part of a Turner seascape, a Pissarro orchard in spring, a medieval village painted by Piero della Francesca.

So many of the great painters, including Constable, Gainsborough and Corot were inspired by the poetry and grace at the back of Nature, as an experience for its own sake. In the philosophy of Corot the soil was a source of wisdom.

Why not develop your instinctive feeling for colour harmony? Don't be afraid of innocence in your approach to the muse. You'll be surprised how appreciation of good pictures deepens the personality, bringing a maturity other people can't help observing.

Rooms are made to be enriched. Always buy a picture you love and think you can live with. After hours of an artist's endeavour an engraving or etching acquires a uniqueness – a real thing with living quality.

Studied with loving care, your selections will help create an atmosphere of serenity and charm – a home after your own personality. Art can be truly a balm for healthier lives in a world of rush and pressure.

I like pictures. I have boxes of beautifully coloured cards collected from the galleries of Europe over the past fifty years. Some are a little faded, others have colours as brilliant as on the day they were printed. No card is too old to bring back some memory of the original.

I have only to close my eyes to see the marvels of Raphael, Michelangelo and Leonardo da Vinci, who lavished their supreme gifts on European culture and who share with me their talent for beauty.

I know I shall never be able to afford a masterpiece, yet the walls of my home are filled with inexpensive yet superb copies – full of colour and character.

I love the Impressionists who brighten a grey corner and flood an empty hall with light. If you have had the good fortune to see the originals in palatial European galleries you are seldom likely to feel lonely or depressed.

At the time of your visit, what is to prevent you storing unforgettable impressions in your mind to recall in moments of leisure? Expect your favourite pictures to spring alive in your mind. Your gallery colour card will assist. Some people spend considerable sums of money on meditational and anti-stress techniques which art and music can produce at little or no cost.

Colour combinations of the Old Masters have a fascination of their very own. More meaningful than a photograph, they have been born out of an overwhelming love of the beautiful.

A picture tells us more than paint and canvas. It is a human document fashioned out of the creative energy of a man's soul. What we need is a mind stored with lovely pictures, a Rijksmuseum full of Rembrandts, a Hermitage with visions of Renoir. As with flowers, the process of dissection is often a process of destruction.

Who could possibly forget the glorious cobalt blues of Fra Filippo Lippi or those gleaming emeralds of Botticelli? Bellini, Correggio and Titian ride high in a sky of lesser stars, depicting the drama of history and the enchantment of Nature's loveliness.

I hope you will make the acquaintance of some of the English painters. Romney, Gainsborough and Turner await your advances if you have not yet discovered them. Do you look for a landscape full of scintillating light as an antidote to ruthless art? Then look at Canaletto. He always painted his scenes in sunshine. He left enchanting views of London, bathing Wren's churches in a Mediterranean radiance.

Even after centuries, some pictures by their colour and poignant appeal stir our hearts as powerfully as ever. I am sure you will not wish to miss the wonderful world of the Old Masters – full of unforgettable impressions that stimulate, educate, comfort and soothe.

Another aspect of art and health is the very real part it can play in convalescence. Art therapy has been a valuable aspect of recovery and convalescence in many hospitals and can be a creative and restoring hobby for the retired and the sick in their home situation.

Good books

I am grateful to the literary giants of history whose intimate thoughts have often been my inspiration. My life is the richer for having caught a glimpse of that burning compassion which has prompted many a masterpiece.

If we have not read any of the classics we may never know what a comfort can be brought into our lives by the world's choicest thoughts preserved in the choicest words. It is like the writer and yourself speaking to each other. Emerson's exciting discovery was that being alive was an almost unbelievable pleasure. He simply had to commit it to writing.

How fortunate for us that he did. At the time he wrote, just after the American Civil War, the country's morale was in the doldrums. Struggling farming communities drew inspiration from his publications when there was no money and little heart to tackle the enormous problems ahead. His words were psychosomatic medicine, especially to those who had lost loved ones in the struggle.

'I embrace life', he affirmed, meaning darkness as well as light, the bitter as well as the sweet, and went on to prescribe thankfulness, joy and cheerfulness.

I know an insatiable globetrotter, who has shared in the thrills of distant lands, has flown over the Grand Canyon and lingered beside the crystal pool of the Taj Mahal. But he is no longer able to do so.

Now, without the fatigue of long journeys, the inconvenience of weighty luggage and the complicated arrangements with travel agents, he has the whole wide world to explore. He has become a great reader. He is one of those rare souls who has not yet lost his sense of 'wonder'. Though he patiently bears in his spine old war wounds sustained in the navy, he is still young at heart.

Seasons come and go; he never seems to change. It is very unlikely that he will ever again ride in a rickshaw or a funicular railway, but from the pages of his ample stock of paperbacks he again hears the song of the palm fronds, and gives himself up to the cool and pleasant breezes of the East Indies. We have never known a man with such a disability get so much out of life.

The world of books is indeed a world of wonder.

The power of music

I am grateful to the great musicians – companions of my solitude. To the listening ear and the sensitive heart they breathe a rhythmic commentary on life. Hum of insect, song of the west wind and the natural inflection of the human voice – the air is filled with the sounds of articulate voices. Cry of seabird, thunder of surf, the mountains and hills – the whole earth is alive with the sound of music.

'There is no mightier art than this', wrote George Sand, 'to awaken in a man the sublime consciousness of his own humanity; to paint before his mind's eye the rich splendours of Nature; the joy of meditation, the national character of a people; the passionate tumult of their hopes and fears . . . Remorse, control, despair, enthusiasm, faith, calm and glory –

these and a thousand other nameless emotions belong to music'. What a boon is music!

I am sure music makes for health and balance. All that is profound in music creates a sense of expansion and liberation. Physiologists tell us it even influences glandular function. If that is so, it is a factor in healing some mental and personality disorders.

Experience confirms that music has the power to calm and strengthen the mind. There is much more to music than we are aware of. It is possible it pierces an unknown dimension within ourselves, releasing powerful energies.

It was Pythagoras who said the movements of the planets make a musical sound. Is it not reasonable to believe that the ancients were right when they referred to the harmony produced by movements of the stars?

Do you recollect hearing a recording of the keynote of the moon when struck by a discarded module at the time of the historic landing? It was a startling experience. The steady vibration pitched an accurate 'middle C' which continued to sound for over an hour.

In his book *The Symphony of Life* scientist Donald Hatch Andrews writes: 'To sum up the nature of this scientific revolution in a single phrase, we are finding that the universe is composed not of matter but of music.'

For relaxation you may wish to play the first movement of Beethoven's *Moonlight Sonata* or his *Pastoral Symphony* (Sixth). If the storm scenes in the latter prove a little too agitating, you may switch off and reach for a Chopin *Nocturne*, Liszt's *Liebestraüm*, or one of Mendelssohn's *Songs Without Words*.

I once knew a surgeon who at the beginning of every day, before leaving for the hospital, listened to Bach's *Air on a G String*. Few pieces are more calming and reassuring. A high spirituality shines through many of the works of Bach.

Think of Pablo Casals, world-famous cellist, to whom music meant so much. 'Every day I am reborn', he said. 'My early morning piece of music is a sort of benediction on the house. It fills me with an awareness of the wonder of life, with a feeling of the incredible marvel of being human. Music is never the same to me. Each day it is something new and unbelievable.'

We should avoid dividing music into 'classical' and 'popular'. There is good and bad in each. There is music for different temperaments. Personally, I love all kinds, especially the shimmering sparkle of a bank of violins – singing strings. But there are hundreds of talented artists all over the world who enliven and inspire by their various styles and instruments.

Musical genius is rare, but with a little encouragement most children and adults can learn to play an instrument for relaxation and fun. Performance, however humble, opens up an exciting new world. You may be one of the fortunates who was taught the elements in childhood. If so, you will know how to strike a few chords and charm your cares away.

Old pianos and other instruments have therapeutic value. When you're depressed, anxious or nervous, there's nothing like a few minutes making your own music. Note how it sends you back into the world in sunny mood.

Simple chords can be easily learnt. Even non-players lose their worries by the soothing sound of a few chords struck in harmony.

Whether we favour the classics, pop or rock, our selection may be one to prepare the body for action or assist in the performance of a task. It is likely that we will want to turn it on for its soothing influence in times of stress.

George Duhamel, novelist, when playing a humble song on his flute, found his painful thoughts going to sleep and a calm serenity steal over him. He writes: 'For a man deprived of the consolation of faith, music is nevertheless a kind of faith. That is to say, it is something that upholds, re-unites, revives, comforts.'

Hobbies

You say you have no talents? Now you know that's not true. Experience and history have convinced us that people possessing the most meagre gifts have changed the world. What they lacked in brains, they made up with perseverance, grit and the ability to see through some distasteful duty to the very end.

Gifts increase our power to give help. They make us more useful citizens. Are you talented in banking or economics? It is your duty to seek service on local government councils and not leave the job to political opportunists with only half the qualifications.

Everybody has a talent. True, we might be quite independent now. Completely self-contained. Yet in a few years the situation may be different. Strength may fail, health may break down through overwork or unwise food combinations. Wealth may disappear overnight as it did for thousands in the 1929 depression. Friends may desert us. Even our much vaunted twenty-first century science may prove of no avail when confronted with the realities of life. In short, we may be thrown upon the chance mercies of the world. We may need a second string to our bow.

Now is the day when you have the greatest power and opportunity to do a good turn to someone far too proud to request your aid. Do it while you may. Do it while you have strength and ability. Do it while your talents are still silvery and shining. Do it with those few pence you have left over after your commitments to the welfare state. What, only a few coppers left? Then you can buy stamps and paper on which to write chatty notes to pen pals in hospitals, prisons and places of confinement. Your talent will be to make people laugh and to leave a trail of smiles in a lonely and thirsty land.

Are you a good mixer? That's a talent indeed. Put it to good use. Thousands of unhappy folk just haven't got that gift. Their lives will be a little livelier for an occasional squirt of the oil of cheerfulness that only *you* can inject into their social gearbox. Good mixing is an art. Many of us have to learn it. If you want to be good at anything you must keep practising it for years.

We may not all be endowed with the specialist skills of the artist, musician, financier or master-builder, but our talents with spade, pen or even a pair of knitting needles may bring rare inner contentment and yield rich fruits, tenfold, twenty fold – not to mention an ever-widening circle of friends.

Meditation

Relief from stress through meditation has become a major culture, commended by the medical profession. A leading physician has said: 'You can throw away your tranquillizers, your diet sheets and your tracksuits. All these are out. Meditation is in. There is a way of coping with stress by conditioning our internal chemical responses, thus maintaining a physical state of peace and calm while relaxing the creative and intellectual powers of the brain.'

Though I do not wholly agree to dispose of diet sheets or tracksuits, as you can imagine, it is clear that there are profound resources to be tapped from the depths of our being in the stillness of meditation. I refer to a simple form of which we are all capable – not transcendental meditation, which is an advanced form as practised by some religions. It is not necessary to have a religious belief to learn to meditate.

Long years ago Tibetan monks demonstrated how an impressive increase in body temperature was possible under Arctic conditions, purely by the power of thought. This led to scientific experiments which revealed how this ancient practice reduces high blood pressure, retards heartbeat, and sedates nerves without the aid of medicines.

Meditation proves valuable to both old and young. Sufferers of arthritis and nerve disorders may long for an alternative to pills and tablets. Classes now exist in most hospitals and clinics, and are one way of helping people forget their pains and discomforts.

Sportsmen say it improves their performance. Others find that the harmony it engenders improves their relationships with other people. Motionless meditation is so restful, and is a means of renewing spent energies and bringing refreshment to mind and body. Those with an exacting job to do find it improves concentration.

To free oneself temporarily from the tumult of our times is to arrest involuntary nerve contractions and nerve waste. We have to 'let go'.

The meditative state is encouraged by sitting in a chair (with your back supported) or lying on your back, relaxing as completely as you can, 'letting go' all of your muscles. Slow deep breaths are taken. The lotus position practised by various schools of meditation, including Zen Buddhism, may be possible.

Of course, we can meditate anywhere, at any time of the day. Your body should not be rigid, but free from tension, with the eyes closed. Distracting thoughts are sure to invade your shell of privacy, but they can be quietly ignored.

With true meditation comes a dawning consciousness that leads us back to Nature. Intuition is sharpened. If we have problems, we perceive more clearly what decisions we ought to make, what action we should take. Guidance becomes practical and positive. But, throughout it all, will throb a heart thankful for all the blessings of this life.

Gardens

'Much of today's social unrest, including student disorders, can be traced in some degree to a decline in gardening,' declares Joseph Ludlow, botanist. He believes that this activity gives anchorage and moral strength. 'We found that truly stable people – surgeons, ministers and airline people were dedicated gardeners . . . in a definite number of cases gardeners imparted a strength and sense of security to their families.'

Joeseph Ludlow was referring to an experiment he carried out with Dr A. Sallyborn, sociologist, when they found that 85% of all men who got divorced were non-gardeners. Also, they found that 90% of serious traffic offenders were non-gardeners.

Money can't buy good health. Right living, right eating and right activity is the secret. And what activity could be more wholesome than planting a garden?

There's nothing to compare with the vitamins and whole natural foods you grow yourself. Every citizen's necessity is fresh, homegrown food, where possible from their gardens without the aid of 'artificials'.

Maybe you need to reclaim your kitchen plot by careful composting. Then you can adopt simpler cooking techniques, where wholesome foods replace the refined foods of the supermarkets. For one thing, your homegrown crops will have the edge over those on sale elsewhere by being at their peak of freshness. This is especially true in the case of vitamin C, which can perish within hours.

Have you ever grown your own strawberries? Is anything more mouth-watering than freshly-picked, homegrown strawberries?

'Healthy crops can only be grown on a well-nourished soil,' wrote the late Dr W. E. Shewell-Cooper from Arkley Manor, Hertfordshire in the UK, home of the Good Gardener's Association, 'and that is why composting lies at the heart of every good garden.'

Compost is the most superior fertilizer in the world. It is a kind of recycling of life. However large or small your garden may be, you can follow the amazing transformation of animal and vegetable 'leftovers', eggshells, orange peel, and anything from calcified seaweed to old boots, into rich dark soil.

Enthusiasts swear by use of the upright wire compost bin, so that you can get at it easily – just dumping suitable residues into the top. Others knock together a rough wooden frame about 1.2m (4ft) high into which they layer kitchen wastes with dead leaves, grass-mowings, even a bit of straw followed by a sprinkling of lime.

This, they cover with a sheet of polythene or wooden slats to hasten the breakdown process. About every month they will give the contents a 'hook-up' with a garden fork to mix thoroughly. At the end of six months your new 'soil' will be a rich humus used as a mulch around your prize peas, roses or asparagus.

Volumes can be written about the delicious flavour of compost-grown crops, their freedom from blight, and the remarkable alternative they offer to garden chemicals, which tend to produce insipid, flavourless vegetables. Organic food culture avoids the use of chemicals on the land, but for crops that need a little extra fillip, there is always bagged organic fish meal.

An ambition of most 'good gardeners' is to grow magnificent cabbages free from caterpillar damage and onions with no white rot. They will want to have the answer to black fly on beans. Health begins with the compost heap, which has been shown to provide a positive answer to many present-day gardening problems. Organic gardening opens up an exciting new world.

I once talked to a small quixotic figure with a huge smile revealing two gold teeth. He told me his hobby was orchids.

'But don't you ever tire of them? What about growing something else for a change?'

'Not on your life! It's a disease. I've got it in my blood. I'm a bus conductor during the day and find people becoming more abusive. But, in my greenhouse I forget time and the passenger who bilked her fare. Outside it may be raining cats and dogs but in here it's always summer in a garden in Spain.'

As I looked around at the egg and cream cartons used as seedling trays I couldn't help envying him. He told me more people were growing tiny trees from the stones of avocado pears and, sure enough, there were some, pointed end up in 15cm (6in) pots of compost and sand.

Are you a pip planter? You transfer tiny trees to the garden when they get too big for the house. For curing her of some vexation of the body, a patient brought me a lemon tree grown from a pip. It was a source of fragrance but grew so large it was found a home in a local conservatory where it still grows happily in a sunny aspect.

As for myself, I love an old-fashioned garden with hollyhocks, tall and stately. In sunshine or shadow your garden offers a safe arbour – a haven of peace. We cannot all have a reproduction of a monastery garden with its border carnations and musk roses; but we can plant flowers beloved by the Elizabethans: gilly-flowers, lilies and violets. With bee plants we can look forward to summer, air vibrant with the beating wings of those 'singing masons building roofs of gold'.

Borage will grow on almost any soil and makes a sovereign drink for the melancholy mood. If you wish to put it to the test, you can always fill a border with aromatic mints, said to disperse nightmares.

How heart warming to see giant angelica (to be crystallized for Christmas) and variegated thymes smelling like 'down in Paradise'. It is reassuring to see them in a garden. You get the sense that nothing has really changed. Their reappearance each sunny June brings its own benediction.

If you have tasted the delights of gardening you will know there is no other joy quite like it.

Under an open sky

In an unpretentious country house in Bellingen, Switzerland, psychiatrist Carl Jung talked about his life.

'I have done without electricity, and tend the fireplace and stove myself. In the evenings I light the old lamps. There is no running water and I pump the water from the well; I chop the wood and cook the food. These simple acts make man simple. How difficult it is to be simple!'

To a remarkable degree our lifestyle has become swamped with a mass culture, mechanized, pragmatic and cheerfully anarchic.

To Paul B. Sears this is a matter of some concern: 'And as we lengthen and elaborate the chain of technology that intervenes between us and the natural world, we forget that we become steadily more vulnerable to even the slightest failure in that chain.

'The time has long since passed when a citizen can function responsibly without a broad understanding of the living landscape of which he is inseparably a part.'

Our new lifestyle is likely to react against the artificial, plastic and meaningless culture into which we drift. Rather it will favour discipline and, at times, self-denial. People are apt to forget how much they rely upon their own efforts for survival and a reasonable standard of health. Do we take too much for granted?

What we need is to rekindle a spark of love for the earth, and a striving to do all in our power to preserve its environment. There are important reasons why we should not neglect frequent contact at grass-roots level. There is a part of our nature which atrophies when denied exposure to the gentle influence of green acres under a wide sky.

The secret laws of Nature are beautiful in operation. They are revealed to the sensitive hearts which seek not to outwit them, or bend them to their will. All nature asks for is that people live humbly and obediently, and in accord with her laws.

> Look to this day! For it is life, the very life of life. In its brief course lies all the varieties, All the realities of existence: The bliss of growth, the glory of action, the splendour of beauty;
>
> For yesterday is always a dream, And tomorrow is only a vision; But today, well lived, makes every yesterday a dream of happiness. And every tomorrow a dream of hope. Look well, therefore, to this day.
>
> Kalisda

At whatever level in society, our personal nest reveals remarkable clues into our taste and character. We have attained to peace in the home when we have learnt to live with others day by day. Home is the place where we have to learn to be nice to each other.

The very word itself kindles confidence – the place where we know we can find welcoming warmth and a relaxed atmosphere in which we and our family feel secure. Security is perhaps our greatest need. Home is also the place where we regain the courage we once had – the place where we find all the things we hold dear – and words from those who understand.

How we need to help preserve the family unit! Does it really pay to abandon moral standards in the name of freedom? Anxiety and stress caused by broken marriages have become the biggest cause of classroom failures. We want the best for our children. The best we can possibly give our children is our time, our interest and our love.

It is natural for a woman to want a career. It is more natural still for a child to want its mother. Improved educational systems are no substitute for a loving and responsible home.

It takes a lot to make a real home. You sometimes have to be a bit of a roamer before you appreciate things you've left behind. Your home will have little to do with possessons or being rich. In fact, a lot of money may spoil your chances of domestic success.

Home's a place for earnest honest toil, where babies are born and which is left by youth to get married. It is where everything is in its place: little shoes, playthings and personal treasures gathered from our travels over the years.

A homemaker can tell in next to no time if every chair and table top has been lovingly cared for. Going into a new house he or she knows instinctively if each room breathes air and light and love. A house takes a lot of living in to make a home where people have lived and loved together.

When people come home from work, they know there's no other place in the world where they don't need to measure their thoughts or weigh their words. Home's a grand place where you can laugh with mother and have fun; where you expect to find all those never-to-be-sold things we were brought up with and never want to forget.

Neighbourliness. I hope you will not overlook an important ingredient of happiness – neighbourliness. To share a cup of tea with that other person across the way is something else that makes life well worthwhile.

The house next door, with a children's swing and a well-worn path to the back door tells us that here is someone on whom we can depend. A good neighbour does not have to tell us he cares. There is a lot of friendship waiting to be tapped in the country, in the town and on new estates.

If you are a stranger you will use the front door, ring the bell and wait for the door to open. But if you are an old friend you will use the back door and walk straight in. There's nothing more stimulating than a Windsor chair in a neighbour's kitchen.

A garden fence is a friendly place to chat across, to keep up-to-date on the price of groceries, to enquire of the cat's kittens and to ask how the children are getting on at school. We can never feel a handshake if we don't hold out ours. 'If you want a friend, be one' runs the adage.

Maybe, you haven't time for all this. 'I haven't a garden fence,' I hear you say. Then at least you can pass on to them a smile. A smile costs nothing but gives much. As an anonymous writer discovered: 'A smile enriches those who receive, without making poorer those who give. It takes but a moment, but the memory of it sometimes lasts forever. None is so rich or mighty that he gets along without it and none is so poor but that he can be made rich by it.

'A smile creates happiness in the home, fosters goodwill in business and is the countersign of friendship. It brings rest to the weary, cheer to the discouraged, sunshine to the sad and is Nature's best antidote for trouble.

Yet it cannot be bought, begged, borrowed or stolen for it is something that is of no value to anyone until it is given away. Some people are too tired to give you a smile. Give them one of yours, as none needs a smile as much as he who has no more to give.'

Reverence for life

If you ever came across a copy of *Out of my Life and Thought* by Albert Schweitzer, you will remember how he wrote most of it out of pain and much weariness after a full day's toil at his jungle hospital.

Your first impression might have been that here was a man whose practical medical and musical skills were sensitized by a philosophy sorely needed today in our material world.

Scholars and ministers may spend a whole lifetime at their teaching posts and pulpits yet miss the essential truth enshrined in their books.

No lifetime study of man-made philosophies can carry half the illumination of one precious moment of truth. Schweitzer was travelling by barge along a river through the deep African wildwood when he recorded this experience.

'Late on the third day at the very moment when, at sunset we were making our way through a herd of hippopotamuses, there flashed upon my mind, unforeseen and unsought, the phrase "reverence for life". The iron door had yielded. The path in the thicket had become visible. Now I had found my way to the idea in which affirmation of the world and of ethics are contained side by side. Now I knew that the ethical acceptance of the world and of life, together with the ideals of civilization contained in this concept, had a foundation in thought.'

In this phrase 'reverence for life' you and I find what we are seeking. Like the words 'God is Love', this marvellous phrase is a lamp shining in a dark place, an open-sesame to the riches of knowledge, a mighty in-rush of water on a dry and thirsty land.

How can we relax?
In the days when I could afford not so much as a glass of ale, weary and faint from walking on stone pavements, and later, in better times, often straight from labours which will never be distasteful, I went to rest my heart with loveliness in the National Gallery in London, or the Greek sculpture galleries in the British Museum. I go still. There the form of limb and torso, of bust and neck, gave me a sighing sense of rest. These have thirsted of sun and earth and sea and sky. Their shape spoke this thirst like mine – if I had lived with them from Greece till now I should not have had enough of them. Sometimes I came in from the crowded streets and ceaseless hum: one glance at these shapes and I became myself. Wherever there is a beautiful statue there is a place of pilgrimage.

Richard Jefferies, *The Story of My Heart*

Attitudes of mind

Many times it has been shown how what you think in your mind tends to reproduce itself in your future experience. Let us identify ourselves with abundance. A regular, daily, adequate food supply is much to be thankful for. To express thanks audibly on rising creates a mental climate in which responsibilities of the day seem less arduous.

If we wish to identify ourselves with success, we must fill our minds with thoughts of success. Fears of failure beget failure. Anticipate meeting new friends, attracting to ourselves new experiences. Let us live in constant expectancy that the best, and nothing but the best, is working out in our lives.

Psychiatrists are coming round to the belief that all thoughts are forces. They have substance, quality and power. By our thought forces we have creative power. Everything first started in thought. Every implement, picture, article of furniture and dwelling had its conception first in the mind of the person who created it. Through unseen thought energy we build castles in the air. Before we can have castles on the ground, we must first have them in the air.

The pattern of our lives is so complex that even secret thoughts play a part in shaping our fate. Constantly, we attract to ourselves conditions similar to those of our own thoughts. Whether we are conscious of it or not, this law is always in operation. Every thought we generate sends out vibrations of a specific frequency. It is now possible to prove that with the birth of a thought, cells of the brain oscillate with a minute electrical charge.

With every thought is an out-going energy. This energy may be constructive or destructive according to the will of the thinker. The perfect vibration, conducive to mental and physical harmony, comes from a motivation of our thoughts by love, joy and peace. Anything less than these spells discord and disease. Good health is very much an attitude of mind. If we live in fear of getting some disease we shall probably end up with it. 'As a man thinketh, so is he'.

Loneliness

It comes to us all at some time or another. We would all cure it if we could.

Perhaps there are different kinds of loneliness. The self-employed businessman may know the loneliness of being different. There are people ahead of their time who feel out of tune with today. They may be shunned by the crowd who regard them as offbeat.

It is one of the enigmas of our times that in the midst of crowded cities millions long for a little solitude, and millions more get too much of it. Loneliness has little to do with social status, being found in all classes.

There are occasions when we sink so low and become so inward looking, that our eyes are clouded in our own dilemma. Few kinds of loneliness approach that where friends reproach us with their eyes; we don't want to be hurt.

If we fail to take ourselves in hand, it is so easy to erect barriers around ourselves and withdraw into a world of our own. When we permit this separation to go on, as in unduly prolonged grief, it somehow gets reflected into the very core of our life, we having less ability to cope.

When we are lonely we need appreciative attention. A musician wants someone with whom he can share his gift. A busy mother with a new baby may yearn for a listening ear into which she can pour her hopes and fears. There are caring groups in most towns and health visitors who would welcome an opportunity to link her with others in similar circumstances.

Some grand-dads are never really old but lonely and shun old boy's clubs. What about young boy's clubs? Club organisers often like to have an older man about the place; it is sometimes good for discipline and advice. Real grannies are at a premium. Who could be more 'wanted' than she who has time to take a child in her arms and read a story? What better sense of security for a child?

We seldom think of children being lonely. Most children love company which they need in order to develop and progress. There will always be 'loners' who shun the crowds, preferring quiet indoor games and long distance running. Such may find emotional satisfaction in pets.

If your child is blessed with a high IQ or special talent he may feel a 'fish out of water' among his peers. He might be encouraged to mix with others of the same interests but of different age groups.

Solitude is not loneliness. Not all people living alone are lonely. Many lead an active life at work and during their leisure hours. Often they will have a full social life, meeting with other people.

I have had patients living alone, openly expressing their preference for the peace and lack of interference into their privacy. They are so busy with their cooking, cleaning and general chores that they have no time to be lonely. 'I can live at my own rhythm', says one.

Parents are usually proud of their children and love to talk about them. There's an opening gambit for you! 'And how's Anne getting on at school?' 'I haven't seen your husband for weeks; I hope he's well.' Appear to be genuinely interested in the family.

Folk also love to talk about their holidays. A leading question may release a torrent of unrepressed enthusiasm which helps to break the ice.

There are many antidotes to loneliness. Some may put their names down for 'Friends of the Hospital' for transport of needy patients. 'Meals on Wheels' is always in need of drivers to convey food to 'shut-ins' and the disabled. In spite of all the materialism around us, there is a wealth of compassion in this society of ours. Keeping in touch with others by regular visits and getting caught up in that mellow world of human kindness adds a new dimension to life.

Almost every family has a lonely person somewhere. He or she may be trying to put a brave face on life. Are we helping by giving a little of our time and interest to that house-bound relative or acquaintance? We have been meaning to call, to write, but our time seems to get filled up with other commitments.

The saddest cases are those who feel they are unloved. There are times when we may feel 'wooden', longing to mingle in a jolly gathering but with-draw because, on that occasion, we just have nothing to say. It may be an act of courage for some to be the first to say 'Hello' to strangers. Whatever our feelings, it is possible for others to be attracted to our side by cheerfulness and sincerity and the ability to crack a joke.

The healing power of reconciliation

How can we be at peace with ourselves and with the world?

First of all, we must be spiritually fit. The basic causes of unhappiness are tension, failure, ill-health, fear and negative thoughts.

Let us remember that all life is generated from within and radiates outwards. 'As within, so without' – in other words, our thought forces and emotions are the causes of effects which manifest in the body as disease (lack-of-ease).

You say you cannot believe in this assertion? Can't you? You are at lunch, at peace with the world, until someone breaks the news that so-and-so has been run down and killed. Your mind communicates the shock to the stomach. The desire for food is arrested. You may even feel sick. It was your mind that signalled the adrenals to release more adrenalin into the bloodstream to arrest the function of all but essential services.

A girl walking home late at night encounters a drunk who stands in her way. She stands trembling with fear, too paralysed to move. And yet you tell me the mind and emotions are unlikely to be the cause of disease? Fear and worry have the effect of closing the paths of nerve energy through the body. The flow of nerve energy has met an obstruction which impairs its circulation.

Prayer for those who are sick
Dear father of all mankind: I realize there is no pathology you cannot correct, no health condition you cannot cure.

I thank you that I am fearfully and wonderfully made and request maintenance of the marvel of normal health. Remind me that I am not alone. Steady my nerves. Quieten my heart. Revive my feeble faith and may it please You to deliver me from this trouble by an intervention of Your grace and Divine Providence.

Remind me that I can do all things through Christ who strengthens me (Philippians 4:13). I ask this in the name of Him who healed the sick and freed men and women from the bondage of ill health.

A woman with a collection of vague pains and pressive headaches had done the rounds from one doctor to another, never carrying out their instructions. In the end, the last doctor in the chain told her flatly he could not cure her. (He had previously been told that this particular woman was at odds with everyone and had few friends.) Her soul was silted up with the toxins of accumulated resentments.

The soul is in the blood – not in some vague chamber of the brain or solar plexus – and her 'sins' were manifesting as high blood pressure and other symptoms. She had not spoken to her brother after a violent argument two years ago. 'I'll get even with him', she told her only friend.

'You're a doctor of reputation,' she retorted. 'I can afford to pay and want you to treat me.'

'I will do so under one condition,' he insisted, 'that you will take what I prescribe for you.'

'What is it?' she asked.

'You will attend church every Sunday morning until you improve. You needn't listen to the sermon, but just sit in that atmosphere of quiet renewal.'

You can imagine with what suppressed fury she slammed the door on her departure. She was determined to write him off forever. However, when venting her rage on her only friend, the suggestion was made that nothing could be lost by putting the doctor's advice into practice. After all, she could always walk out of the service when it was too boring.

She relented. Attending the church the doctor recommended, she was fidgety and the old antagonisms held. After a week or two, she didn't mind going, feeling more relaxed than at any other time during the week.

The practitioner was not the only one aware of the peaceful emotions and healing influences aroused in such surroundings. At first the sermon was double-Dutch but she soon found herself listening and actually understanding what it was all about. Interest kindled in what now appeared to her to be common sense, she made it up with her brother. Other people found her tongue less abrasive and her manner changed.

Within weeks, she lost those curious flitting pains all over her body, health improved and blood pressure returned to normal. Now brother and sister cannot do without each other. Now she has many friends.

There is potent healing power in the act of saying we are sorry. Repaired broken relationships mean so much. Do you have similar problems? If so, here is one of the ways you can obtain a firmer grip on life.

Don't be too hard on yourself. It's not what you eat, but what eats you! So many times, in anger or impatience, an unkind word is spoken. We wish we had not said it. But . . . too late. The damage has been done. A friend has been wronged, and forgiveness alone can repair the torn affection.

Yes, to ask forgiveness is one of the most difficult tasks. But it is worth every gram of self-abnegation, to express an apology honestly and sincerely. We have to learn to give and receive affection. When we do this the tendency is for us to recover naturally from our illnesses – physical or emotional.

Emotional illness arising from a lack of tolerance or forgiveness comes from an iron curtain between our conscious and unconscious mind. This so often means a barrier between ourselves and other people. Perhaps the other person is the Christian who stands a good chance of breaking down such a barrier in the early stages because he/she believes that 'God is Love'. It then becomes easier to love and to be loved – to forge a friendship or be a friend.

You will be quick to perceive that the balance-wheel of your new creative lifestyle is not a technique to be learned, but a gift to be received.

Do you love yourself? We must take care not to hate ourselves, which is so often the reason why we are irritable, impatient and fault-finding at the office or at home.

Love is the ultimate creative force in the world – in giving and receiving – life is never the same again. It's this absence of love which brings us days of depression and guilt, nervousness, frustration and rejection. So when you feel useless, lose weight and get physically sick, remember love is medicine for the sickness of the world.

A loving attitude can bring healing to our minds and bodies. Sometimes it is almost impossible to love, especially when someone has committed to us a grave injury. It is then that we have to realize our limitations and take it to God in prayer.

Strength and stay

To me, life is a miracle. I am grateful for the privilege of being born into this world. I can never tell what next the Creator has in store for me. My tiny capsule of time – some three score years and ten – what is it? It is a drop in the ocean; a single star in a galaxy of billions. Yet His hand is on me, as it is on you. There is a purpose behind your life and mine.

Every morning, as I walk along the clifftops overlooking a tranquil sea in summer and the crash of waves in winter, I need someone to thank for that delicate moment when a Lenten lily in my garden reaches perfection, and for every occasion when I encounter the rare warmth of human friendship. I need to express my gratitude for all the goodness of life.

'Man does not live by bread alone,' are words with which we are all familiar. Sooner or later, we realize that spiritual guidance is an important ingredient of life. It is when we rely on these that we lay the true foundations of health and happiness.

The Creator is ever present and ever ready to help us on our pilgrimage through this world. The simple secret is belief. If you share the conviction that you are not alone you will find that all the wisdom, intelligence and power of the universe is right where you are. Change your belief and you may change your health. It will not be long before you become conscious of strength being given to solve most problems and bring the best out of every situation.

Expect good health. Have a real expectation of God's goodness in every part of your being and added vitality will come to you. Anticipate happiness. Go forward in confidence. Let faith clear your mind of doubt and uncertainty. The power that swings the planets in the spheres can keep you fit in every sense of the word.

> Whatsoever things are true, whatsoever things are honest, whatsoever things are just, whatsoever things are pure, whatsoever things are of good report, if there be any virtue, and if there be any praise, Think on these things.
>
> St Paul, *Philippians 4:8*

Endnotes

1 Pritikin, Dr Nathan. *The Pritikin Program for Diet and Exercise* (Grosset & Dunlap)

2 Greer, Rita. *Easy Gluten-Free Cooking* (Thorsons)

3 Forman, Brenda. *Vitamin B15, Miracle Vitamin* (Grosset & Dunlap, New York)

4 Pauling, Dr Linus. *Vitamin C and the Common Cold* (Pan/Ballantine)

5 Shute, Dr Evan. *Your Heart and Vitamin E* (Devin-Adair)

6 Tobe, John. *Guideposts to Health* (Modern Publications, Canada)

7 Arnold, Dorothy Musgrave. *Dorothy Kerin* (Hodder & Stoughton)

8 Grant, Doris. *The Sunday Times Real Bread Book* (Rodale Press)

9 Jarvis, Dr D. C. *Folk Medicine* (Pan Books)

10 Davis, Adelle. *Let's Cook it Right* (Allen & Unwin)

11 Ibanez, Prof. Julian Sanz and Prof. Adolfe Castellanes, The Cajal Institute, Madrid

12 Royal Lee, Dr. *Sesame Seed* (Lee Foundation for Nutritional Research, Milwaukee, Wisconsin, U.S.A.)

13 Purchas, Dr Samuel (1575–1626). *A Theatre of Political Insects*

14 The Koran. Honey (Penguin)

15 Heyerdahl, Thor. *The Kon-Tiki Expedition* (Allen & Unwin)

16 Carson, Rachel. *The Sea Around Us* (Cassells)

17 Kordal, Lelord. *Healthy Horizons* (Canada)

18 Scott, Cyril. *Crude Black Molasses* (Thorsons)

19 Wade, Dr Carlson. *Natural Food News*

20 Lindlahr, Dr Henry. *Natural Therapeutics* (C. W. Daniel)

21 Thompson, Walter. British Acupuncturist

22 Hunt, Roland. *Seven Keys to Colour Healing* (C. W. Daniel)

23 Gimbel, Theo. *Healing through Colour* (C. W. Daniel)

24 Krieger, Dr Dolores. *Therapeutic Touch Imprimatur of Nursing* (American Journal of Nursing, 1975)

25 Thomson, Dr William A. R. *Spas that Heal* (A & C Black)

26 *See* 7

27 Mackarness, Dr Richard. *Not All in the Mind* (Pan Original)

28 Smythe, Benjamin Roth. *Killing Cancer – The Jason Winters Story* (Vinton Publishing, Nevada, U.S.A.)

29 Scott, Cyril. *Crude Black Molasses* (Thorsons)

30 British Herbal Medicine Association. *British Herbal Pharmacopoeia*, 1996

31 Thomson, Dr William A. R. *Herbs that Heal* (A & C Black)

32 Harriman, Sarah. *The Book of Ginseng* (Pyramid Books, New York)

33 Hyde, F. Fletcher. Hydes Herbal Clinic, Leicester

34 Herbst, Josephine. *New Green World-Story of the Two Bartrams, John and William* (Weidenfeld & Nicholson)

Further Reading

Acupuncture

Points of Chinese Acupuncture. Dr J. Lavier. (C. W. Daniel Co. Ltd.)
Acupuncture Vitality and Revival Points. D and J. Lawson Wood. (C. W. Daniel Co. Ltd. 1976)
The Layman's Acupuncture Handbook. George T. Bewith. (Wellingborough 1981)
Acupressure Technique (For self-treatment and minor complaints). Dr Hans Ewald. (Thorsons)

Aromatherapy

The Art of Aromatherapy. Robert B. Tisserand. (C. W. Daniel Co. Ltd.)
Aromatherapy. Raymond Lautie, D.Sc. and Andre Passebecq, MD. (Thorsons)

Chiropractic

Chiropractic: A Modern Way to Health. J. Dintenfass. (Pyramid, NY 1977)

Diet

Improve your Health with Zinc. Ruth Adams, and Frank Murray. (Larchmont Books, New York)
Let's Eat Right and Keep Fit. Adelle Davis. (Allen & Unwin)
Nutrition and National Health. Dr Robert McCarrison (C. W. Daniel Co. Ltd.)
The Pritikin Program. Nathan Pritikin. (Grosset & Dunlap)
Vitamin B6: The Doctor's report. Dr M. John Ellis. (Harper & Row, New York)
Your Daily Food. Doris Grant. (Faber & Faber)

Herbalism

American Indian Medicine. Virgil J. Vogel. (Norman, University of Oklahoma Press)
A Modern Herbal. Mrs M. Grieve. (Dover Publications 1931)
Australian Journal of Medical Herbalism. Quarterly publication of the National Herbalists Association of Australia (founded 1920). Deals with all aspects of Medical Herbalism, including latest medicinal plant research findings. Regular features include Australian medicinal plants, conferences, conference reports, book reviews, rare books, case study and medicinal plant review. National Herbalist Association of Australia, 33 Reserve Street, Annandale, NSW 2038, Australia
Back to Eden. Jethro Kloss. (Beneficial Books 1971)
Books by Mrs Hilda Leyel. *Herbal Delights, Heartsease, Elixirs of Life, Compassionate Herbs* and others
Common and Uncommon Uses of Herbs. Richard Lucas. (Arco Publishing Co. NY, 1979)
Encyclopedia of Herbs and Herbalism. Malcolm Stuart. (Orbis, 1979)
Green Pharmacy Barbara Griggs. (Jill Norman & Hobhouse)
Greenfiles. A quarterly newsletter of research extracts for herbal and other holistic practitioners who want to keep up with new developments in research and complementary/alternative medicine. A must for the practitioner. Address: 138 Oak Tree Lane, Mansfield, Nottinghamshire NG18 3HR, UK

Herbal Medicine. Diane D. Buckman. (Gramercy 1979)

Healing Plants. W. A. R. Thomson. (Macmillan, 1980)

Herbal Remedies. A practical beginner's guide to making effective remedies in the kitchen. Christopher Hedley and Non Shaw. (Parragon Book service)

Herbs that Heal. W. A. R. Thomson. (Macmillan, 1980)

Indian Herbology of North America. Alma R. Hutchens. (Merco, Ontario, Canada)

Leaves from Gerard's Herbal. Arranged by Marcus Woodward. (Thorsons)

Potter's New Cyclopedia of Botanical Drugs and Preparations. R. C. Wren, FLS. (C. W. Daniel Co. Ltd.)

School of Natural Healing. Dr John R. Christopher. (Biworld, 1976)

The Herb Book. John Lust. (Bantam Books, 1974)

The Home Herbal. Barbara Griggs. (Jill Norman & Hobhouse)

Homoeopathy

The Patient, not the Cure. M. Blackie. (Macdonald & Jane's, 1976)

The Prescriber. Dr John H. Clarke. (C. W. Daniel Co. Ltd.)

A Physician's Posy. (C. W. Daniel Co. Ltd.)

Magic of the Minimum Dose. (C. W. Daniel Co. Ltd.)

Arnica, the Wonder Herb. Phyllis Speight. (C. W. Daniel Co. Ltd.)

Before Calling the Doctor. Phyllis Speight. (C. W. Daniel Co. Ltd.)

Miracles of Healing. Ellis Barker. (John Murray)

Natural healing (Naturopathy)

Everybody's Guide to Nature Cure. Harry Benjamin. (Thorsons, 1980)

Natural Therapeutics. Dr H. Lindlahr. (C. W. Daniel Co. Ltd.)

Practical Encyclopedia of Natural Healing. Mark Bricklin. (Rodale Publications)

Arthritis and Common Sense. Dale Alexander. (World's Work)

Better Sight without Glasses. Harry Benjamin. (Thorsons)

Your Heart and Vitamin E. The Shute Brothers. (Devin-Adair, U.S.A.)

Practical Hydrotherapy. Home Guide to Water Cure Treatment. Gerhard Leibold. (Thorsons)

Osteopathy

Manual of Osteopathic Technique. Alan Stoddard. (Hutchinson London, 1980)

You and Your Back. D. Delvin. (Pan, 1977)

Prescription for living

The Power of Positive Thinking. Dr Norman Vincent Peale. (World's Work)

Enthusiasm Makes a Difference. Dr Norman Vincent Peale. (World's Work)

The Holy Bible.

The Infinite Way. Ralph Waldo Trine.

Grace magazine, A Quarterly magazine devoted to 'Nature's Way'. To help us to live. Positive lifestyle, spiritual refreshment. Healing by natural methods. To give expression to thoughts which the publisher believes will contribute to social and spiritual development. Publisher: Thomas Bartram, Grace Publishers, Mulberry Court, Stour Road, Christchurch, Dorset BH23 1PS. Website: www.gracepublishing.net Email: gracepublishers@mulberrycrt.freeserve.co.uk

Useful Organizations

Acupuncture

The British Acupuncture Council,
63 Jeddo Road, London W12 9HQ
Tel: +44 (0) 20 8735 0400
Fax: +44 (0) 20 8735 0404
Website: www.acupuncture.org.uk

The Chinese Medicine & Acupuncture Research Centre,
2nd Floor, 322–324 Nathan Road, Kowloon, Hong Kong.

Chiropractic

Anglo-European College of Chiropractic,
13–15 Parkwood Road, Bournemouth, Dorset
Tel: +44 (0) 1202 436200
Fax: +44 (0) 1202 436312
Website: www.aecc.ac.uk

Palmer College of Chiropractic,
1000 Brady Street, Davenport, IA 52803, USA
Tel: (800) 722–3648
Website: www.palmer.edu

Herbalism

National Institute of Medical Herbalists,
Elm House, 54 Mary Arches Street, Exeter EX4 3BA
Tel: +44 (0) 1392 426022
Fax: +44 (0) 1392 498963
Website: www.nimh.org.uk
An independent body concerned with the training of practitioners and research into herbal medicine. These activities are carried out at the School of Herbal Medicine. Members (MNIMH) (FNIMH). The institute is the oldest professional organization of herbal practitioners in the world, being founded in 1864.

British Herbal Medicine Association,
1 Wickham Road, Bournemouth, Dorset, BH7 6JX
Tel: +44 (0)1202 433691
Fax: +44 (0)1202 417079
Website: www.bhma.info
The objects of the BHMA can be summarized: (1) To defend the right of the public to choose herbal remedies and be able to obtain them. (2) To foster research in herbal medicine and to establish thereby standards of safety which are a safeguard to the user. (3) To encourage the diffusion of knowledge about herbal remedies and do everything possible to advance the science and practice of herbal medicine and to further its recognition at all levels.

Research Council for Complementary Medicine.
At the time of press, the offices were relocating.
Website: www.rccm.org.uk
The aims of the council are the dissemination of research findings, to collect reviews and disseminate research-based information about complementary and alternative treatments and philosophy, in order to provide the public, government researchers and practitioners an evidence base with which they can take a more informed view about complementary and alternative medicine in prevention.

The Swedish Herbal Institute,
Gruvgatan 37,
SE-421 30, Västra Frölunda, Sweden
Tel: 46 (0)31 339 66 80
Website: www.shi.se

Homoeopathy

British Homoeopathic Association,
29 Park Street West, Luton, Bedfordshire LU1 3BE
Tel: +44 (0) 870 444 3950
Fax: +44 (0) 870 444 3960
Website: www.trusthomeopathy.org
Primarily for laymen to spread knowledge about homoeopathy. Works in close cooperation with the Faculty of Homoeopathy, members of which are statutorily registered health care professionals. Provides a list of homoeopathically trained doctors, dentists, pharmacists, podiatrists, nurses and vets.

The Royal London Homoeopathic Hospital,
Greenwell Street, London W1W 5BP
Tel: +44 (0) 20 7391 8833
Fax: +44 (0) 20 7391 8865
Website: www.uclh.org

Glasgow Homoeopathic Hospital,
1053 Great Western Road, Glasgow, Scotland G12 0XQ
Tel: +44 141 211 1600
Fax: +44 141 211 1610
Website: www.homeoint.org

Tunbridge Wells Homoeopathic Hospital,
Church Road, Tunbridge Wells, Kent TN1 1JU
Tel: 07771 522235
Website: www.trusthomeopathy.org

Homoeopathic Pharmacies
Ainsworth Pharmacy,
36 New Cavendish Street, London W1G 8UF
Tel: +44 (0) 20 7935 5330
Fax: +44 (0) 20 7486 4313
Website: www.ainsworths.com

Nelsons Homoeopathic Pharmacy,
73 Duke Street, London W1M 6BY
Tel +44 (0) 20 7629 3118
Website: www.nelsonshomoeopathy.co.uk

American Foundation of Homoepathy,
Suite 428–431 Barr Building,
910 17th Street,
NW Washington DC, 20006, USA

Naturopathy

British College Osteopathic Medicine,
Lief House
120–122 Finchley Rd, London, NW3 5HR
Tel: +44 (0) 20 7435 6464
Fax: +44(0) 20 7431 3630
Website: www.bcom.ac.uk

Dietetics, fasting, light, water treatments, exercise, psychological and structural adjustment. Members (ND, DO and MBNOA).
National College of Naturopathic Medicine,
049 SW Porter St, Portland, OR 97201, USA
Tel: 503 552 1555
Fax: 503 499 0022
Website: www.ncnm.edu

The Icelandic Nature Health Society,
Laufasvegi 2, Reykjavik, Iceland

Osteopathy

The British School of Osteopathy,
275 Borough High Street, London SE1 1JE
Tel: +44 (0) 20 7407 0222
Website: www.bso.ac.uk
Founded 1915.The only school in the Commonwealth offering a full-time four-year course to qualify for membership of the Register of Osteopaths (MRO) and Diploma of Osteopathy (DO). An out-patient's clinic operates, where some 500 treatments a week are given.

American Academy of Osteopathy,
3500 DePauw Boulevard, Suite 1080, Indianapolis, IN 46268, USA
Tel: 317 879 1881
Fax: 317 879 0563
Website: www.academyofosteopathy.org

Others

Health Food Institute

Gothic House, Barker Gate, Nottingham NG1 1JU

Tel: +44 (0) 115 941 4188

To increase public awareness of the guarantee of expertise and high professional standing of its members, who qualify by examination.

The American Botanical Council

6200 Manor Rd, Austin, TX, 78723 USA

Tel: 800/373-7105, x 1189

Website: www.herbalgram.org

Is the leading non-profit education and research organization using science-based and traditional information to promote the responsible use of herbal medicine. Founded in 1988, the member-supported Council works to educate consumers, health-care professionals, researchers, educators, industry and the media on the safe and effective use of medicinal plants.

Herbalgram – Quarterly Journal published by the American Botanical Council (ABC). A benefit at all levels of membership in the ABC.

Herbal Suppliers

The following supply herbs, roots, barks, dried flowers, fluid extracts, tinctures, essential vegetables and oils of aromatherapy. All are experts in the field and offer a mail order service.

Avicenna,
Bidarren, Cilcennin, Lampeter,
Ceredigion SA48 8RL
E-mail: avicenna@clara.co.uk
Website: www.artemisherbs.co.uk

G. Baldwin & Co,
171–173 Walworth Road,
London SE17 1RW
E-mail: sales@baldwins.co.uk
Website: www.baldwins.co.uk

Bio-Health Ltd,
Culpeper Close, Medway City Estate,
Rochester, Kent ME2 4HU
E-mail: info@bio-health.co.uk
Website: www.bio-health.co.uk

Butterbur & Sage Aromatherapy Oils Suppliers,
7 Tessa Road, Reading,
Berkshire RG1 8HH
E-mail: info@butterburandsage.com
Website: www.butterburandsage.com

Culpeper Ltd,
Head Office, Hadstock Road,
Linton, Cambridge CB1 6NJ
E-mail: info@culpeper.co.uk
Website: www.culpeper.co.uk

The, Herbal Apothecary,
103 High Street, Syston,
Leicester LE7 1GQ
E-mail: herbaluk@aol.com
Website: www.herbalapothercary.net

Kingfham Herbs,
Langston Priory Mews, Kingham,
Oxfordshire OX7 6UP
E-mail: sales@kinghamherbs.co.uk

Neal's Yard Remedies,
15 Neal's Yard, Covent Garden,
London WC2H 9DP
E-mail: mailorder@nealsyardremedies.com
Website: www.nealsyardremedies.com

Phytoproducts,
Park Works, Park Road,
Mansfield Woodhouse,
Nottinghamshire NG19 8EF
E-mail: info@phyto.co.uk
Website: www.phyto.co.uk

Potter's Herbal Supplies,
Leyland Mill Lane, Wigan,
Lancashire WN1 2SB
E-mail: info@pottersherbals.co.uk
Website: www.pottersherbals.co.uk

Proline Botanicals Ltd,
Meadow Park Industrial Estate,
Bourne Road, Essendine, Near Stamford,
Lincolnshire PE9 4LT
E-mail: tony.carter@fpisales.com

Rutland Biodynamics Ltd,
Town Park Farm, Brooke,
Rutland LE15 8DG
E-mail: sales@rutlandbio.com
Website: www.rutlandbio.com

Shirley Price Aromatherapy,
Essentia House, Upper Bond Street,
Hinckley, Leicestershire LE10 1RS
E-mail: info@shirleyprice.co.uk
Website: www.shirleyprice.co.uk

Points of Call

Age Concern England,
Astral House, 1268 London Road,
London SW16 4ER
Tel: +44 (0) 0800 009 966
Website: www.ageconcern.org.uk

Allergy UK,
3 White Oak Square, London Road,
Swanley, Kent, BR8 7AG
Tel: +44 (0) 1322 619864
Website: www.allergyuk.org

Alzheimer's Disease Society,
Gordon House, 10 Greencoat Place,
London SW1P 1PH
Tel: +44 (0) 20 7306 0606
Website: www.alzheimers.org.uk

**Arthritis and Rheumatism Council
for Research,**
Copeman House, St. Mary's Court,
St. Mary's Gate, Chesterfield S41 7TD
Tel: +44 (0) 1246 558 033
Website: www.arc.org.uk

Arthritis Care,
18 Stephenson Way, London NW1 2HD
Tel: +44 (0) 20 7380 6500
Website: www.arthritiscare.org.uk

Breast Cancer Care,
Kiln House, 210 New Kings Road,
London SW6 4NZ
Tel: +44 (0) 20 7384 2984
Website: www.breastcancercare.org.uk

British Chiropractic Association,
Blagrave House, 17 Blagrave Street,
Reading, Berkshire RG1 1QB
Tel: +44 (0) 118 950 5950
Website: www.chiropractic-uk.co.uk

British Heart Foundation,
14 Fitzhardinge Street,
London W1H 6DH
Tel: +44 (0)20 7935 0185
Website: www.bhf.org.uk

British Lung Foundation,
73–75 Goswell Road,
London EC1V 7ER
Tel: +44 (0) 20 7688 5555
Website: www.britishlungfoundation.com

Cruse Bereavement Care,
126 Sheen Road,
Richmond TW9 1UR
Tel: +44 (0) 20 8939 9530
Helpline: +44 (0) 870 167 1677
Website: www.crusebereavementcare.org.uk

Diabetes UK,
10 Parkway, London NW1 7AA
Tel: +44 (0) 20 7424 1000
Website: www.diabetes.org.uk

Hearing Concern,
4th Floor, 275–281 King St,
London, W6 9LZ
Tel: +44 (0) 20 8743 1110
Helpline: +44 (0) 845 0744600
Website: www.hearingconcern.com

Help the Aged,
207–221 Pentonville Road,
London N1 9UZ
Tel: +44 (0) 20 7278 1114
Website: www.helptheaged.org.uk

Macmillan Cancerline,
Macmillan Cancer Relief,
89 Albert Embankment,
London SE1 7UQ
Tel: +44 (0) 808 808 2020
Website: www.macmillan.org.uk

Migraine Trust,
2nd Floor, 55-56 Russell Square,
London, WC1B 4HP
Tel: +44 (0)20 7436 1336
Website: www.migrainetrust.org

National Asthma Campaign,
Providence House, Providence Place,
London N1 0NT
Tel: +44 (0) 20 7226 2260
Website: www.asthma.org.uk

National Back Pain Association,
16 Elmtree Road, Teddington,
Middlesex TW11 8ST
Tel: +44 (0) 20 8977 5474
Website: www.backcare.org.uk

National Osteoporosis Society,
Camerton, Bath BA2 0PJ
Tel: +44 (0) 1761 471 771
Helpline: +44 (0) 845 4500 230
Website: www.nos.org.uk

Parkinson's Disease Society,
215 Vauxhall Bridge Road,
London SW1V 1EJ
Tel: +44 (0) 20 7931 8080
Website: www.parkinsons.org.uk

Royal National Institute for the Deaf,
19–23 Featherstone Street,
London EC1Y 8SL
Tel: +44 (0) 808 808 0123
Textphone 0808 808 9000
Website: www.rnid.org.uk

Stroke Association,
Stroke House, 240 City Road,
London EC1V 2PR
Tel: +44 (0) 20 7566 0300
Helpline:+44 (0) 845 3033100
Website: www.stroke.org.uk

The Migraine Action Association,
Unit 6, Oakley Hay Lodge Business Park,
Great Folds Road, Great Oakley,
Northamptonshire NN18 9AS
Tel: +44 (0) 153 6461 333
Website: www.migraine.org.uk

The Society of Chiropodists and Podiatrists,
1 Fellmonger Path,
Tower Bridge Road,
London SE1 3LY
Tel: +44 (0) 20 7234 8620
Website: www.feetforlife.org

Index

Index

Index

Index